DIMENSIONS OF NURSING MANAGEMENT

DIMENSIONS OF
NURSING MANAGEMENT

S. W. Booyens
(editor)

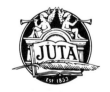

1993
Juta & Co Ltd

First published 1993

© Juta & Co Ltd
PO Box 14373, Kenwyn 7790

ISBN 0 7021 2988 7

Edited and set by Dr D. E. Michael, Kenilworth

Printed and bound in
the Republic of South Africa by
Creda Press, Eliot Avenue, Eppindust

ACKNOWLEDGEMENTS

A number of people gave generously of their time, knowledge, and expertise to make this book possible and their contributions are greatly appreciated. They are: S. Kingsma, a personnel management consultant; J. Dednam, C. V. Folscher, H. Reeve-Saunders, and C. Stegman of the Cape Provincial Administration, Hospital and Health Services; D. Edwards, F. Horwitz, R. Kirsch, and J. P. van Niekerk of the University of Cape Town; D. Gowdie of Foschini; L. Helman of the University of Stellenbosch, T. Koorts, A. E. Lambrecht and N. Venter of Panorama Mediclinic; P. A. van Aarde, B. Verster and E. Vismer of Rembrandt; F. Mountford, A. Bester and P. T. Vurgarellis of the Department of National Health and Population Development; G. M. Mashope of Shell South Africa; and A. Brand, P. Burger, P. Chaffey, A. Coyle, S. Kabat, B. van den Berg, M. J. van den Berg, M. J. van der Schyf, A. van der Walt, and J. Wheway of Groote Schuur Hospital.

The following people are also thanked for their assistance, input, and encouragement: Mr K. Howie of F. G. G. Architects, Durban, and Dr R. Neethling of NPA Health Services. A special word of thanks is addressed to Mr Hennie du Toit and Dr Cobus Scholtz for their contributions.

PREFACE

Dimensions of Nursing Management attempts to describe the many dimensions of the task of the nurse manager in a health service organization.

The nurse manager's role involves a wide range of activities and is strongly influenced by the structure and functions of the organization in which she is working. The major aspects of her role will depend on the type of service in which she is employed. It is not, however, possible for a book of this nature to cover the managerial requirements of all the different health services; instead it examines those aspects of a nurse manager's role that are important in a wide range of settings.

Dimensions of Nursing Management was originally a medium-size project. Gradually, however, more authors joined and it grew to the sizeable volume that you are now holding. The participation of each new author was welcomed as each contributed a particular area of expertise, with the result that such important aspects as quality assurance and improvement, strategic health manpower planning, the design and commissioning of health service facilities, group dynamics, labour relations, job evaluation, leadership, staff development, and financial management could all be dealt with in detail.

Initially, the book was intended to meet the needs of those students who already possessed their basic nursing qualifications and who were studying at a tertiary institution with a view to qualifying for registration with the South African Nursing Council as nurse administrators. As the project evolved, though, it became clear that it could be of use to a number of other health care workers, namely student nurses, practising nurse managers, professional nurses in charge of units, hospital administrators, physicians in managerial positions (especially those working closely with nurse managers), nurse educators, and others who work in close collaboration with nurse managers and professional nurses in supervisory posts.

The book is organized in five parts which correspond to the five main aspects of the management process: planning, organizing, staffing, leading and control. As all administrators or managers should know, however, these five aspects are usually intertwined and often cannot be clearly distinguished. This fact comes to the fore throughout.

A philosophy of participative leadership and management, and a belief in the value of employees taking part in decisions regarding the running of an organization, are regarded as essential for good quality management. This point emerges in a number of chapters. This approach to management, the basic managerial skills which the modern nurse manager must possess in order to lead a nursing service, and the background necessary for the acquisition of these skills, are all described in depth. It is hoped that the readers of this book will thus gain considerable knowledge of nursing management from it.

S. W. Booyens

LIST OF CONTRIBUTORS

S. W. Booyens B.Cur (I et A) (Pret), MA(Cur), D.Litt et Phil (Unisa), RN, RM, RCN, RNA, RIN, RT
Professor, Department of Nursing Science, Unisa, Pretoria.

L. June du Preez RN, RM, DOTNS, DNed, DNA
Former Deputy Director, Nursing, Groote Schuur Hospital, Cape Town.

Renée du Toit B.Soc.Sci Hons (Univ. OFS), DAN (Unisa), RN, RM, RPN, RNA
Health Care Facility Planner, Johannesburg.

S. Koch MA(Cur), D.Litt et Phil (Unisa), RN, RM, RCN, RNA, RT
Senior Lecturer, Department of Nursing Science, Unisa, Pretoria.

M. H. Hart BA(Cur) (Unisa), DNed, DNAd (Witwatersrand), RN, RM, RNA, RCN, RT
Lecturer, Department of Nursing Science, Unisa, Pretoria.

J. H. Roos B.Cur (Pret), MA(Cur) (Unisa), RN, RM, RCN, RNA, RPN, RT
Lecturer, Department of Nursing Science, Unisa, Pretoria.

C. M. Nel B.Cur(I et A) (Pret), MA(Cur), D.Litt et Phil (Unisa), DNE (Pret), RN, RM, RCN, RNA, RT
Professor, Department of Nursing Science, Unisa, Pretoria.

K. Jooste MACur (Unisa), RN, RM, RCN, RNA, RT
Lecturer, Department of Nursing Science, Unisa, Pretoria.

R. Troskie MA(Cur), D.Litt et Phil (Unisa), RN, RM, RCN, RNA, RT
Associate Professor, Department of Nursing Science, Unisa, Pretoria.

M. C. Bezuidenhout B.Cur(I et A) (Pret), M.Cur (RAU), DNE & DCN (Pret), Dip Renal Nurs (Aus), RN, RM, RCN, RIN, RNA, RT
Senior Lecturer, Department of Nursing Science, Unisa, Pretoria.

M. E. Muller M.Cur, D.Cur (RAU), RN, RM, RCN, RNA, RIN, RT
Professor, Department of Nursing, Rand Afrikaans University, Auckland Park, Johannesburg

CONTENTS

PART THREE: STAFFING

PART FOUR: LEADING

PART FIVE: CONTROL

PART ONE:

PLANNING

CHAPTER 1

STAGES OF HUMAN RESOURCE PLANNING IN HEALTH CARE

June du Preez

CONTENTS

INTRODUCTION

Strategic human resource planning is driven by an organization's overall strategic plan and strategic objectives. It is generally recognized that there are advantages in using a planning method which has a comprehensive and co-ordinated approach. This enables plans to be effective, and allows economical use to be made of scarce and expensive human resources.

The main objectives in health care are:

- clinical care;

- education;

- training; and

- research.

The planned development of management has been neglected in the health services. There has been inadequate planning, poor management practices, and a high degree of centralization of decision-making and control. This has resulted in inefficient and expensive duplication, and lack of effective communication and understanding. Personnel administration has been problematic, with wastage and loss of potential due to cumbersome centralized personnel administration systems, and inadequately planned staff development and retention of personnel. Under these conditions the health service has been vulnerable and has declined over the past two decades.

South Africa is experiencing unprecedented and radical socio-economic, political, demographic, technological, and epidemiologic change which is placing increasing and overwhelming demands on the overburdened and weakened health services. This is happening in the face of inadequate and dwindling resources and outdated, ineffective management systems.

The introduction and management of change, and the survival and reconstruction of the health services, depend on managers and personnel who are appropriately qualified, whose careers are properly developed, and who continually update their knowledge and skills. The introduction of human resource planning and human resource management departments into larger organizations, possibly by changing the existing staff and personnel administration sections and having them headed by qualified and experienced human resource managers, would be an advantage. In each of the smaller institutions there needs to be at least one person who is qualified or experienced in human resource management.

Strategic planning and its subcategory, strategic human resource planning, are management tools that have been developed to deal with change. Their application would be the first step in introducing the wide spectrum of activities that go to make up effective, comprehensive, and co-ordinated human resource management. This would provide a base from which to introduce change in personnel management in the health services.

STRATEGIC PLANNING

Strategic planning and forecasting methods were introduced in the 1960s as part of a quest for ways of managing increasingly rapid and complex change. Scenario planning made its appearance twenty years later. Techniques for planning continue to be developed. In the process of strategic planning, the mission of the organization is formulated, the external and internal environments are analysed, objectives are set, strategies are devised, and action plans are drawn up for achieving the objectives of the mission statement. The plans are implemented, and progress is monitored and evaluated. The results are then fed back into the system as shown in figure 1.1.

The strategic planning exercise is costly and it results in raised expectations regarding the solving of organizational problems. Success requires the commitment of top management. All the stages of the strategic human resource planning process must be worked through. The process must be applied on an ongoing basis, with strategic thinking being promoted among all the personnel. Each manager and staff member should understand that the onus is on every individual to work according to the plan in order to bring about the required changes in their organization. Without such commitment nothing will change.

STRATEGIC HUMAN RESOURCE PLANNING

Strategic human resource planning is a subcategory of the strategic planning process. It should be linked to, and activated by, the strategic plan and strategic objectives of the organization. Nkomo defines strategic human resource planning as 'the process used to establish human resource objectives' (Nkomo 1988: 67).

Figure 1.1 shows the five stage model of the strategic human resource planning process. It is an example of a structured and comprehensive approach to human resource planning. The stages are:

- investigating;

- forecasting;

- action planning;

- implementation; and

- monitoring.

Figure 1.1: The strategic human resource planning process

NOTE: This process is activated by the corporate strategic plan

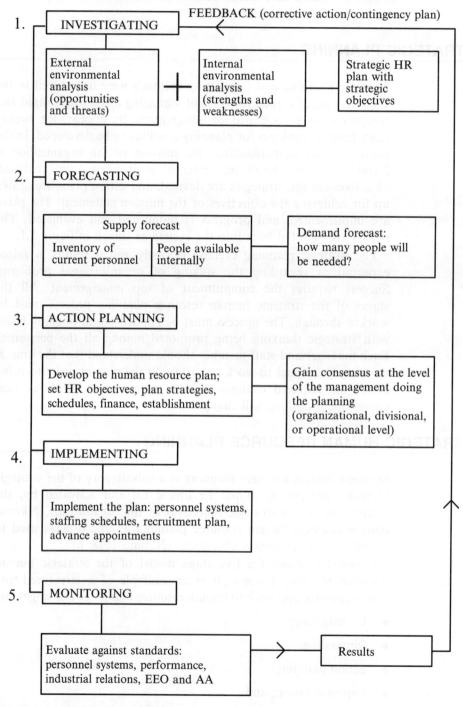

(adapted from Walker 1980.)

The process is applied at three levels in the organization (see table 1.1):

- the corporate or organizational (top management) level;
- the divisional level;
- the operational level.

Each of the levels of management carries out the stages relevant to its own functional level.

Strategic human resource planning objectives at the three levels

Corporate level

Development and succession planning programmes at top management level are essential in order to develop 'an organization-wide human resource strategy which supports the overall corporate mission' (Nkomo 1988: 69).

Divisional level

Planning is required here in order to acquire the correct mix of adequately developed and qualified personnel with the required skills in sufficient numbers to achieve the objectives of the division. It involves:

- designing policies and programmes for staffing, training, and development in the operational areas;
- carrying out management development and succession planning; and
- designing policies and programmes for the operational areas of staffing, training, and development (Nkomo 1988: 64).

Operational level

At the operational level, it is necessary to carry out human resource plans in terms of divisional policies and programmes. This involves:

- deploying staff;
- hands-on care;
- supervision;
- teaching;
- developing and appraising staff;
- evaluating progress; and
- providing feedback for the divisional level.

Table 1.1: The three strategic planning levels

LEVEL	KEY QUESTIONS, AREAS FOR DECISIONS AND ACTION
A. Corporate or organizational	What is our business? 1. Develop statements of philosophy, mission, and vision. 2. Formulate organizational strategic objectives. Note: 1. and 2. activate divisional planning.
B. Divisional/ departmental or unit	What must we do to help achieve the organizational mission and strategic objectives? 1. Statements of divisional philosophy, mission, and vision. 2. Decisions/objectives. What: — disciplines should be in the division? — communication systems? — spectrum of care? — technology? — ethics? — standard of practice? — quality assurance methods and programmes? — scope of education, teaching, training, and research?
Human resource management functions with divisional management	Human resource management with divisional managers: planning personnel needed to accomplish divisional objectives; finalize manpower plan by consensus; provide programmes for staff development; management of performance and management of careers.
Administrative service and services	Provide administrative, clerical, and logistical support.
C. Operational	What must we do to contribute to achieving the divisional mission and objectives? 1. Operational objectives and goals. 2. Provide organized information for input at divisional level and receive information and feedback.
Human resource management with operational managers	Actions: hands-on clinical care and procedures; standards of care/practice; ethical standards; use of technology; resource planning, deployment, and control; procedure manuals. Policy manuals; optimum staffing levels (multi-disciplinary); teaching programmes; personnel appraisal and development; industrial relations.

Human resource management departments

The management of people in the workforce is a line function which should be carried out by line managers, supported by personnel administration or human resource management. As organizations have grown in size and complexity, however, human resource management and planning departments have developed, staffed by personnel qualified in this discipline.

An example of the mission of a human resource management department is:

to support the company in the achievement of its strategic objectives by providing a professional and effective service which will support line managers in their resourcing, management, and development of people to ensure effective and efficient staffing of the business, and a motivated and productive workforce . . . support is provided in strategic human resource planning; workforce planning; succession-planning and career development; selection and recruitment; training and development; compensation (rewards); industrial relations; corporate social responsibility; and employee counselling. (Human 1991: 261)

The operational managers and supervisors remain responsible for managing, planning, and directing their personnel.

Essential functions and duties of managers at all levels are:

- promoting the development of staff;

- team building;

- promotion of the development of skills, including multiskilling;

- promotion of productivity.

With bottom-line management it is recognized that remuneration should be linked to productivity. The development of multiple skills results in an individual having a broader career path. As a result she is able to make a greater contribution to the organization.

THE FIVE STAGE PROCESS OF STRATEGIC HUMAN RESOURCE PLANNING

Figures 1.1 and 1.2 and table 1.1 show this process. A broad strategic plan and the strategic objectives for the organization are produced by the top management team. The team should be representative of all the divisions, and should include human resource management. The organizational strategic plan activates the human resources planning process.

Stage one: investigating

The corporate mission and objectives should be kept in mind when the divisions undertake external and internal environmental analyses related to human resource needs.

The analyses are carried out from the perspectives of the different divisions — eg medicine or surgery — in conjunction with human resource planning.

The following shows some parameters which are useful in structuring environmental analyses for the health care field. Each organization will decide on the issues relevant to its own particular field. Note that Foster (1988) advances an overall information framework. The environmental analysis may be carried out according to this. He stresses the importance of arranging the information in minimum data-sets. Foster's work is useful because the writings and parameters in his framework relate specifically to health services.

ENVIRONMENTAL ANALYSES

External environmental analysis
(Opportunities, threats and trends will be defined from this analysis.)

Parameters

Geographic
Demographic

Epidemiological	indications of type of care needed and skills required from personnel are gained from these two parameters
Technological	
Social services	eg availability and cost of transport and accommodation, community infrastructure, and facilities such as creches and recreational facilities
Labour	availability of transport, accommodation and facilities
Competitors	eg competitors for patients/clients in the private sector and scarce funding in the state services
Legal	laws and regulations relevant to conditions of service, patient care, safety, statutory professional legislation and regulations
Industrial relations	union organization and activities, and current labour legislation. Note implications for professional practice and ethics
Political	government policy
Financial	

Internal environmental analysis
(Strengths and weaknesses within the organization will be defined from this analysis.)

Parameters

The workforce

- Employee demographics
- Skills and potential
- Performance
- Attitude

Management development and competence

- Organization
- Climate of the organization
- Structure
- Job analysis programme
- Work activities
- Quality of work life
- Absenteeism
- Turnover
- Effectiveness of human resource programmes (after Nkomo 1988: 70).

During analysis, each parameter is debated in detail by those involved in the strategic human resource planning exercise. Each person comes well prepared, with relevant statistics and in-depth information from his field of expertise. A great deal of information is generated, prioritized, and refined.

Opportunities and threats in the external environment are defined, as are internal strengths and weaknesses. Once these factors have been prioritized, thought is given to converting threats into opportunities and weaknesses into strengths.

Strategies are designed to exploit opportunities and deal with threats in the external environment, and to capitalize on internal strengths while remedying internal weaknesses.

A broad strategic human resource plan with three components will be drawn up from the analysis (Nkomo 1988: 67). The components are:

- The immediate need for personnel with particular skills.
- Longer term needs for staff.

- What human resource programmes can be designed to deal effectively with environmental contingencies and pressures?

The divisional managers and human resource managers use the information as a basis for stage two — forecasting.

Stage two: forecasting

The interpretation of the external and internal environmental analyses is used to define trends and forecast internal needs in terms of divisional objectives. A *needs forecast* is then formulated and presented.

The personnel budget is one of the most costly items in the total budget. Forecasting is important in the planning and control of staffing and the related costs.

Strategic human resource planning makes it possible for the organization to timeously provide an adequate number of appropriately qualified personnel with the desired mix of skills. Such planning addresses the full spectrum of staff categories, from the general assistants right through the professional categories.

Planning is geared to the achievement of the longer-term strategic objectives of the organization, and not simply to the replacement of personnel.

In their strategic planning, management may decide to introduce new or updated systems. Orientation, induction, and in-service education programmes would be required to support these. The programmes might necessitate an increase in the staffing establishment, which should be included in the forecast. This is a controversial issue in view of the scarcity of resources. Development plans may be curtailed due to lack of finance. The aim should be to enhance productivity while reducing costs. Such issues should be borne in mind in order to produce a realistic needs forecast.

Walker describes an integrated process of six components which he regards as necessary for effective forecasting (Walker 1980: 102). The six components are:

1. *Environmental analysis.* Analysis of external and internal environmental conditions enables one to consider their impact on human resources, and to assess what will be needed in order to achieve the mission and objectives of the organization.

2. *Inventory of current talent.* Most organizations have a computerized personnel information system with full details of individual staff members.

3. *Projected future human resource supply*. Milkovich and Boudreau divide the supply analysis into two sections, internal and external

(Milkovich and Boudreau 1988). As regards the *internal* supply analysis, turnover patterns may be seen from records. The following are recorded:

- attrition;

- resignations;

- terminations;

- retirements;

- mobility;

- promotions;

- demotions;

- skills utilization;

- transfers.

Listings give details of numbers of staff, experience, abilities, race, and sex. The *external supply analysis* is carried out using the external environmental analysis, taking into account all aspects which directly affect the availability of human resources: demographics, educational institutions, the supply forecast, and legal provisions.

4. *Current human resource requirements.* Organizations are seldom ideally staffed. This is due to various factors such as financial constraints, lack of suitably qualified applicants, the number of posts available, and the planning of an extension to an existing facility or a new facility. The analysis of current demand and the projection of optimal current staffing provide the baseline for planning future demand. The different techniques for making projections, and the use of computer technology for this activity are described in the literature (Milkovich and Boudreau 1988; Walker 1980).

5. *Projected future requirements (demand analysis).* This involves the analysis of organizational changes and conditions, marketing plans (see the section on marketing), financial plans (see appendix 1, notes on finance), operational plans (see table 1.1, section C, operational level), and technological plans (see table 1.1, sections B and C).

6. *Needs forecast/presentation.* The projections for demand and supply are balanced. The results indicate those human resource

needs which may be met within the organization and/or from outside. A *human resource needs forecast* is drawn up and presented, indicating immediate and longer-term needs, with the matching phasing. Proposals are included to suggest how the needs may be met by means of such activities as recruiting, reorganization, reallocation, development, and better use of personnel. The financial implications are to be included with the needs forecast.

The following documentation is required for needs forecasting:

- a schedule of the establishment of required posts indicating categories and phasing;

- an organizational structure diagram showing the arrangement of posts;

- a schedule showing the current and planned distribution of posts;

- a schedule of the state of the current establishment, indicating posts filled (appropriately and inappropriately) and vacant;

- a schedule of planned phasing and priorities for the creation of posts;

- financial estimates indicating phasing and priorities;

- documents indicating the procedure for procuring finance (see appendix 1: 'note on finance').

Stage three: action planning

The objective of action planning is to formulate detailed plans for realizing the divisional objectives.

The heads of divisions will have received input regarding operational level objectives and personnel needs from their staff at the operational level. The human resource planners/ co-ordinators will plan ongoing work-groups with divisional and departmental heads, ensuring their active involvement in the planning process, and working towards consensus. The co-ordinators will provide guidelines for the work-groups, will work with the groups, and will set dates for the submission of completed documents. They will also set dates for priority and planning meetings with peers and top-level management.

The strengths, weaknesses, opportunities, and threats in relation to human resources will be determined from the results of the environmental analyses (external and internal). Strategic human resource issues such as amended legislation, introduction of new technology, trade union activities, and the closure or extension of facilities, will be pinpointed and taken into consideration when planning.

The human resource co-ordinators will, in consultation with the divisions, compile a schedule of the personnel required by each division for the carrying out of their respective plans. The completed divisional action plans, together with financial estimates, will be incorporated in the corporate strategic planning as the action plans of the whole organization once they have been approved by top management.

Figure 1.2 depicts the three levels of planning and the support function of human resource management for managers throughout the organization.

Action plans (see figure 1.1) are central to the development of the human resource plan. These are necessary to produce and execute the programmes for the management of performance and careers.

Performance management

Performance management is concerned with 'improving the performance of individuals and the organization as a whole' (Walker 1980: 10). This comprises both personnel and organizational development.

Approaches to the management of employees' productivity, motivation, and performance are changing and evolving.

> Companies are strengthening vital supervisory skills, equipping employees to manage their own work better, and modifying the structure and environment of work in ways that promote performance improvement. (Walker 1980: 16)

The aim is currently to empower managers (who have undergone development) at all levels by structuring the organization in order to allow them greater autonomy and freedom to make decisions in their own units and departments.

Walker sets out three areas which management has control over and where management can introduce changes to motivate personnel and promote productivity and quality of performance (Walker 1980):

1. The organization

Work activities: understanding on the part of the employee of his role and commitment; relationships (interpersonal as well as between people and the organization)

Responsibilities: qualifications, knowledge, skills, abilities, competence (job specifications)

Standards: performance standards required: professional practice and ethical standards of professionals

Quality of work life: consideration of the needs of the individual and the organization

Figure 1.2: Management structure — the three levels of strategic planning at institutional level

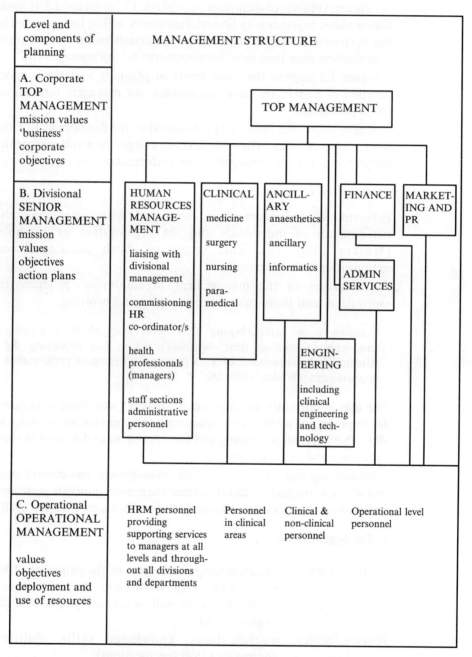

NOTE: In this figure human resources management is shown as a department which functions throughout the organization, and is on the level of a division. Its function is to support the managers in the planning and management of human resources.

2. Performance appraisal

- Individual goal-setting and planning with review of progress and appraisal of performance.

- Training for managers and employees in appraisal, and coaching and counselling for employees in appraisal techniques.

- Evaluation: the measurement of individual performance against required performance standards. Evaluation influences management decisions regarding such matters as salary, promotion, termination, and opportunities for training.

3. Reward structures

Compensation: What is a job worth? Job evaluation is used to determine this.

Merit: Merit awards are once-off amounts paid in recognition of good performance. These amounts are not part of the salary.

Incentives: There are a variety of incentives. Incentives are paid for performance. This system does not operate in the state health service.

Benefits: Pension, insurance, medical benefits, leave.

Career management

This involves 'activities to select, assign, develop and otherwise manage careers in an organization' (Walker 1980: 10).

A shortage of developed human resources has led to increasing efforts to retain staff, and these are backed by the identification, planning, and development of career paths as a part of career management.

Walker divides the required career management programmes into four categories (Walker 1980: 11):

1. Policies and systems
   — Recruitment
   — Selection and placement
   — Promotion and transfer
   — Development and training
   — Termination and retirement

2. Individual assessment
   — Position requirements
   — Replacement charting
   — Succession planning
   — Tracking career progress

3. Career opportunities
   — Job requirements
   — Career paths
   — Career communications

4. Individual career planning
   — Self analysis
   — Personal career plans
   — Development of action plans

In the context of this discussion, the planning of the programmes is linked to the organization's strategic objectives and the related human resource needs. The programmes are designed to meet *current* needs, and there is regular monitoring. As circumstances and needs change, programmes are amended or discontinued.

Needs of the organization and the individual

When applying human resource principles and systems to an organization, one should aim to achieve a balance between meeting the objectives and needs of the organization and meeting those of the individual. Lovemore Mbigi maintains that, in order to address the challenges of human resource management in South Africa, a model is required that suits the situation in the country.

He proposes the *Unhu or Ubuntu developmental human resource model* (Mbigi 1992). This involves setting up management practices which focus on development issues in order to meet the challenges in Africa — 'a poor continent facing tremendous development challenges' (Mbigi 1992). The model focuses on the continuous improvement and development of people, products, systems, structures, markets, productivity, quality, and performance (Mbigi 1992).

The principles apply particularly in health services where the product is the health of the community (which comprises not only patients and the wider community but also care-givers and all who work in the services). Health services generate large numbers of jobs in communities. The services carry responsibility for development of their personnel.

Planning the required resources

The following remarks by Gerber et al. (1987: 126) are important:

> The nature of the job that the individual must do in the enterprise forms the basis of all the activities of manpower planning. Before any decisions can be made about the type and number of people necessary to do the job the task that enables the enterprise to achieve its goals must be studied.

Job analysis

Milkovich and Boudreau have stated that:

> Job analysis is a systematic process of collecting data and making certain judgements about all of the important information related to the nature of a specific job. Results of the job analysis serve as input for many human resource activities.

Work analysis (also referred to by other terms such as 'work study' or 'job analysis') is regarded as essential for effective manpower planning. It is a detailed and expensive activity, but is correspondingly valuable.

Job design entails the integration of the content of the job with the qualifications required to perform it and the returns and rewards for performing it in a way that will ensure that the work is accomplished to the satisfaction of the organization. The employee should also experience job satisfaction. The aim should be the meeting of both organizational needs and the needs of employees. Job design has implications for productivity, related costs, and motivation.

A *job description* is 'a written statement of what the job holder actually does, how he or she does it, and under what conditions the job is performed' (Dessler 1984, in Gerber et al. 1987: 127).

A *job specification* is defined as 'a statement of those human qualities thought necessary to perform a job' (Gerber et al. 1987: 128).

With a comprehensive *job analysis programme*, ongoing development and control of the essential functions would be possible. Programmes would need to be developed for each component.

Planning of organization structure and human resource planning

1. Use analytical methods: research, systems analysis, work study (refer to the literature regarding this complex activity);

2. arrive at a manpower plan and budget;

3. determine posts required through job analysis;

4. compile costing;

5. develop organizational structure.

The full range of the work to be accomplished in the undertaking must be defined. Tasks are then grouped to form jobs by using analytical methods.

The parameters of the job are measured using job analysis. These parameters might include work output, cost-benefit indicators, level of effort required, tasks/activities performed, education, knowledge, skills and experience, level of decision-making or problem-solving, and the number of subordinates reporting to a particular manager (Walker 1980: 153). This information is used to decide the number and type of posts required. The jobs or posts which must be created are then planned and arranged in order, usually from the lowest to the highest levels. The jobs may also be arranged to form specific teams in order to facilitate efficiency and productivity. The relevant conditions of service are applied to each post, job descriptions are required for the posts, and job specifications are desirable.

The foregoing steps are essential for human resource planning. Operational and managerial level personnel should be fully involved in the planning.

Existing job descriptions or position summaries may be used as examples. Care should be taken to design for the organization in question and not to transplant job descriptions, structures, and systems directly from one organization to another.

Action planning is a comprehensive function. Action plans provide specific and detailed direction and objectives for personnel, enabling them to work in a goal-directed manner, using their creativity in working towards the achievment of the objectives of the organization as they implement the action plans. 'The value of human resource planning depends on effective implementation' (Walker 1980: 47).

Stage four: implementation

Implementation is the conversion of the divisional human resource action plans into action. It is accomplished through the practical application of the programmes for human resource management — eg recruitment, selection, and appointment — as well as the programmes for individual performance appraisal and development. Human resource management will ensure the insight, commitment, and co-operation of the managers who will be responsible for implementing the planning, especially level C line managers (see table 1.1).

When human resource plans are implemented, change is introduced. There may be new policies, systems and programmes, new members of staff, new equipment, and new technologies as planned by the managers in the divisions. The effective introduction and management of change, and of people caught up in change, is the main challenge that managers will face.

The line managers implement the plan which they have designed, supported by the human resource management or personnel section staff. An essential function of human resource management is to maintain good relationships with and among the managers, countering resistance to change by supporting and motivating personnel.

The line managers are responsible for ensuring good staff relationships and communication — especially good industrial relations — during the period of change. Implementation will follow the human resource plan. Progress, phasing, and finance will be monitored, evaluated, and controlled. More information is given in the section on commissioning in chapter three. The basic principles apply to established undertakings as well as those being commissioned.

Recruitment

Career management and development have become more important because of the general lack of an adequate number of applicants with the required standard of education and the lack of developed human resources. In answer to the need for better use of existing personnel, internal recruitment and retention programmes are increasingly receiving attention. This is particularly relevant when commissioning redevelopments or new organizations.

The greatest deficit is at the levels of management and professional and skilled workers. Management succession planning and planned programmes for the development of individuals are essential (Walker 1981: 17).

Implementation of a human resource plan for nursing

The nursing establishment is usually the largest part of the organization. It is also complex and expensive. A heavy load of staff work is generated in the management of the nursing function. When implementing the plan it is essential to involve the operational nurse managers and support them. An effective exchange of information is vital.

An effective way of co-ordinating and controlling the implementation of the human resources plan was devised in the nursing division of an academic hospital under redevelopment. It involved setting up a *nursing division establishment committee*. The committee functioned in liaison with the routine commissioning work groups. Once established, the committee remained to develop its functions as a permanent structure in the nursing administration. The aim of the committee was the overall control and co-ordination of functions relating to the establishment of posts. Its members included the regional deputy director of nursing (who served as chairman), and nurse managers responsible for all departments (personnel, clinical, education and nursing information systems). (Administrative and other categories of personnel may be co-opted as required for planning and problem solving. There should be regular liaison between committee members, the staff office, and commissioning staff.)

The main functions of the committee were as follows (Du Preez 1986):

- the application of policy in respect of establishment;
- the continued planning of establishment, short- and long-term;
- organizing establishment, especially in respect of the redevelopment project (this included organizational development);
- monitoring financial aspects:
- submission of schedules of priorities (of posts) in accordance with the phasing of the project;
- devising procedures for management of establishment — eg for advertising posts, recruiting, interviewing, selection, placement, applications for study opportunities, providing policy and procedure manuals;
- monitoring the state of establishment (with costing, including costing of vacant posts with a view to saving, especially during financial cuts);
- control of the staffing function (movement of people into, within, and out of the organization, according to the personnel administration systems);
- liaison with personnel development and education sections (these sections include amongst their functions orientation, induction and training, and industrial relations);
- organization and co-ordination of selection committees (appointments, promotions, continuing education);
- management (and development) of the information system, and computerization;
- co-ordination of the inputs and outputs of the establishment information system.

The effective establishment committee promotes controlled implementation of the human resource plan. Monitoring and evaluation of progress are carried out with feedback. The committee initiates and/or carries out contingency planning.

Stage five: monitoring

The final stage of human resource planning involves continuous monitoring of the detailed human resource plans and programmes — eg recruiting, training, and development — by observing and recording results and progress. Results are evaluated against the objectives that have been set, and the information is fed back into the system at stage one (investigating — figure 1.1). In the case of deviations, contingency plans may be devised.

Elements of a formal evaluation and review procedure

Nkomo (1988: 71) states that a formal evaluation and review procedure should involve the evaluation of the results of human resource programming activities and the correction of any deviations that are found. Such a review should include at least the following:

- actual versus planned staffing requirements;

- productivity levels versus established goals;

- actual personnel flows (turnover, absenteeism, promotions, etc.) versus desired rates;

- actual personnel programmes versus planned programmes;

- the actual costs of labour and personnel programmes versus budgeted amounts;

- ratios of programme results (benefits) to programme costs.

A research-based, disciplined approach and a well-planned, comprehensive, computerized information system are required for effective monitoring, evaluation, and feedback of results. These functions are often neglected. New methods and programmes may be designed and implemented as availability of resources (including the knowledge and expertise of the human resource manager) permits.

Monitoring is discussed further in the section on commissioning in chapter three.

CONCLUSION

The management of rapid and radical change is a challenge to mangers in the overstressed health service. Strategic planning provides direction for the undertaking and promotes understanding of external pressures and opportunities as well as the resulting conditions within organizations. This permits more effective management of personnel caught up in change. Strategic human resource planning is activated by the strategic objectives of the organization and is linked to them. The main thrust is development of human resources. In the comprehensive concept of Ubuntu, development is advocated not only in the workplace but in the community at large. The greatest need in South Africa is for the development of people.

Strategic human resource planning and management are at the very heart of goal-directed, people-orientated management. These skills are a powerful means for managers to manage change and to promote the development of people and organizations. The necessary knowledge and expertise are available in the qualified and experienced human resource managers whose skills are needed in the continuing development of the health services.

References

Du Preez, L. J. (1988). Groot Schuur Hospital nursing division establishment committee. Reference J/44 1986, revised 1988.

Foster, D. (1988). A dynamic approach to strategic planning. *Hospital Development Journal,* May 1988.

Gerber, P. D., Nel, P. S., Van Dyk, P. S. (1987). *Human Resources Management.* First edition. Southern: Johannesburg.

Mbigi, L. (1992). Unhu or Ubuntu. The basis for effective HR management. *People Dynamics,* volume 11, number 1, pp. 20–6.

Milkovich, George T. and Boudreau, John W. (1988). *Personnel/Human Resource Management: a Diagnostic Approach.* Fifth edition. Business Publications: Plano, Texas.

Nkomo, Stella M. (1988). Strategic planning for human resources. Let's get started. *Long Range Planning,* volume 21, number 1, p. 67.

Walker, James W. (1980). *Human Resource Planning.* McGraw-Hill: New York.

CHAPTER 2

KEY ISSUES IN PLANNING AND ADMINISTRATION OF HUMAN RESOURCES

June du Preez

CONTENTS

INTRODUCTION

New approaches to the planning and administration of health manpower have emerged. In the past, health authorities did not think it necessary to consider issues such as affirmative action, AIDS, and the empowerment of workers. The health service managers of today, however, are faced with a number of different issues concerning the administration of human resources — employee assistance programmes, formulation of policy regarding AIDS in the workplace, equal employment opportunities, and the active development of all employees, to name but a few issues.

ORIENTATION, INDUCTION, AND EDUCATION/TRAINING

Seen against the concept of human resource management:

> for induction and training in industry to be optimally effective they should be approached against the background of a clearly defined, integrated personnel policy. If an organization does not give the necessary attention to, for example, selection, placement, supervision, etc. even the best induction and/or training system will not provide optimum results. (Retief and Koorts 1976: 1)

Structured human resource and training departments have important functions to perform in acting as change agents, developing people, and promoting organizational development. Creative ways need to be found to accomplish necessary changes under conditions of scarce resources. It is believed that the human resource function would be more effective in organizations where it is carried out comprehensively by a human resource management department, co-ordinating for the whole organization rather than in piecemeal fashion.

The successful functioning of an organization depends on effective orientation, induction, and education/training of personnel. The philosophy, mission, policies, procedures, systems, technology, equipment, and standards of care should be understood and accepted to ensure that facilities are used optimally and according to plan. Current policy and procedure manuals, with relevant position summaries or role analyses, form the nucleus of the learning/teaching material. The criteria and objectives against which regular evaluations of the organization and personnel are carried out are contained in these.

Finance needs to be made available for the ongoing orientation, induction, and education programmes and for co-ordinating of personnel. Records of attendance, which are taken into account in staff appraisal, are kept by the line manager or the tutor in the individual staff records.

AFFIRMATIVE ACTION (AA) AND EQUAL EMPLOYMENT OPPORTUNITY (EEO)

Affirmative action (AA) has not always been introduced with success. Human sees affirmative action as a means to an end — ie equal employment opportunity (EEO):

> The organization has to recognise people development as a key strategic objective as reflected in both its values and reward systems. The development of people is a line responsibility.
>
> Promotion and development from within, and hence workforce succession and career planning, are vital for the development and motivation of people. Top management must be committed to people development.
>
> Affirmative action should take place at the selection and recruitment stage only and thereafter all employees should be promoted on merit.
>
> Selection and assessment of potential should move away from the traditional 'formal education and experience' approach to an approach which more adequately addresses the actual requirements of the job. (Human 1991: 324)

Equal employment opportunity can be facilitated by the eradication of racism and sexism through affirmative action. In the process, opportunities are created for women and black men. *White men should not be excluded.* The system should be objective (Human in discussion 1992).

Olivier believes that, in order to have a successful affirmative action programme, planning should take place on a more long-term basis, either feeding into a quota system or enforcing equal employment opportunities. By providing post profiles for all posts in an organization, career ladders may be designed to enable individuals to plan and follow their own career paths. Succession planning should be introduced at the lower levels. There should be access to information on career planning. Management should create a climate of open and effective communication. Recognition of potential in employees, and the development of career paths, should be linked to the predicted strategic human resource requirements (Olivier 1922: 22).

Organizations should plan affirmative action and equal employment opportunity programmes which should be monitored and evaluated regularly.

EMPOWERMENT

Empowerment should go hand-in-hand with the development of people. It may be achieved by a move away from centralized, bureaucratic systems and structures. This should empower personnel by enabling them to take responsibility for the functioning of their units. Empowerment of blacks and the economic empowerment of women are topical issues requiring attention, particularly with regard to their influence on recruitment.

WOMEN IN THE WORKPLACE

Employers are going to have to look increasingly to employing women in order to obtain the skills that they need, and they are going to have to cater for the roles of women as mothers as well as breadwinners (Gon 1992: 3).

The majority of personnel in the health services are women. It is therefore necessary for management to focus on their needs. Appropriate policy should be formulated and introduced into the human resource management system.

The following are areas requiring attention:

- the prevention of discrimination in respect of gender and race;

- promoting full use of women;

- providing access to job opportunities and promotion;

- providing education and development;

- assisting women to reach their full potential;

- developing women as managers;

- ensuring equitable conditions of service;

- formulation of policies on maternity leave which are fair to both employers and employees;

- the provision of information on conditions of service and personnel policies for prospective staff at interviews;

- the formulation of policy on sexual harassment.

PERSONS WITH DISABILITIES

Health care organizations should formulate policy regarding employment of people with handicaps. Organizations may even need to make ergonomic adjustments to assist them in their work. Special training programs may be required. Policy is required to ensure that promotion takes place in accordance with qualifications and productivity.

AIDS

According to a World Health Organization statement on AIDS in the workplace (27–29 June, 1990), an HIV positive employee has no obligation to inform his employer. 'This should only be the case if the illness has job performance implication' (Gon and Pellinet 1992: 29).

In the health services there are policies and protocols for dealing with HIV positive persons and those suffering from AIDS. Policy in respect of personnel is required in all organizations. This would include a health education programme. Objectives of such a programme would be to inform staff about the disease, to prevent its spread, and to prevent discrimination against sufferers.

AIDS in the workplace: IPM guidelines for members for policy formulation

The establishment of a multidisciplinary task force should include all appropriate company departments and business functions. Some recommended business functions and their suggested roles in such a task force are given below:

Function	Area of responsibility
Personnel	Problem resolution, work practices, reasonable accommodation, termination issues, counselling services.
Industrial relations	Co-operation with union(s), employee relations.
Legal	Compliance with legislation, protection against unfair dismissal, and unfair labour practices.
Non-discrimination	Recruitment.
Selection	Selection policies, pre-employment screening.
Personnel administration	Alternative health care benefit coverage, disability benefits, death benefits, pension benefits, health care cost containment.
Medical/ personnel	Counselling, testing, education, return to work.
Public relations	Establish credibility, use all available channels, liaise with community and local media.
Trade unions	Joint formulation of policy and action plans with management, representing employees' views as

part of task force; protection of employees' rights; referral of employees to counselling services where appropriate; access to employees.

AIDS — some resources

- Training and Information Centre: The South African Institute for Medical Research, PO Box 1038, Johannesburg 2000. Telephone: (011) 725 3009

- Department of National Health and Population Development, Regional Offices.

Counselling services for HIV positive persons and those suffering from AIDS and their families are provided by various organizations as well as by psychologists and social workers.

EMPLOYEE ASSISTANCE PROGRAMMES

Employee assistance programmes include assistance for employees with problems relating to alcohol, substance abuse, ill-health, and also with family matters and emotional and work-related problems. Supervisors are encouraged 'to concentrate on job performance concerns, and not attempt to diagnose the nature of the problem' (IPM Fact Sheet 182: 1989: 2). The employee assistance programmes are comprehensive, covering all factors affecting work performance. Confidentiality is of prime importance.

Information on employee assistance programmes for the enlightenment of all personnel is essential to ensure management support and to encourage general use of the programmes. Agreement between management and the representatives of the workers is desirable in ensuring the success of employee assistance programmes.

The need for employee assistance programmes will no doubt increase in proportion to the rate of change occurring in organizations. These programmes should be put in place timeously when new facilities are brought into use, as this is a period characterized by an intense degree of change and stress (IPM Fact Sheet 182).

MARKETING

Marketing involves the use of a combination of social, economic, and management theory, applied in special ways to meet needs. With skilled application, marketing can help raise the standard of health care through its emphasis on consumer needs, patient outcomes, and quality of service (Alward 1991: 3).

Marketing management is increasingly recognized as essential in non-profit organizations and health care undertakings.

Professionals have seen marketing as being at variance with professional ethics. This view is changing, however, as a result of the increase in complex pressures affecting professionals in their work. There is competition as the numbers in a profession increase. Today the public, clients, and patients are more critical of health services, health care professionals, and the associated rising costs. More information is required before the public makes its choices.

In order to introduce planned marketing into an organization, a framework based on the following six questions may be used (Sinclair and Beaton 1987: 81–2):

1. What will marketing do?

2. Who will control and monitor the various activities?

3. How much time needs to be allocated to it?

4. How much money must be spent?

5. Which systems of control are necessary?

6. How will the staff remain involved and in touch with the programme?

In view of current conditions, and especially the rapid and radical changes being experienced today, administrators in the health services in the private and public sectors should consider the need for introducing marketing with their management systems. Effective marketing is necessary whenever there is a highly competitive, resource-constrained environment (Alward 1991: 3).

INDUSTRIAL RELATIONS

The Labour Relations Act (1956) does not apply to the public service. This precludes public servants from negotiation with a view to making binding agreements, as well as the right to strike. The result has been increasing conflict and labour unrest, particularly in the state health services.

The Labour Relations Act should apply to the entire economy, but the right to strike poses a problem when those involved in essential services such as health care and the police are concerned.

[Increasing] penetration of the trade union into the public sector ... cannot be avoided. It would be wise for the public sector to be pro-active and prepare for this development as soon as possible by creating the necessary collective bargaining machinery in the public sector. (Wiehahn 1988: 71)

Both workers and employers should have a right to protection in the workplace. Management should be encouraged to bring about a greater involvement of employees in negotiation, and should train them to acquire negotiating skills. Programmes for training and development in industrial relations are essential for all levels of personnel.

Handling grievances

An employee with a grievance should discuss this initially with her supervisor. If necessary the matter may need to be taken further, bringing in a worker representative. The employee should eventually have access to the highest authority in the organization in an effort to find a solution to a problem.

Disciplinary procedures

Disciplinary action is any action initiated by management in response to unsatisfactory worker performance or behaviour. Policies and procedures regarding disciplinary action should be made known to all concerned. Provision should be made in the procedure for employees to be accompanied by a colleague or representative of their choice at a formal hearing. There should be a right of appeal against disciplinary action.

In terms of the Public Service Act (No. 111 of 1984) and the Public Service Staff Code, provision is made for dealing with inefficiency and misconduct (chapter VI). Chapter VII of the Act covers grievance handling and disciplinary procedures.

Industrial relations and nursing

During public sector hospital strikes, nurses carrying out their duties have had to run a gauntlet of intimidation, assault, death, and the destruction of their homes, but they have had to keep on and do the work of the strikers in order to provide safe care for their patients.

In South Africa, nursing services are not at present defined as essential services in terms of the Labour Relations Act, 1956 (LRA). Essential services are not entitled to use strike action as a form of dispute resolution. Where the Nursing Act, 1978 previously prohibited strikes by nurses, it is now (since the removal of the no-strike clause from the Act) in theory possible for nurses in the private sector to embark on a legal strike. However, nurses abandoning their patients remain professionally liable in terms of the SA Nursing Council's rules regarding the acts or omissions in respect of which the Council may take disciplinary steps. Nurses in the public sector, on the other hand, are subject to public sector legislation, which effectively prohibits strike action. The fact that nurses are denied this right, however, places an onus on the community and the employer to afford them access to other fair and equitable means of resolving disputes. (Nursing News 16:8:1)

The South African Nursing Association (SANA) and ten other employee organizations meet with the Commission for Administration in the Public Service Joint Forum to discuss matters of concern.

In the private sector, communication between SANA and employers is informal or occurs by way of recognition agreements. There is now a 'trade union leg' of the association to make provision for those members (in the local authorities) for whom it is 'necessary to have a registered trade union to negotiate on their behalf'. Membership of the union is not compulsory (Nursing News 16:8:10).

HUMAN RESOURCE INFORMATION SYSTEMS (HRIS)

The following is a definition of a human resource information system:

> An HRIS is a systematic procedure for collecting, storing, maintaining, retrieving and validating certain data needed by an organization about its human resources, personnel activities and organisation unit characteristics. (Milkovich and Boudreau 1988: 296)

Organized, retrievable information is an essential resource that is necessary for reasoned decision-making. Certain information is required in terms of legislation.

Information systems are specialized, organization-specific, and expensive. They may be computerized. Information is required for all human resource management functions, not least for human resource planning, through all five stages as set out in figure 1.1.

When commissioning a reopened or newly-opened part of a facility, or a new organization, staff work may need to be undertaken in large batches. Where the recruitment, selection, appointment, transfer, and deployment of large numbers of personnel is involved, computerization facilitates the work and simultaneously produces the required records.

Human resource planning must proceed in accordance with the management control plan and the phasing and contingency plans. This can be done effectively with computerization. An important aspect regarding nursing staffing when opening new areas is the need to indicate the total number of personnel and the amount of nursing time available as this limits the number of beds that can be commissioned (see figure 3.2 — projected staffing status computer printout.) The schedule in figure 3.2 was used during commissioning as a planning tool for the allocation of personnel to areas that were being commissioned.

Innovation and progress have resulted in a wide selection of new software programs. The market should be scanned in order to procure the best and most cost-effective. There are many advantages in planning one's own programs as these are tailored to individual needs. With bottom-line management having come into prominence, more sophisticated programs have been devised which are particularly useful in nursing management. There are nursing staff scheduling packages which enable the nurse manager to cost individual shifts, receive information on workloading, and redeploy personnel without delay to where they are needed. Records are kept of finance and allocations.

PERSONNEL ADMINISTRATION IN THE STATE HEALTH SERVICE

The state health services fall under the Department of National Health and Population Development. The following legislation applies:

- the Health Act, 1977 (No 63 of 1977);

- the various acts applying to health care and the allied professions;

- the National Policy for Health Act 1990 (No 116 of 1990);

- R158 of 1 February, 1980, in terms of Section 44 of the Health Act (No 63 of 1977) applies to private hospitals and unattached operating theatre units;

- the Defence Act (No 44 of 1957) applies to health service in the military services. This is in addition to other legislation relating to the health professions, its practices and the provision and management of health services.

Personnel administration for the public service — which includes health service — is centralized in Pretoria under the Minister for Administration and Economic Co-ordination. The Public Service Act (No 111 of 1984) is relevant to personnel administration.

The Commission for Administration (CFA) is the top policy-making and policy-controlling body.

The large hierarchically-structured state health service thus falls under two state departments, each with its own minister and legislation. This perpetuates the problems of centralized control in the health services. Long-standing and continuing problems are experienced by professionals functioning within the bureaucracy, caught between the conflicting professional and institutionalized bureaucratic value systems.

In terms of the Public Service Act the Public Service Staff Code contains details relating to the organization and establishment of posts, employment and career control, training and language proficiency, general conditions of service, personnel structure and remuneration, and other functions relating to the Commission for Administration and its powers.

The personnel administration standards (PAS), which should be read in conjunction with the staff code, provide detailed information on designation of posts, post classes, establishment, salaries and prescribed 'job contents' (the latter being abbreviated basic job descriptions used for the purpose of establishing levels of posts).

Despite the existence of statements of 'job contents', position summaries still need to be provided in health care institutions. There is room for creative thinking when planning position summaries in the state health care system.

The National Plan for Health Service Facilities provides a guide to estimate the required staffing for local authority community health centres and midwife obstetric units, based on the ratio of health worker to population in the categories of health visitor, clinic sister, nursing auxilliary, doctor, dentist.

Nursing

The manual for the provision of posts for nursing staff was released by the Commission for Administration in July, 1982. The guidelines are intended to serve as a basis for the development and refinement of the guidelines for staffing and have been applied and tested in practical situations.

The guide is detailed and provides comprehensive parameters of nursing care, including time factors and the desired ratios of registered nurses to enrolled nurses and nursing auxilliaries.

Medicine and allied professions in the academic hospital

The traditional functions of the academic hospital are patient care, education (teaching and training), and research. At this time there are no known norms. Attempts have been made to define guidelines.

THE PRIVATE SECTOR

The doctors are the clients. They use the facilities financed by private enterprise and thereby generate income for the organization. There are no norms.

COMMENT ON GUIDELINES/NORMS FOR NURSING

Methods other than those described in the Commission for Administration's guidelines are being introduced in different countries in the face of the scarcity and the escalating costs of the professional nurse. Manthey, the initial exponent of primary nursing in 1966, introduced her system of primary nursing during a period when there was a critical shortage of nurses, to provide for the maximum use of the available nursing resources for hospitalized patients. The system of primary nursing was designed:

1. to allocate 24-hour responsibility for each patient's care to one individual nurse, and

2. to give the nurse responsibility for the actual provision of her patient's physical care whenever possible (Manthey 1980: preface).

Decentralized decision-making, and full involvement of the relevant nurses in implementing the system, were considered essential for the system to succeed. Ever since this major breakthrough, conditions regarding resources have continued to become more difficult and, with repeated budgetary cutbacks, nurse managers are devising research-based methods of improving the quality of care and productivity with fewer personnel. They are also providing support for the professional nurse at the bedside to free her to devote maximum time to nursing care.

Models may be based on patient classification, according to acuity, by means of a workloading index and computer-based information systems. Helt and Jellinek demonstrated improved productivity and quality of care in spite of cost-cutting in their study carried out in a group of USA hospitals in the Medicines National Database where effective information systems were provided (Helt and Jellinek 1988: 36–48).

THE PRO ACT (PROFESSIONALLY ADVANCED CARE TEAM)

The 'alternative practice model' at Robert Wood Johnson University Hospital reduces the workload for professional nurses by providing support for the professional nurses at the bedside (Tonges 1989: 31–7).

At one South African hospital, a system of patient classification for determining workload was introduced in 1982 and was developed over time (Van der Walt 1990). Standard times for nursing interventions provided the basis for calculating the mean number of care hours per patient class. The model has proved useful for:

1. the determination of workload;

2. developing staffing patterns to ensure safe standards of nursing care delivery;

3. developing the skill mix combinations required for nursing care delivery by different categories or levels of nursing staff;

4. using the information obtained as a basis for long-term manpower planning.

Planning of the system of performance management in health care needs to take into account standards of care and practice. In the complex milieu of a health service, with a high percentage of professionals on the staff, standards of care and practice are governed by the statutory law of the professions, by professional ethical codes, by the norms of the community, and by morality. The aim is to strive for acceptable, safe standards of practice. Medico-legal hazards result from certain acts or omissions which may result in harm or injury to the patient or even death (Du Preez 1988).

The organization should have an efficient information system, with organized information on personnel and records of legally required registration, experience, skills, abilities, and competence. Job specifications should be available.

Standards should be set for all aspects of the organization, not least for hands-on care. Up-to-date policy and procedure manuals are required to assist personnel as they deal with the many legal and ethical aspects of care-giving. Research, teaching, medical, and surgical interventions add further parameters. This all presupposes the setting of standards along with the institution of the necessary quality assurance and risk management programmes.

A system of peer review of individual performance within the organization is required in order to set and enforce standards. The professions organize this within their own ranks. Peer review currently takes place mainly through the statutory professional councils and their disciplinary bodies at national level.

Ethics committees have been established in some health care organizations. An ethics committee and a disciplinary committee were set up in the nursing division of one academic hospital. Ethical issues were debated through the ethics committee. The setting of standards was influenced by this. It also served as a learning forum. Peer review was exercised through the investigation of those incidents which could be referred to the disciplinary committee. At this level a detailed investigation was carried out, and this was followed by appropriate action from the committee. This action included such measures as discussion, counselling, a decision to provide remedial education, a warning and, when necessary, a report to the South African Nursing Council (Du Preez 1988).

CONCLUSION

Use of the strategic plan provided at national level by the Department of National Health is a necessity when it comes to giving direction in the planning and management of the health services throughout the country. Attention to the key issues in strategic human resource planning are of extreme importance in developing a healthy workforce.

References

Alward, R. and Camunas, R. (1991). *The Nurse's Guide to Marketing*. Delmar Publishers.

Du Preez, L. J. (1988). Deputy director: nursing, Groote Schuur Hospital. Memorandum N/F/4/3/1. 18 July, 1988.

Du Preez, L. J. (1988). Protecting the patient. *Nursing RSA,* volume 3, number 7, pp. 17, 21–7.

Gon, S. and Pellinet, L. (1992). AIDS and dismissal. *People Dynamics,* volume 10, number 8, p. 29.

Helt, Eric H., and Jellinek, Richard C. (1988). In the wake of cost cutting, nursing productivity and quality. *Nursing Management,* volume 19, number 6.

Human, Linda (1991). A people development process. In Human, Linda (ed.) *Educating and Developing Managers for a Changing South Africa.* Juta: Cape Town.

IPM (1988). *Grievance Handling and Disciplinary Procedures,* fact sheet 105.

IPM (1989). *Employee Assistance Programs,* fact sheet 182, p. 2.

Manthey, Marie (1980). *The Practice of Primary Nursing*. First edition. Blackwell Scientific Publications.

Milkovich, George T. amd Boudreau, John W. *Personnel/Human Resource Management: A Diagnostic Approach.* Fifth edition. Business Publications: Plano, Texas.

Nursing News (1992). SANA's policy statement on nurses and structures. *Nursing News,* volume 16, number 8, p. 1.

Olivier, A. A. (1992). A practical option for affirmative action programmes. *People Dynamics,* volume 10, number 11, pp. 21, 24–5.

Pensegrouw, Gustav (1985). Strategic human resource management — an emerging dimension. *IPM Journal,* volume 4, number 5, pp. 22–8.

Retief, T. and Koorts, J. T. (1976). *Induction and Training in Industry*. National Institution for Personnel Research: Johannesburg.

Sinclair, R. and Beaton, G. (1987). *Marketing in Practice for the Professions*. First edition. Southern: Johannesburg.

Tonges, M. C. (1989). Redesigning hospital nursing practice: the professionally advanced care team. *JONA*, volume 19, part 7.

Van der Walt, A. *Patient Classification in the Groote Schuur Hospital Region, Republic of South Africa. Paper submitted for publication.*

Wiehahn, N. (1988). Civil service should have a collective bargaining process. *HRM Yearbook*.

CHAPTER 3

PLANNING FOR, AND MANAGEMENT OF COMMISSIONING

June du Preez

CONTENTS

INTRODUCTION

The planning and commissioning of health facilities is a complex undertaking. It involves strategic planning, detailed human resource planning, and a series of actions when commissioning takes place.

PLANNING AT NATIONAL LEVEL

It is necessary to use the strategic plan of the Department of National Health and Population Development at national level for the initiation of effective planning in health care organizations countrywide. This formulates the mission, philosophy, values, strategic objectives, strategies and service plans of the department for the country as a whole. It gives direction to planning at all other levels in the public sector health services, including the military health service. Planning in the private sector is influenced by national planning.

Public sector projects are approved by the Minister of Health and Population Development, the treasury, and the provincial executive committee. In private health-care top-level planning is carried out by the board of directors.

CAPITAL PLANNING FOR A NEW INSTITUTION AND/OR REDEVELOPMENT

Strategic planning for a proposed new project or redevelopment in the public sector will be undertaken at top level by the relevant provincial, state or military authority, with the local regional management team or equivalent. The resulting motivation will be submitted to the Department of National Health and Population Development. In the private sector the board will carry out the corporate strategic planning.

The first two stages of the five-stage planning process described in chapter one were *investigating* and *forecasting*. These two stages of the process comprise the *feasibility* study (see figure 1.1). This will consist of the statement of mission and objectives, external and internal environmental analyses, and schedules of:

- required physical facilities;
- equipment;
- posts.

Detailed financial estimates will be attached to the three schedules. In addition, a manpower forecast (forecasting demand and supply) will accompany the schedule of required posts.

Once the project has been approved, the commissioning team will be established. This may occur one or two years after the feasibility study was submitted with the initial manpower plan and estimates. Thus there may be a considerable time lapse between forecasting (stage two of the five-stage planning process), action planning (stage three), and the development of the human resource plan as set out in figure 1.1.

COMMISSIONING AND HUMAN RESOURCE PLANNING

Millard describes commissioning as bringing the hospital building, plant, and equipment to a state of operational readiness, with suitable numbers of staff trained to work using systems which match the design (Millard 1981: 18).

The commissioning team works together with the hospital management team and the project and design teams. A major function of the commissioning team is to produce the human resource plan in conjunction with the hospital management and the provincial branch or the directors.

The members of the team who are responsible for co-ordinating human resource planning will liaise with medical, nursing, administrative, and other categories of personnel and the staff section for the project. In the absence of a qualified human resource manager, a senior and experienced nurse member of the team may be delegated to take responsibility, working with a member of the administrative staff who has experience in staff work and finance. She will liaise with the head of the institution, the project team, divisional and departmental heads, heads of the services, and line managers.

Due to the size of the planning task, it is usual for personnel to be made available by the health authority to undertake the detailed human resource planning with the managers and the co-ordinators. When the stage of appointing staff is reached, additional personnel will be required to deal with the suddenly increased workload. With regard to the nursing division (which characteristically comprises the largest total number of personnel in any service, accounts for over 40% of the budget, and requires detailed organization) it is usual for the tasks to be delegated to experienced nursing personnel and clerks who work in co-operation with the head of nursing.

The impact of a new facility on the size of the establishment

In forecasting the needs for human resources for a new health service or redevelopment, planners need to be aware of opportunities for introducing creative change in clinical medical practice and procedures through the introduction of sophisticated technology which requires new skills. Usually more space is provided in new buildings with different spatial configurations. In one new hospital floor space almost doubled. The number of beds increased by 35% in wards and by 45% in intensive care units.

New systems are introduced, updated, and expanded in fields such as informatics, materials handling, and management. Orientation, induction, and in-service education programmes are required in support. These invariably necessitate an increase in the staffing establishment. This is a controversial issue in view of the scarcity of resources. Plans may be curtailed due to lack of finance.

In carrying out strategic human resource planning and management during commissioning, the five stages of the strategic human resource planning process are again used.

Figure 3.1, which shows the relationship between human resource planning and commissioning, provides guidelines indicating (in the first column) the three phases of commissioning with key activities (Millard 1981: 10). Phase one sees the establishment of the commissioning team immediately the project has been approved at top level. Phase two is a long period in which buildings are erected. During this time there is detailed planning of the human resource programmes and the management systems that will enable people to carry out their appointed work within the buildings as they were planned.

In phase three of the commissioning process, the time for handover approaches — buildings are completed and handed over. This is a period of accelerated activity for commissioning teams and for the personnel who will be moving their departments into the new facility after handover, according to the commissioning management control plan.

In column two of figure 3.1, the activities undertaken in human resource planning are set out against the three phases of commissioning. Column three contains the related human resource tasks. These fall into the categories of action planning and implementation (ie stages three and four of the five-stage process as shown in figure 1.1).

Monitoring and evaluation of the manpower plan in relation to the commissioning management control plans is done at top management and departmental levels in order to measure progress in the implementation of the human resource plan. In some projects, commissioning may continue for several years, depending on the phasing of the project.

In the case of a decanting operation, when a section moves from its existing area into a temporary area, monitoring is essential. The information that is recorded is evaluated against the standards that

Figure 3.1: Human resource planning in relation to commissioning

Phases of commissioning	Human resource planning activities	Comment SHR planning activities as shown in figure 1.1
Phase 1 Establishment of commissioning team	Develop the manpower plan	Set HR objectives, plan strategies, schedules, posts, and finance
Phase 2 Building and preparation period	1. Design personnel systems and organizational structures.	This starts when building has commenced, with development of operational policies and management systems, documentation and planning of equipment and supplies.
	2. Preparation of staffing schedules	
	3. Consultation and preparation of recruitment plan	Consultation with department heads. Gain consensus. Make detailed schedules with costing for each department.
	4. Advance appointments of senior personnel	Stage IV. Implementing. Timeous, carefully-worded advertisements. Considered selection. Planned dates of appointments, neither early nor late.
Phase 3 Approaching handover, completion of buildings and opening	1. Recruitment, advertising, selection, and appointment.	Prepare staffing. Evaluate progress. Contingency plans in case of changes in MCP budget for the recruiting programme.
	2. Staff transfers.	
	3. Orientation, induction, and training.	

(Phases one, two, and three of commissioning and functions in column two from Millard 1981: 10) have been set. Methods that are found to be satisfactory are applied in the next decanting operation and the unsatisfactory ones are eliminated. It has been found that, in a series of decantings, the performance of personnel improved as each group incorporated the lessons learned from previous groups. The attitudes and motivation of personnel improved each time.

In this period of upheaval for staff and patients, all aspects are monitored and information is recorded. This should be managed in such a way as to obtain the maximum opportunities for learning and teaching from the exercise. Staff and patients receive support from the human resource management or personnel development staff and counsellors.

The human resource programmes for performance and career management should be planned and instituted from the beginning in order to ensure the effective and timeous acquisition, employment, and utilization of people (Walker 1980: 10). The programmes should be monitored, evaluated, and developed for the short- and long-term.

Regardless of whether an organization is established or in the commissioning state, management has a duty to facilitate the management of careers and performance. The development of people in their careers should not be interrupted, suspended, or jeopardized because they are involved in commissioning. The line managers should carry out routine staff appraisals from the beginning and should facilitate development of human potential by educating, guiding, and counselling regarding career paths and planning. The needs of the organization and of the individual should be weighed-up, and personnel should be counselled in order to prevent them being sidelined. Records should be kept of interviews and decisions.

We shall now deal with specific aspects to be monitored and evaluated against the detailed manpower plan during phase three of commissioning — handover and practical completion prior to opening.

Recruitment

This is the forerunner of selection. Recruitment practices and the wording of advertisements have both positive and negative effects on the attitudes of the public and of personnel. This applies particularly where the issues of equity, opportunities for minorities, and affirmative action are concerned. The recruitment programme should be monitored, evaluated, and amended as necessary to ensure an adequate number of the desired type of applicants. Likewise, the policy regarding affirmative action and equal employment opportunity should be applied, monitored, and evaluated from the start. Progress with the programme may be audited. An adequate budget should be planned for the recruiting programme.

One of the aims of recruiting should be to bring in individuals with the appropriate qualifications, qualities, and potential who will be needed for promotion at a later stage. This should be monitored as a criterion for judging the effectiveness of the recruiting programme.

Selection

Choosing the right person for the job is important for an organization. Human resources make the organization what it is, and good staff selection also enables the individual employee to be productive and achieve job satisfaction. The line manager should play a major part in the selection of his staff. Selection tests may be used as well as the interview and selection committee methods.

Monitoring and evaluation of selection methods are important to the organization in order to ensure satisfactory appointments. They are also important for the public, who note fairness or otherwise in an organization. If the impression is negative, recruitment by an organization could be badly affected. Conversely, a positive impression could promote recruitment.

Appointment

Decisions will be taken in consultation with senior management about advance appointments of key senior staff and those to receive special training for new technology or procedures.

The advertisement should indicate a closing date. Numbers permitting, there will be shortlisting of applicants who will be interviewed and appointed if satisfactory. Time may be needed for appointees to work a period of notice before being able to commence work. This must be considered in relation to the management control plan when making appointments and making placements according to the staffing schedules.

Staff should be deployed according to the detailed plan for each department and section. Monitoring, evaluation, and control can be facilitated by introducing a schedule of staffing which gives information on the number of staff available, the total number of beds, and the maximum number of beds which can be staffed with the available staff complement. One academic hospital applied the policy that wards would not be opened until to do so was safe for the patients. The level of nursing staffing was a key variable.

A tool — the schedule of projected staffing status — was designed in order to enable managers to resist pressure to open required numbers of beds with too few staff. Figure 3.2 shows a computer printout of the projected staffing status for a number of intensive

Figure 3.2: Projected staffing status

NORM USED = 32.82 HRS PER PATIENT PER WEEK *
RATIO USED 40:40:20

GSH NURSING DIVISION
PROJECTED STAFFING STATUS
FOR NGSH

REF: NJ/32

MONTH: DECEMBER
YEAR: 1988

WARDS	BEDS	RATIO: CATEGORY STAFF REQ. FOR 24 HR SERVICE				ALLOCATION OF PERSONNEL				DEFICIT/EXCESS				HRS OF CARE AVAILABLE	
		RN	EN	NA	TOTAL	RN	EN	NA	TOTAL	RN	EN	NA	TOTAL	HRS	%
C13	14	5	5	2	11	3	2	2	8	-1	-2	0	-4	22	66.0
C5	32	11	11	5	26	7	5	5	17	-3	-5	-1	-9	22	66.0
C9	12	4	4	2	10	3	2	2	7	-1	-2	0	-3	22	66.0
C22	30	11	11	5	27	11	8	7	25	0	-3	1	-2	34	93.1
C23	15	9	9	5	23	9	7	6	21	0	-2	1	-2	56	93.1
J7	20	7	7	4	18	7	5	4	17	0	-2	1	-1	34	93.1
D26	23	8	8	4	21	8	6	5	19	0	-2	1	-1	34	93.1
C27	20	36	36	18	90	35	26	22	84	-1	-10	4	-6	167	93.1
E26	3	5	5	3	13	5	4	3	13	0	-1	1	-1	167	93.1
		0	0	0	0				0	0	0	0	0	0	0
D12	14	25	25	13	63	25	18	16	59	-1	-7	3	-4	167	93.1
D13	6	9	9	5	23	9	7	6	21	0	-2	1	-2	140	93.1
D22	13	23	23	12	58	23	17	15	54	-1	-6	3	-4	167	93.1
E12	7	11	11	5	26	10	8	7	24	0	-3	1	-2	140	93.1
F4	10	15	15	8	38	15	11	9	35	0	-4	2	-3	140	93.1
C12	28	10	10	5	25	10	7	6	23	0	-3	1	-2	34	93.1
F17	30	10	10	5	25	7	5	4	16	-3	-5	-1	-8	22	66.0
TOT	277	199	199	99	497	185	139	119	443	-13	-60	19	54		

J7 = 36 HRS   TOTAL BEDS 1288

NORM USED FOR C22 = 36 HRS
C23 = 60 HRS   D9 = 36 HRS
C17 = 60 HRS   D26 = 36 HRS
D13 = 150 HRS   E12 = 150 HRS
F4 = 150 HRS   D22 = 179.76 HRS
F19 = 36 HRS   C27 = 179.76 HRS
D27 = 36 HRS   D12 = 179.76 HRS

EXCLUDED FROM TOTALS = S/N AND P/N
OT = RN = 85 EN NA 81
ED = RN = 33 EN = 2
OPD = RN = 97 EN = 27 NA = 67
PCU = RN = 4 NA = 1
OTHER = RN = 17 EN 1 NA 6

care units. Details are given of the number of patients, wards, beds, norms used to determine the nursing complement, and allocation of available staff. Staff deficits or excess numbers and categories of staff are indicated. The hours of care available are given in the last column, indicating the percentage of the total hours of care required.

The appointment of staff may need to be accelerated or slowed down in order to have staff deployed when required. Control and co-ordination of the completion of buildings, the equipment and preparation of buildings, and the appointment and induction of personnel are essential. Without this, the personnel may be appointed too early, become demotivated, and leave. Industrial action may be triggered by discontented staff. If buildings are equipped too soon or too late, they may be left standing vacant. This can result in valuable assets not being used and deteriorating. Vacant buildings may be vandalized and equipment may be damaged or stolen. The provision of security to prevent this is expensive, and may not have been included in the initial financial estimates.

Staff transfers

This discussion concerns staff transfers in the context of the reorganization of a health care facility, which may be a redevelopment or a new facility within the region of the health authority involved. The work of Roe (1981) contains detailed information.

Management should be committed to providing job security for personnel. The principles and policies governing staff transfers should be planned, approved, and written down, taking into account the objectives of the organization and the legal provisions relating to conditions of service.

The establishment of posts, both local and in the region as a whole, should be reviewed. This makes it possible to keep posts open for transfers and the redeployment of personnel. Policies should be formulated to ensure fairness. Posts should be advertised in accordance with accepted procedures. A programme of individual interviews should be drawn up to fit in with the recruiting programme. Staff may wish to bring a colleague or representative with them. Personal records should be discussed in order to arrive at decisions regarding transfer or other outcomes. There could be changes in delegation and status such as promotion, retirement, specialization, or further study to gain new skills that will be required for future programmes (clinical, technological, or administrative). Detailed and accurate records of interviews should be kept. Counsellors should be on hand. A positive attitude should be fostered towards the new organization at all times.

There may be applications for early retirement, routine retirements, and resignations. These could result in cost-saving if posts are frozen or abolished.

Redundancy may occur as a result of the curtailment or closure of a service or through severe financial cuts. Every effort should be made to avoid this. In the case of alternative employment not being available, policies should be in place to ensure fairness in selection for redundancy. Personnel who are affected should be treated with empathy. Staff counsellors should be available to give support. The grievance-handling procedure may be invoked by personnel who do not accept their selection for redundancy.

From the initial project planning stage of a facility, the personnel need to be kept informed of matters which may affect them. Information should be provided about the proposed project and the proposed timeframes. Regular updates are essential, especially regarding:

- consultations about the proposed closure or change of use;

- arrangements to mitigate the effects of the changes on staff;

- the agreed method of transfer of staff (Roe 1981).

Accurate, continually updated information and records must be kept of the state of the establishment together with the post list, the register of staff for transfer, and the commissioning management control plan.

The foregoing are important aspects of the implementation of the human resource plan. In this country, existing methods for dealing with transfers and redundancy need to be assessed with a view to planning and introducing improvements. This applies not only to the commissioning of health care facilities but to reorganization as well. In periods of change, with changes in government policy and changing economic conditions, no effort should be spared in husbanding human resources. Staff should be able to make their contribution to the community through their labour for as long as possible, and not become a liability to the community either economically or healthwise.

CONCLUSION

The commissioning of a new facility is a complex and detailed operation. The acquisition of sufficient skilled staff members to run the new service was discussed, as well as the planning of these human resources in relation to commissioning.

References

Millard, Graham (1981). *Commissioning Hospital Buildings*. A King's Fund Guide. Third edition. King Edward's Hospital Fund for London: London.

Roe, J. W. (1981). *Policy on Arrangements for Staff Following a Closure or Change of Use of Premises*. Department of Health and Social Security: London.

Walker, James W. (1980). *Human Resource Planning*. McGraw-Hill: New York.

CHAPTER 4

PLANNING AND COMMISSIONING OF HEALTH CARE FACILITIES

Renée du Toit

CONTENTS

INTRODUCTION

The planning of hospitals and clinics offers an exciting challenge to the nurse manager.

Health care buildings are complex. It is therefore important to realize that the planning, implementation, and operation of health care buildings can easily give rise to expensive mistakes (Kleczkowski and Nilsson 1984: 4).

In view of the ever-increasing pressures on the budgets of health care organizations, it is enormously important that health care buildings should be planned, built, commissioned, and operated in the most efficient manner. To ensure that this takes place, the correct people should be involved at the appropriate stages of a building project. The multidisciplinary team involved in the planning and commissioning of buildings must understand the process that is to be followed, as well as the input that each member of the team has to provide in each of the different stages.

Nurses have gained much experience in the commissioning of hospitals and clinics. Their involvement in preparing the completed building for operation has always been accepted as essential. The opportunity for them to influence the outcome of a new or redeveloped building is, however, minimal at the commissioning stage. It is therefore essential that nurses become involved during the planning stage if they are to make any significant impact on the design and facilities that will be provided.

Involvement in planning is also one of the duties of registered nurses, viz. 'the establishment and maintenance, in the execution of the nursing regimen of an environment in which the physical and mental health of a patient is promoted' (SANC 1984).

This chapter examines the process of establishing hospitals and clinics and identifies the members of the multidisciplinary project team and their functions. Specific guidelines are given to enable nurses to participate meaningfully. The health care building process is described in three major stages, namely *planning, construction,* and *commissioning.* Emphasis is placed on the planning stage.

Examples will be given to illustrate the process, but specific guidelines or 'tips' for the design of particular departments will not be given. The references may be helpful in this regard, especially those on ward and ICU design in appendix 3.

PLANNING

The word 'planning' has different meanings for different people involved in the planning process. A closer look at the process from the perception of a need for a new facility (or a change to an existing one) to the point where it has been designed on paper will identify four steps, all of which form part of the planning process. These steps are:

- strategic health care planning;

- need identification and approval;

- briefing; and

- design.

Strategic planning

The structure of the National Health Services Facilities Plan (NHSFP) for the RSA (Republic of South Africa 1981) consists of six levels, as shown in figure 4.1.

Figure 4.1: National Health Services Facilities Plan structure

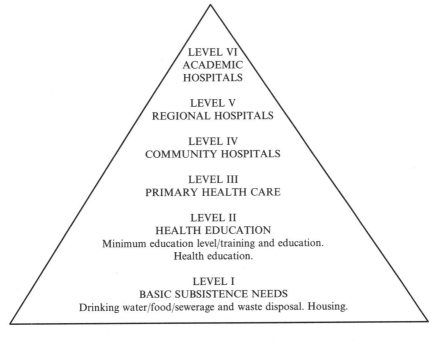

As can be seen, it is necessary to provide services in a logical progression from Level I upwards for an efficient and effective health care system.

Much emphasis has lately been put on the improvement of community health facilities in an endeavour to deliver health care more efficiently — ie to improve access to preventive, promotive, and curative health care that is close to communities and that is delivered at appropriate levels. There is also an attempt to reduce the pressure on regional hospitals which are currently overloaded with patients using them for primary health care (Hospital Supplies 1992: 4). The inappropriate use of health care facilities is costly in terms of manpower and technology.

Strategic health care planning in South Africa has been complicated significantly by the political system which has created a great number of role-players. This, however, changed to a certain extent when the 'own affairs' health departments amalgamated into the Department of National Health and Population Development.

Various bodies have been created at local, regional, and national levels in an attempt to co-ordinate health care delivery. The development of new buildings or the redevelopment of existing facilities must form part of the strategic health care planning process. Reference will be made to some of these bodies when discussing the process for the approval of needs.

Identification of needs and approval of public facilities

The planning process for capital projects — ie for new buildings or the redevelopment of existing buildings — starts with the identification of needs. This determines the level and type of health care functions — ie whether at primary, secondary, or tertiary level, space or area needed in a particular place, and the cost allowed for it.

In the public sector, health care buildings must conform with certain guidelines or 'norms' ('need norms', 'space norms' and 'cost norms') — the so-called South African Hospital Norms or 'SAHNORMS', laid down in the National Health Services Facilities Plan (NHSFP) (Republic of South Africa 1981). Different norms apply to academic and regional hospitals, community health centres, and staff accommodation. The norms are instruments for measuring the funds that are allocated for the achievement of given health care objectives within affordable limits. 'Need' refers to the need for the health service that is envisaged, ie the objective, whilst 'space' and 'cost' norms define maximum amounts of space and expenditure allowed for a building needed to provide the health service. New space and cost norms for community health centres, and for maximum security and closed ward units in psychiatric hospitals, have been established (Republic of South Africa 1992) but the need norms for these are still described in the NHSFP.

The norms serve as a framework within which planners must satisfy needs. They set limits.

The need norm either uses existing patient statistics (eg patient turnover) to determine the 'planning units' or uses the population to be served to determine the required staff. This, in turn, determines the planning units. Planning units (PUs) include, for example, examination rooms for outpatient services, beds for obstetric and day care units, and operating rooms. The number of planning units is used to calculate the space/area guidelines and cost limits of the facilities in which the services are to be rendered.

The establishment of the appropriate norms appears to be a difficult task to begin with, but with the relevant SAHNORMS at hand, and with the examples given in tables 4.1 and 4.2, it becomes an exciting challenge! Note that, although nurse managers are not generally required to do the calculations, a general understanding of the norms will give insight into the process.

The identification of needs, and the motivation for a capital project, has to be carried out within the strategic health plan of a given authority. A community profile would be of great value in drawing up the motivation and placing the project in perspective. The aim is to make the most effective use of expensive technology and manpower and to provide an efficient service to a community. A fundamental choice must be made in the selections of interventions (or services) that can realistically be expected and provided within the epidemiological and resource profile of a given community (Tjam 1992: 405): one has to decide how sophisticated the service is to be, whether the equipment needed can be operated and maintained, and whether staff can be found to run it. Trends such as the increasing possibility of conducting advanced medical procedures such as laser surgery, on an outpatient basis, rather than on an inpatient basis, are also important and will be discussed below.

Abbott (1992: 20–2) lists factors that have to be taken into account when drawing up a profile of the community for which a facility is being planned.

- demographics — population growth, morbidity, migration, etc.;

- health profile or epidemiology;

- the availability and accessibility of existing health services;

- the extent, nature, and quality of existing health care;

- the availability and training of medical, nursing, and paramedical staff;

- legal factors;

- the availability of capital and operating funds;

- the policies of the health service;

- the transport and roads infrastructure, enabling access to health care.

Table 4.1: Need, cost, and space norm calculation for CHC outpatient service

STEP	EXAMPLE
1. Establish population to be served.	30 000 people
2. Calculate expected patient visits. (a) Curative visits — 2.16 per person/ year. (b) Preventive visits — 1.5 per person/ year. (Norm visit figure often higher than recorded/actual visits.)	(a) 2.16 × 30 000 = 64 000 (b) 45 000
3. Work back to number of visits per type per day (250 days per year).	(a) 64 800 ÷ 250 = 259.2 curative patients per day (b) 180 preventive patients per day
4. Nurse can see 35 curative patients per day or 50 preventive patients per day.	(a) 259.2 ÷ 35 = 7.4 nurses (b) 3.6 nurses a + b = 11 nurses
5. Doctor will see 15% of curative patients and 10% of preventive patients. Sees 50 patients per day.	(a) 38.88 patients (b) 18 patients a + b = 56.88 patients per day
6. Calculate number of nurses (curative and preventive) and number of doctors.	Nurses 11 Doctors 1 (56.8 ÷ 50)
7. Provide one planning unit (PU) per staff member. (Examination room is the PU for outpatients.)	12 PU = 12 examination rooms
8. Area guideline AA/PU 58 m^2 AA:GA = 1:1.61 (AA = assignable area, calculated in nett m^2. GA = gross area, includes all areas of the building, circulation, and walls.)	12 × 58 = 696 m^2 nett 696 × 1.61 = 1120.56 m^2 gross area
9. Cost limit R/PU (at April 1990) is R117 642/PU	R117 641 × 12 = R1 411 692

With this information, appropriate health service goals and the strategies for meeting these goals can be drawn up. These direct the calculation and specification of the need norm for a specific project.

Note that this first step, the identification of needs, is often the most difficult and it directs the rest of the process. The population profile is constantly changing and often unpredictable. Population Statistics produced by the Bureau of Market Research, UNISA, are recommended. The Department of Health has also recommended that facilities should not be erected for an area unless the influx of people takes place in an ordered and well-calculated manner. Temporary services, such as mobiles, should therefore be provided for areas such as new squatter areas until a clear picture emerges to direct meaningful planning for permanent services.

Table 4.1 illustrates the calculations for the outpatient services at a Community Health Centre.

The space norm imposes a maximum area per planning unit. The cost norm also imposes a maximum. The cost of the project should be as far below the cost limit as possible.

The management of a particular service typically identifies a need, draws up the initial motivation for the project, and channels it to the planning division of its authority. This then verifies the need by visiting the existing facility and confirming the appropriate statistics, and calculates the planning units. The area and cost norms can then be applied.

The process is relatively straightforward for new buildings. When existing facilities have to be extended or redeveloped, one has to use the applicable statistics directed by the relevant need norm, eg that for community health centres, to establish the corresponding planning units which, in turn, dictate a certain area. The difference between the allowed area and the existing area is calculated. If the existing space is in excess of the norm allowed, then the planned alteration may not go ahead. The norm is accurate enough for one to assume that the facility is either badly managed or poorly designed; one then has to explore a management solution, or a redevelopment of existing space by moving internal walls etc., and this should be planned within the minor works budget.

Table 4.2: Examples of norm applications for regional hospitals

Department	Planning unit	Need norm	Area m^2 (gross)	Cost norm
Casualty	Patients in 3 hour peak period	Determine likely number of patients per 3 hour period	430 m^2 per 60 patients plus 100 m^2 for each additional 50 patients.	R378/m^2
Delivery unit	Delivery room	One delivery unit per 8–15 obstetric beds.	1 d.r. = 200 m^2 ×1 2 d.r. = 140 m^2 × 2 3 d.r. = 120 m^2 × 3 or more.	R78 700 R55 000 R47 200
Intensive therapy	Bed	4.5% of total general acute beds	40 m^2	R16 400

If an existing hospital, for example, requires additional delivery rooms, the need norm must first be applied to establish if any increases are possible. The need norm allows one delivery room per 8–15 obstetric beds (see table 4.2). If there are two existing delivery rooms but the number of beds has increased to 45, therefore, the need norm allows for a total of three delivery rooms — ie an increase of one room. The space norm is now applied: for a total of three delivery rooms 120 m^2 × 3 = 360 m^2 is allowed. Note that the area/m^2 allows for a delivery room and the necessary support facilities. The existing space is then calculated and compared with the allowed space. The combination of the existing space and the new/planned space may not exceed 360 m^2.

It has to be remembered that, prior to 1981, facilities may have been planned without regard for norms. Where space has been used inefficiently it may be more economical to provide additional new facilities, even if they do go over the allowed norm space, rather than carry out costly redevelopments of existing facilities just to remain within the norm. The overriding consideration should always be the provision of appropriate health services facilities rather than a slavish adherence to the norms.

If the project is possible in terms of the need and space norms, the capital and running costs are calculated as well as the effect of the project on present facilities. The planning division then submits this whole motivation to the head of the relevant authority (eg the Executive Director: Health Services, Provincial Administration). The project is then placed within the health priorities of the department/authority.

If approved, the planning division then forwards the motivation to the controlling authority (eg the Executive Committee of the Provincial Administration). This ensures that the authority has the funds and the means (including staffing and funds to meet running costs) to carry out the project and that it fits in with the overall priorities in relation to the other responsibilities of the relevant administration such as roads or education.

The calculation of running costs is often neglected at this stage, and this may result in facilities being built but not occupied for lengthy periods. This has tended to happen where one authority/body provides the capital funding and another meets the running costs — the problem should improve as health care structures become more rational. Note that the running costs overtake the capital (building and equipping) costs within two to three years for hospitals (Cowan and Louw 1985) and within about one year for clinics and community health centres.

After approval, the application is submitted to the Regional Health Co-ordinating Committee (RHCC) which consists of all relevant health role players and is constituted differently in each region. This debates all planning requests for the region and makes recommendations by consensus. Undecided matters can be referred to the National Health Policy Council, constituted in terms of the National Policy for Health Act, No. 116, of 1990. Note that all proposed facilities, whether planned by the private sector, the Independent Development Trust, local or provincial authorities, or national states, have to be discussed by the RHCC.

The relevant authority then applies to the Department of National Health and Population Development in Pretoria (DNHPD) for approval, and includes the recommendations of the RHCC. This allows the DNHPD to carry out its controlling and co-ordinating role, and ensures that the project conforms to SAHNORMS. If approved, this approval constitutes a 'licence to proceed with planning'. The Department of National Health uses seven health care regions in its planning — these overlap to a certain extent with the generally-used nine official Regions for Development Planning designated by the Department of Constitutional Development and Planning.

There are various parameters that determine whether further approvals are needed. Some of these are: the value of the project, whether new construction is involved, and whether existing norms are being exceeded by more than 10%. In general, projects under R5m require minimal approval, and projects between R5m and R20m require approval of the Treasury Committee for Building Norms and Cost Limits. Projects over R20m require the additional approval of the Treasury Capital Priorities Committee. Mechanisms have recently been developed to co-ordinate projects within a five-year Central Capital Planning System, where each large government authority and department is represented.

Note that the Treasury approvals do not guarantee the availability of funds and are merely a 'licence' to spend money which should be budgeted for in the normal way.

The Health Services and Works Department will then prioritize the project. The Works Department can then administer and manage the project, appointing consultants and putting the project out to tender.

It may take a year or more to have the project approved in principle. When it would be built is determined according to the priorities and strategic plan of the region and available funds. The importance of adequate documentation by the original motivators is therefore clear!

Identification of needs and approval of private facilities

The need for, or perceived viability of, a private hospital or clinic may be identified by any person with or without health care experience. A project may be started by a group of doctors or a private developer, for example. Establishment of private hospitals is governed by requirements laid down in the Regulations Governing Private Hospitals and Unattached Operating Theatre Units (R.158, Government Gazette number 6832, 1 February 1980, as amended). The routes and stages of approval are illustrated in figure 4.2.

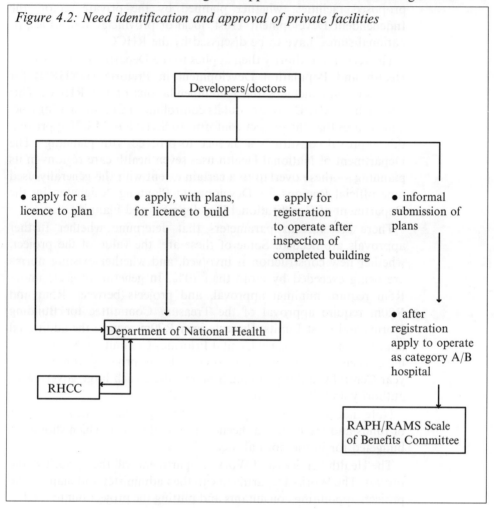

Figure 4.2: Need identification and approval of private facilities

The SAHNORMS are loosely applied when plans are studied by the DNHPD. It should, however, be noted that the Regulations (R.158) sets minimum standards as guidelines to planners and designers. This can lead to the provision of inadequate space when decisions are based mostly on cost rather than a close look at the functions and operation of the facility. The minimum space requirement for a central sterlizing department (CSSD) is a case in point. The regulations under R.158 are badly documented and are applied with interpretations that are open to question. The regulation is currently under review.

The briefing stage

This starts once the need, space, and cost norms have been approved — ie once permission has been granted to take the project to the design stage.

It is recommended that the brief be presented to, or developed with, the designers as a structured document. This increases the likelihood that requirements will be considered as an integrated whole rather than as isolated departments or services. It is useful to view the hospital as an open system. Figure 4.3 gives a broad outline of the types of input, throughput, and output to be found.

It is crucial that nurses, and all service providers, participate in the briefing stage as the possibility of them influencing the design and functioning of the building is greatest during this stage (Kleczkowski and Nilsson 1984: 20).

There is a great temptation to do the 'real planning' only when a plan has been developed and one has 'something to look at'. This approach is, however, detrimental to the development of buildings and services. Briefing leads the briefing team to consider the hospital/clinic as a whole and to use the brief as a checklist during the design stage. Briefing also saves time in that the plan does not have to be redesigned every time that some important aspect which has been neglected is suddenly remembered. The brief can be augmented during the design stage, but the initial development of a holistic brief allows for realistic integration of changes at a later stage. Planning a facility without a proper brief is rather like trying to do a puzzle where many of the pieces are missing.

The brief should therefore present a clear picture of the intentions of the client and will be used as a checklist once plans have been drawn.

The briefing documents

The brief consists of three documents:

- the schedule of accommodation;

- the operational narrative;

- the room descriptions.

The schedules refer to the list of rooms and their proposed sizes per department, as shown in table 4.3. The operational narrative describes the overall concept and the purpose of the facility, as well as the intended objectives, functions, and relationships of each department. The room descriptions detail the functions to be performed in each type of room, and the services, fittings, and equipment needed to fulfil these functions.

Figure 4.3: The hospital as an open system

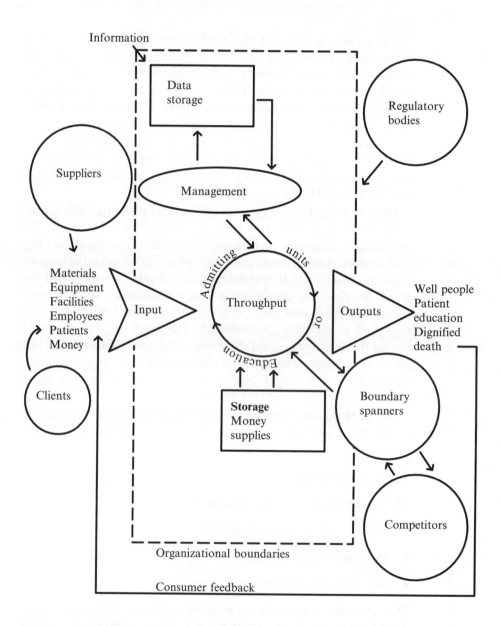

Information

Data
storage

Regulatory
bodies

Suppliers

Management

Materials
Equipment
Facilities
Employees
Patients
Money

Input

Admitting   units

Throughput

or

Education

Outputs

Well people
Patient
education
Dignified
death

Clients

Storage
Money
supplies

Boundary
spanners

Competitors

Organizational boundaries

Consumer feedback

Sullivan and Decker 1988: 18

Table 4.3: Schedule of accommodation

NEW GROOTE SCHUUR HOSPITAL

		Date: Sept 79					
		Rev. Sept 82	0	1	0	1	0

TYPICAL WARD
ACCOMMODATION FOR
30–32 BEDS

NUMBER			DEPARTMENT	Area m²			
				Nett	S/total	Gross	Remark
01			ADMINISTRATIVE FACILITIES				
	1.1		Offices outside ward:				
		1	Head of firm office 1/ward	12			
		2	Senior lecturer's office 2/2 wards @ 20 m²	10			
		3	Matron's office 1/4 wards @ 12 m²	3			
		4	Social worker/sister tutor/dietitian				
			1/2 wards @ 10 m²	5			
		5	Consultants part-time 1/2 wards @ 12 m²	6			
		6	Consulting room 1/4 wards @ 8 m²	2	38		
	1.2		Offices within ward				
		1	Registrar	11.5			
		2	Interns/student interns office	17.5			
		3	Laboratory adjacent to office	4			
		4	Relatives interview	10			
		5	Ward secretary 1/2 wards @ 16 m²	8			
		6	Sister's office	12	63		
02			TEACHING FACILITIES				
	2.1	1	Seminar room 1/2 wards @ 32 m²	16			
		2	Nurses training room 1/2 wards @ 13 m²	7	23		
03			INPATIENT FACILITIES				
	3.1	1	6 bed rooms × 4 @ 60 m²	240			
		2	1 bed room × 6 @ 12 m² +	72			
			4 bed rooms × 1 @ 40 m² (88)				
		3	Day/dining room 1/2 wards @ 35 m²	17.5	329.5		
04			INPATIENT ANCILLIARIES				
	4.1	1	Nurses' station	16			
		2	Treatment room	20			
		3	Dirty utility/HMC/flowers	16			
		4	Clean utility	4			
		5	Bedpan sluice	8			
		6	Bedpan sluice 1/2 wards @ 8 m²	4			
		7	Stores 1 @ 15 m²				
			1 @ 10 m²				
			1 @ 6 m²	31	99		
	4.2		Ablution and toilet facilities				
		1	Hospital type bathroom	7			
		2	Shower/WC/Whb × 8 @ 4 m²	32	39		

New Groote Schuur Hospital			Date: Sept 79				
			Rev. Sept 82				
		Pg. 2	TYPICAL WARD ACCOMMODATION FOR 30–32 BEDS				

NUMBER			DEPARTMENT	Area M²			
				Nett	S/tot.	Gross	Remark
05			**SERVICE FACILITIES**				
	5.1	1	Housekeeper's office 1/2 wards @ 10 m²	5			
		2	Central kitchen 1/4 wards @ 32 m²	8			
		3	Collection return goods + HMC 1/4 wards @ 12 m²	3			
		4	Laying-out room 1/4 wards @ 12 m²	3			
		5	Patient reception area 1/4 wards				
			— waiting area @ 8 m²	2			
			— kit room @ 14 m²	3.5			
		6	Tea room 1/4 wards @ 20 m² = 5 m² *		24.5		*On duty
06			**STAFF AND PUBLIC FACILITIES**				
	6.1	1	Nurses' chng. rm & toilets × 2 @ 8 m²	16			
		2	Domestics' WC 1/4 wards @ 4 m²	1			
		3	Labourers' WC 1/4 wards @ 4 m²	1			
		4	Staff M + F 1/2 wards @ 4 m²	4			
		5	Public M + F 1/2 wards @ ± 5 m²	±5			
		6	Sleep-in 1 ward @ 8 m²	8			
		7	Ablutions for sleep-in 1/2 wards @ 4 m²	2	37		
					653		
			+ 45% gross factor		293		
						946	

The schedule of accommodation

This is a complete list of the space required by each department. The schedule for a typical ward, developed for the New Groote Schuur Hospital project, is shown in table 4.3. The total gross area of the hospital or clinic may not exceed the space norms specified for the facility. The gross area is the floor area calculated to the exterior of the containing walls, while the nett area is the area of the floor calculated to the interior of the containing walls (Kleczkowski and Nilsson 1984: 78).

The total *nett* area allocated to a department is the total area within all the listed rooms. The department's total *gross* area is the total area occupied by the whole department, including wall thickness and circulation space such as corridors and staircases. Flexibility should be maintained when planning within the gross area.

The nett areas are usually calculated first and a grossing factor, often 45%, is added to this to arrive at the gross areas. This allows the architect a certain flexibility. If a department — for example a ward — can be designed to fit into less than the total gross area, the opportunity arises for either creating more rooms in the department, or transferring the area gained to another department in need of more space (if practically possible) or, of course, effecting a cost saving by not building more rooms. It must be remembered that the space norms determine the maximum space allowed and that an efficient plan could be developed in less space. The transfer of space between departments should be controlled by the policy-makers and architects but in consultation with the users — the individual departments usually have their own interests at heart whereas the policy-makers should have a co-ordinating function.

In order to develop an understanding of space it is advisable to use scale models or to do a mock-up and physically measure an area in order to establish the required space. It is preferable to base this on a room where the intended functions are presently being performed so as to prevent any misunderstandings and to eliminate guesswork. It is also useful to measure a room that one is familiar with, such as an office or the room in which planning meetings are held, and to use this as a point of reference.

Most mock-ups can be simple and inexpensive. To determine the recommended space in a consulting room, for example, one would use an existing one, with the existing or intended furniture, and set up a few activities requiring space — for example, interviewing the patient and/or escort, physical examination, x-ray viewing, etc. The floor area required is then marked with masking tape or chalk and measured. Loose screens should be used to indicate walls, if needed, as this helps to define the space. It is important to be as realistic as possible and identify an absolute minimum space and perhaps make allowance for more working space if there is additional space available. Figure 4.4a shows the space required at the bedside — the tape on the floor represents the cubicle curtains. A model of a consulting room is shown in figure 4.4b.

Note that the schedule of accommodation is a guideline and room sizes may change as the design develops.

The operational narrative

This tells the 'story' of how a department is intended to function. It should be written so that a non-clinical person, for example an architect or engineer, can develop an understanding of the

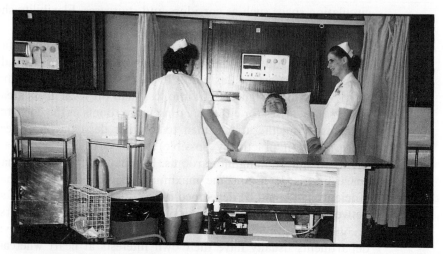

Figure 4.4a (above): Mock-up of bedspace

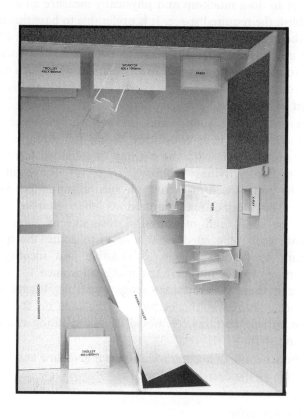

Figure 4.4b (left):

Model of consulting room

Table 4.4: Guidelines for writing an operational narrative

I PHILOSOPHY AND OBJECTIVES OF SERVICE

As an introduction, give a general and concise description of your department or area: the aims, activities, and workload. (Try to do it in such a way that you clearly explain to an outsider what your department is all about.)

II POLICIES

1 *Population* involved, daily statistics of categories of patients seen, students taught or operations done etc. Also state exclusions and how these are dealt with.

2 *Hours of work* for different categories of staff and timespan during which the service will be provided.

3 *Admissions policy* eg patients admitted to ICU on referral by consultant of referring department.

4 *Relationships:* external and internal.

4.1 *External relationships:* giving reasons, expand on the desired relationships with other departments. Bear in mind that the hospital has to work as an integrated whole; in the end you may not be located in the ideal position but in a functional one. Use diagrams to illustrate intention (refer to diagram 1).

4.2 *Internal relationships:* briefly explain the relationships of rooms or areas **within** your department. Refer to diagram 2.

5 *Flow patterns:* explain the desired flow pattern of patients, staff, supplies, food, refuse, etc. Give a brief description and an illustration. Refer to diagram 3.

6 *Support systems/services:* describe the desired systems applicable to your department, eg portering, catering, cleaning.

7 Communication and mechanical and electrical services, eg telephone, intercom, computer, steam supply — in general terms only. Specific needs will be described later, per room.

8 *Physical environment:* state only unusual or specific needs, eg in ophthalmology wards patients may prefer dark rooms, or a piece of equipment may require structural support or certain levels of humidity or temperature.

9 *Staff involved:* list categories, numbers and facilities required. A work study assessment will verify needs later on.

III ROOM FUNCTIONS

Give a specific description of all activities performed in each room. At a later date facilities needed to fulfil these functions will be drawn up and these may be described in various documents.

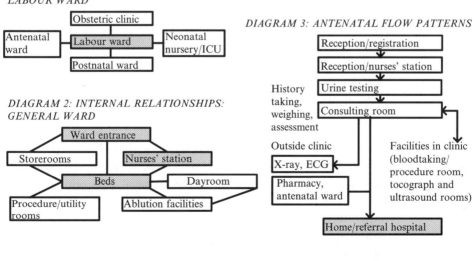

DIAGRAM 1: EXTERNAL RELATIONSHIPS: LABOUR WARD

DIAGRAM 2: INTERNAL RELATIONSHIPS: GENERAL WARD

DIAGRAM 3: ANTENATAL FLOW PATTERNS

department's aims, objectives, and functions. The process of writing it allows one to consider all aspects and to decide whether to continue current practices or to introduce change. It may be easier for staff to plan for change in a new environment.

Table 4.4 may be used as a guideline. It has three major sections. Firstly the philosophy and objectives of the department, secondly the policies, and lastly room functions.

The philosophy is a broad statement of intent, and the objectives should provide an overview of the department.

The policies describe the way in which the department is intended to function with regard to the population (eg type of patients seen), or the work involved (eg operations done). Hours of work, admission policy, and relationships follow.

External relationships refer to the department's association with other areas — for example the labour ward, the ante- and postnatal wards, and the nursery should be close to each other while the obstetric clinic should not be too far away. (The need for an operating room within the labour ward depends on the size of the facility, its patient turnover, and the available staff.)

It is essential to give reasons for requests because if the architect understands them he is far more likely to develop a logical master-plan which would locate departments in the most practical positions.

Internal relationships in a department refer to the relationship of the rooms within the department. Reasons should again be given why one room should be associated with another or perhaps why it should be kept away from others.

A description of the flow patterns of patients, staff, supplies, refuse, etc. provides further background for developing the sketch plan. The need for support systems such as portering, catering, etc. should be identified by each department. The systems themselves should be described separately in their entirety. Table 4.5 gives a list of services and systems to be considered — the systems are initially referred to when drawing up the brief for their associated departments, but are detailed only during the design stage. Systems should never be adopted from another facility without analysing the implications for the intended facility.

The communication, mechanical, and electrical service needs such as steam, intercoms, and bedhead services, should be referred to in general terms only as they are detailed later in the room descriptions.

Special requirements regarding the physical environment should also be identified — for example, if specific levels of humidity or temperature are required, perhaps in a nursery.

Staff categories, numbers, and facilities should be listed — detailed work study assessments will be done later on, with reference to the design of the building.

Table 4.5: Services and systems to be considered

CLINICAL SERVICES

Hospitals and clinics may have any combination of the following clinical disciplines and services may be rendered at a general practitioner or specialist level for inpatients and/or outpatients.

MEDICAL
General medical
Cardiology
Immunology
Nephrology
Neurology
Dermatology
Haematology

SURGICAL
General surgery
Orthopaedics
Cardiac surgery
Thoracic surgery
Urology
Ophthalmology
Otorhinolaryngology
Neurosurgery

INTENSIVE SERVICES
Medical emergency
Trauma
Intensive care
Renal dialysis
Labour ward
Burns unit

OBSTETRICS AND GYNAECOLOGY
Ante- postnatal clinics and wards
Labour ward
Nursery
Infertility
Family clinic

PAEDIATRICS

Neonatology

ALTERNATIVE MEDICINE
Chiropractor
Homeopath
Herbalist
Traditional healers
Traditional birth attendants

PSYCHIATRY
Psychology
Psychiatrics

ANAESTHETICS
Pain clinic

ONCOLOGY

CLINICAL SUPPORT SERVICES

These services support inpatient and outpatient departments and include:

Administration:

Information/computer, inpatient and outpatient administration, staff administration, typing, revenue, registry, boardroom.

Radiology
Radiography
Radiotherapy
Nuclear medicine
Pathology:

Chemical/bacteriology, virology/antenical, microbiology/haematology

Blood bank
Physiotherapy
Occupational therapy
Speech and hearing therapy
Social work
Dietetics
Community health
Stomatherapy
Dental clinic

GENERAL SUPPORT SYSTEMS *(Table 4.5 contd.)*

Catering	Security
Materials handling	Maintenance
Linen handling/cleaning	Central medical technical department
Waste handling	Orthopaedic workshop
Pharmacy	Mortuary
Central sterile supplies	Messenger/pneumatic tube
Infection control	Transport
Sewerage/water supply	Parking
Portering	Signage

MECHANICAL AND ELECTRICAL SERVICES

Building management
Boilers
Incinerators
Bulk and reserve oxygen
Fire detection and protection

Electrical:	Standby
	UPS
	Lighting
Communications:	Telephone
	Intercom
	Nurse and emergency call
	Computer
Air conditioning:	Heating
	Ventilation
Medical gas:	Medical gas
	Air installation
	Vacuum installation
	Plant rooms and bulk storage
Lifts	

AUXILIARY SERVICES

Education:	Medical school
	Nursing college
	Lecture rooms

Creche
Chapel
Banks
Building societies
Post office
Public telephones

Library:	Staff/patients

Volunteer services
Religious counsellors

Recreational facilities:	Indoor/outdoor

Residential facilities
Laundromat
Staff clinic
Hospital school
Restaurant/cafeteria/vending

In the third major part of the operational narrative, room functions should be described in detail. There is usually not enough time at the outset of a project to include detailed room descriptions as part of the initial brief. If this can be done, however, the room functions need not be included in this part of the narrative but can be briefly referred to in the section describing internal relationships.

As mentioned, systems should be drawn up separately — refer to table 4.5. The same preparation and process is followed as is used for briefing in order to arrive at the correct system. Systems planning is rooted in a departmental or service area, but pervades all parts of the hospital. Cleaning equipment and staff may, for example, be based in the central cleaning department but teams would go to all departments. Some facilities, such as slophoppers to dispose of dirty floor water, would, however, be provided within or close to particular departments within the hospital. Systems develop logically from the briefing documents and should be under discussion as sketch plans are developed.

Systems are finalized through the combined efforts of the briefing and design teams. Having first identified the need for various systems in the operational narrative, the developer is responsible for analysing the management and operational implications of a system while the design team focuses on the design implications. The client retains the authority to approve or reject the system.

Nurses are particularly affected by the efficiency of the support systems and must be involved in planning them. Principles should be laid down at the outset to serve as guidelines for the detail to be developed. When handling linen, for example, the principle that as few people as possible should handle dirty linen has to be followed up with a policy that contaminated linen should be sluiced centrally by a machine rather than by nurses or domestics at ward level.

The schedules and narrative for each department should develop alongside each other and should be in balance. One could, for example, start by listing the rooms one supposes would be needed and then describe the department. The schedules would then be adjusted as the functions to be performed are detailed.

The team preparing an operational narrative must be flexible and must include as many relevant disciplines as possible. An architect with specialist knowledge may, for example, give an important input at this early stage.

Completing the operational narrative is, however, of the utmost importance as it leads the planners to analyse the various medical, nursing, and other functions to be carried out, and the requirements in terms of space, fixtures and equipment needed to carry out the functions. It is appropriate to assess current practices and plan for changes which may be needed when drawing up the operational narrative. It is often easier to adopt new practices when the whole environment changes.

The room descriptions

This last section of the brief contains the detailed description of requirements for every type of room in each department. It is essential to describe the functions to be performed in a room before listing the facilities or equipment.

The description of a function logically directs the choice of facilities and equipment needed to fulfil that particular function. These facilities include:

- finishes — eg wall and floor coverings;

- mechanical and electrical services — oxygen, power, etc;

- fittings — eg worktops and cupboards;

- environmental standards — air-handling, temperature, and noise control;

- sanitary ware — basins, showers, etc;

- fixtures — mirrors, grabrails;

- equipment.

Any format can be used to document room descriptions, but the information should be collected and presented in a standardized manner to allow for easy reference.

It is helpful to first draw up a master set of room descriptions — for one ward, for example — and then to adopt these for successive departments.

The brief is therefore used to guide the designers, and plans can be checked against it. The brief is also eventually used during the commissioning stage in order to develop the operational policies and manuals for every department — ie for translating the original intentions into policies for the hospital or clinic. Staff should then be trained to ensure that the facilities are used as planned.

Development of the brief

Overall responsibility for the development of the brief and for the participation of relevant staff members during the various stages usually lies with the medical superintendent or the manager of the hospital or clinic. The nurse manager is similarly responsible for organizing the input of the nursing staff, as are other heads for their departments. Multidisciplinary input is as essential in planning as it is in clinical practice.

Nurses, in particular, have an important role to play in integrating information from different departments since they work in most departments and have detailed knowledge of the functions, services, and equipment needed and the interrelationships between various departments. They are also the only professional staff members who personally attend to patients over any length of time and can observe their reactions to their environment in the activities of daily living and treatment.

It is furthermore important to consult all categories of staff in the planning of a department, including, for example, domestics and porters, as each staff category has a different and important contribution to make.

Preparation for planners to participate meaningfully involves the appointment of appropriate staff, followed by reading, visiting other facilities, and analysing both current and future practices.

Appointing or allocating staff specifically for planning is probably the most productive and cost-effective way to organize staff participation in the planning process. Even for smaller projects, where full-time commitment is not necessary, specific people should be allocated planning tasks and their work schedules should be rearranged to allow for this.

The appointment of an overall co-ordinating body, usually called a planning and commissioning unit (PCU), is essential. Such a unit can be at hospital or head office level and should at least include medical, nursing, and administrative representatives.

The planners should be able to analyse clinical and managerial functions, and should have the ability and authority to take decisions and make recommendations at the appropriate levels. Planners at managerial level principally co-ordinate and elicit information from the staff (users) in various areas. The users are the up-to-date experts in their fields, able to relay important aspects of their practice, as well as trends.

The appropriate individuals to draw up the briefing documents vary from project to project. The medical superintendent or general manager is usually responsible, but may delegate the work to individual heads of departments. Any category of the health team may then be designated within each department to draw up the documents for approval by the head.

What is important is not who establishes the documents but rather how the decisions recorded in the documents are made.

The most meaningful way in which to make planning decisions is to have multidisciplinary meetings. The appointed departmental planner, or head of department, or PCU member, could chair the meetings. The advantages of multidisciplinary meetings are, firstly, that everyone has the opportunity to listen to and understand the needs and viewpoints of the other participants and, secondly, that much time is saved by not having to go back and forth between different groups.

Brief development meetings should therefore have representatives from:

- people working in the department — medical, nursing, and other specific users;

- hospital management or PCU — policy-makers;

- support and maintenance services, as appropriate;

- professionals with appropriate experience.

The meetings for the development of the brief lead to design meetings where plans, based on the brief, are tabled and discussed. The design meetings remain multidisciplinary but now include design team members as appropriate — ie architects and/or relevant engineers.

The briefing documents (and plans) must be approved by all sections of the client body. For public projects, this would include the user (head of department — medical and nursing), the medical superintendent/representative at hospital/clinic level, the planning division of the Director of Health Services, and the Department of Works. Time and effort may again be saved if representatives of all these sections are present at briefing meetings and later design meetings. The way in which planning decisions were made at strategic, middle management and operational level for the New Durban Academic Hospital serves as a specific example (Du Toit 1990: 27–33).

The client body (eg Department of Health Services, Department of Works, and users) is responsible for the brief, including the room descriptions. It can, however, benefit the project if the client and members of the design team are brought together when the room descriptions are drawn up. This combined process works well as the client/user can state the functions and equipment that are intended for the rooms whilst the designers can suggest the most appropriate and economical facilities needed to fulfil the functions — ie the finishes, services, and fittings.

The design team will also have a greater understanding of the needs and functions of the health care workers if they participate in the meetings to establish room details. This understanding enhances the development of a plan that meets the needs of the department. The advantage of good communication between briefing and design teams cannot be overemphasized.

Note, again, that the representatives of the different sections should have the authority to make decisions at the meeting. They must also be in a position to convey the opinions of their managers or heads of departments and colleagues and, in turn, should act as a source of information to them. Much time, effort, and energy may be wasted if a significant change is made at the end of a period of discussion because someone was not fully informed.

Continuity of the people involved in the project is very important. This should be borne in mind when appointing staff for planning. Planners should, as mentioned, have general clinical and management experience, but a general understanding of the principles involved and enthusiasm for the project is as important.

Having appointed or designated planners as required at the various levels, it is essential that everyone involved be clearly advised of their functions — for example, at operational level they should be given a format for drawing up the briefing documents. Everyone should also be made aware of the importance of preparing for a meeting — agendas should therefore be circulated in advance. Good record-keeping is also absolutely essential in order to document the development of decisions.

Once all departments have completed their briefing documents, the planners at middle management level or the PCU should prepare an integrated brief for the project.

One set of health care facility users who are usually ill-represented are the patients. A novel approach was used during the new Derbyshire Children's Hospital project (Butler 1992: 33–5).

They used children in groups aged 4–7, 7–11 and 11–14 years, drawn from various schools, as well as parents and the staff of the existing hospital. Seven workshops were held over the five year period and were started before any design work, but after a site and the budget content had been decided on.

The workshops were run by a group of community artists who formed a bridge between the designers and the users, were independent of each, and freed designers and users to participate in the discussions (they would otherwise have been tied up or distracted by chairing meetings, record-keeping, or providing sketches during the discussions).

The project and design teams felt strongly that they knew what the users wanted and what they needed to get right in the building. The strength of the design also convinced the users that the new building would retain the best elements of the old — a crucial factor in maintaining user interest over the project period.

The planning and construction of clinics and community health centres was recently funded by the sale of strategic oil reserves — the 'Central Economic Advisory Service clinics project'. Specific directions were issued by the Director General of the Department of National Health and Population Development to consult and involve the communities for whom the facility was to be built (Slabber 1991; Meijer 1992). Figure 4.5 shows a model for community involvement in the clinic, developed by project managers DLV (a firm of consulting architects and engineers) in Pretoria (Van der Merwe 1993). The community participated in the planning and construction of, for example, Ivory Park Clinic and has developed a proud association with the 'ownership' of the clinic. Note specifically the development of the various subcommittees, such as the job creation and allocation committee, shown in figure 4.5. The committee helped to identify people within the community who had appropriate skills and could be employed during the building phase.

It is time-consuming to involve the community but the benefits make this process essential. It is a learning process for all involved.

The identification of the people who will participate firstly in briefing and then in design assessment completes the first step towards meaningful participation by planners. This has to be followed by reading, visiting, and evaluating practices and trends, as explained below. Designers would obviously require similar preparation.

Reading about hospital and clinic planning in general and about individual departments, such as the ICU and CSSD, should be done critically. An architectural journal recently featured a host of clinic and small hospital projects. It merely gave descriptions of the facilities provided, with no comment as to how functional the buildings actually were. One clinic's plans showed the examination couches placed so that one would have to examine from the left hand side. These mistakes can easily be repeated if one assumes that just because something is published it must be correct!

Note that the planning and design guides of the Department of Health and Social Services in the United Kingdom describe requirements and solutions in great detail and are of great assistance (Battersby 1983). The Appropriate Health Resources and Technologies Action Group also has guides of particular interest to smaller facilities. The Building Technology section of the CSIR has developed planning and design guidelines for wards, theatres, CSSDs and Community Health Centres.

Visiting as many similar facilities as possible teaches one what to repeat and what to avoid. Most people are happy to share their experiences in the knowledge that future patients and staff can benefit. These visits must, however, be focused, and should be written up to remain of any value, as one quickly forgets essential details. Guidelines for visits are shown in table 4.6.

It is important to *analyse current practices and functions* as well as the facilities and equipment associated with them. Functions have to

Figure 4.5: Model for project co-ordination which includes community participation

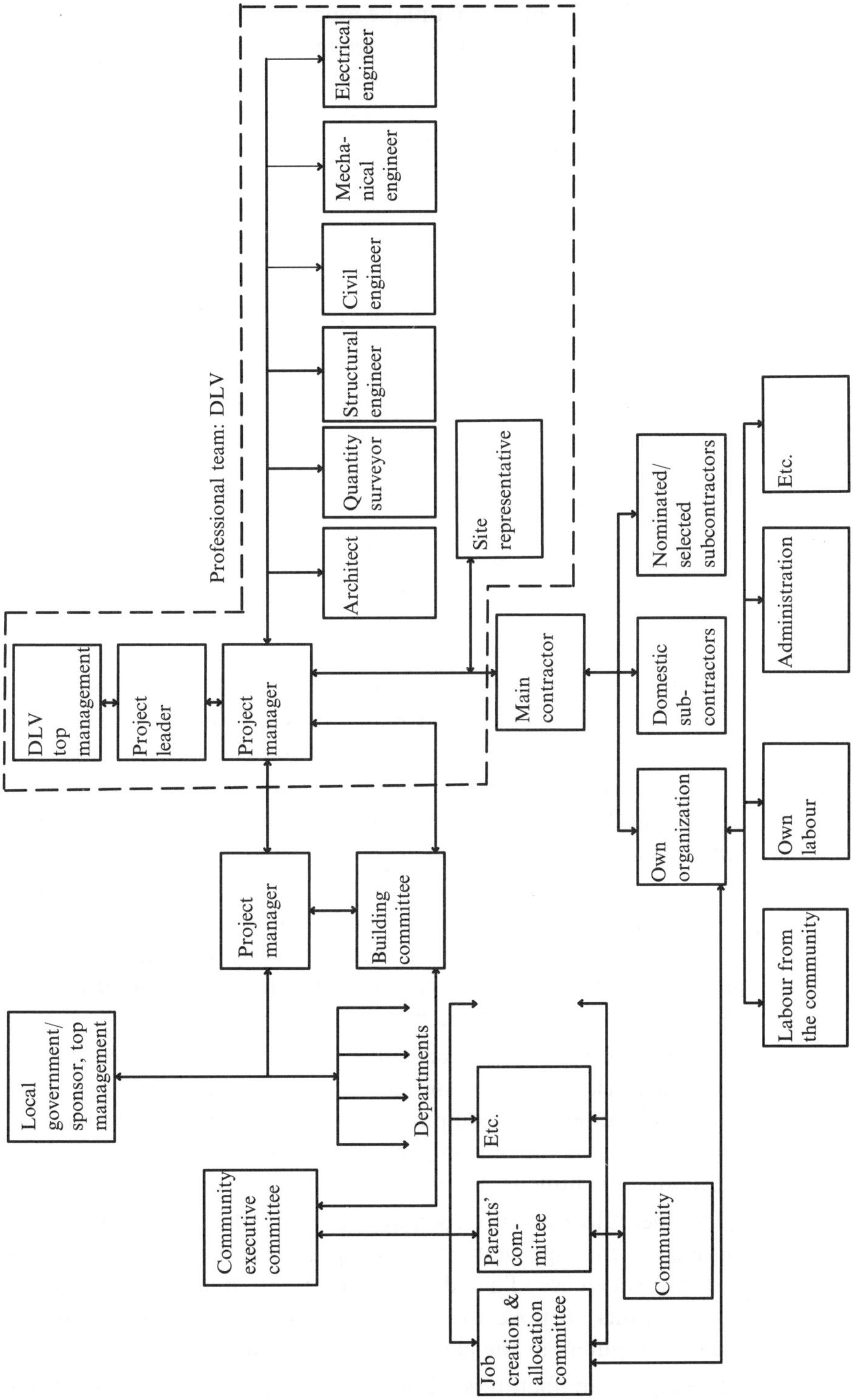

be analysed objectively to decide the best place and person to perform them. This is a unique opportunity to change to more streamlined work-systems — for example, to reallocate non-nursing duties such as reception and clerical work to a ward clerk. Note that an observational study of registered nurses reported that they spent 34.2% of their time on clerical duties and 7.1% on other duties, leaving 53.7% of their time for nursing care (Van Tonder 1988: 6–11).

Table 4.6: Guidelines for visits

- Focus on the area you are planning.
- Interview all categories of staff and patients.
- Ask for their comments and reasons for statements.
- Record similarities, deviations, special features and innovations — relate their use, reasons for differences from own practice.
- Record advantages, disadvantages of the facilities, equipment and support systems.
- Complete a written and photographic record as soon as possible and distribute where appropriate.

The efficiency and durability of current facilities and equipment should also be evaluated. The maintenance staff or Central Medico-Technical Divisions can make valuable contributions in this regard.

It is important to *consider expected developments and trends* in both practice and facilities in order to ensure that the new building will remain functional for as long as possible and that the service will be cost-effective.

An example of how clinical practice influences planning may be found in orthopaedics where external fixing of fractures is now preferred to splinting which requires much longer hospitalization and also more space around the bed.

Colleagues have to be consulted as far afield as possible and research work has to be assessed to identify likely trends as well as the new facilities and equipment that these trends may require. In clinical medicine the time lag between the invention of a method and it becoming routine is, for the most, at least ten years.

The identification of trends applies not only to the clinical field, but also to management principles, practices, facilities, and support systems/services. The development of health maintenance organizations, a move towards participative management, and the use of computers in the clinical field, are examples.

Leading manufacturers of health care products should also be contacted to ascertain their projected developments and the implications of these in terms of space, services, and manpower — new training or maintenance programmes or new categories of staff may have to be established. Decisions made during the planning stage influence and direct the later design and commissioning stages.

Once these preparations have been made, the briefing documents can be written. The preparation time must be balanced against the time available to produce the brief. It is no use spending so much time researching the requirements that too little time is left to set them out in writing!

Should one go to all this trouble for small projects? Yes! The same process should ideally be followed for small and large projects, and for public or private hospitals. Obviously, if a central planning and commissioning unit or private developer deals with many projects, standards are developed and this saves time.

It is important to develop a brief for smaller projects, such as private hospitals or clinics. In practical terms, however, it may not be possible for the planning team to do this at hospital/clinic level because of a lack of planning information and experience or time. It may also be likely that the planning team is incomplete. For private hospitals it is, for example, common to have either a developer or a directing planner such as a medical doctor but no nursing or administrative planners at the outset. In such instances it is particularly important to have an experienced design team.

A further problem in establishing a brief prior to design is that it is imprudent for the client or professional team to tie up resources by commencing planning prior to a license being granted.

A condition of the license is that plans have to be submitted for approval within three months. During this period, the final brief must be established and sketch plans must be prepared and developed into detailed plans in consultation with the users, leading up to the submission of plans. These are basically preliminary working drawings.

This is a fairly tight programme but it does not take into account the fact that, during this period, the developer must establish the feasibility of the project in order to commit the necessary investments. The financial commitment can only take place after the preparation of sketch plans that are sufficient to allow the accurate estimation of cost. This usually involves a period of some weeks whilst the investments are committed.

This break in the design process renders the allotted three month period impractical and can result in undue pressure on the design team to continue work without being paid for it in the hope of being appointed should the project go ahead, and in some instances inappropriate plans are submitted purely to meet the deadline.

To compound this problem, developers (usually those without a clinical background) may not have the specialist knowledge required for the planning and evaluation of designs or a professional design team may be appointed that does not have the insight and knowledge needed to develop the design whilst a brief evolves. This can lead to inappropriate design. By the time that mistakes are noticed it could be too late to rectify them, which results in problems in the future running of the facility. As an example of this, a recent design for a small hospital had no pharmacy! These problems are often highlighted in the design of a CSSD. In a number of instances the CSSD had conformed with the minimum requirement of 12 m^2 laid down by R.158, which is totally inadequate for meeting the needs of a theatre suite and can, in fact, hinder the development of the theatre to full capacity.

The responsibility for developing a meaningful brief — ie schedules and operational narratives — is shared by planners and designers. It can be developed through a series of meetings, with the most experienced party giving direction. It is essential that all disciplines be represented at the outset, even if staff have to be seconded or borrowed from other existing facilities. If not, errors of judgement or understanding made during the early planning stages may be difficult or impossible to correct later on.

Once the brief is developed, it is handed to the appointed design team as a formal guide to design of the hospital or clinic. The brief is then thoroughly assessed and verified through discussions between the briefing and design teams. The various members of the project teams are shown in figure 4.6. A glance at the variety of disciplines involved will show that a structured approach to projects is essential in order to co-ordinate and integrate the facilities of each.

The design stage

This is the exciting stage during which the architects and engineers translate the ideas and proposals contained in the accommodation schedule, operational narrative, and room descriptions into visible plans. The project brief is also finalized through discussion. The layout and design of the building are completed and the method of construction is determined for approval by the relevant authorities. The information needed by the construction teams (ie working drawings, specifications, and bills of quantities) is completed and arrangements are made for obtaining tenders for construction (Kleczkowski and Nilsson: 81).

The design stage is usually subdivided into three sub-stages: master plan, sketch plan, and working drawing stages. Approval by the client is sought at the end of each stage. Assessment and approval

Figure 4.6: People involved in a building project

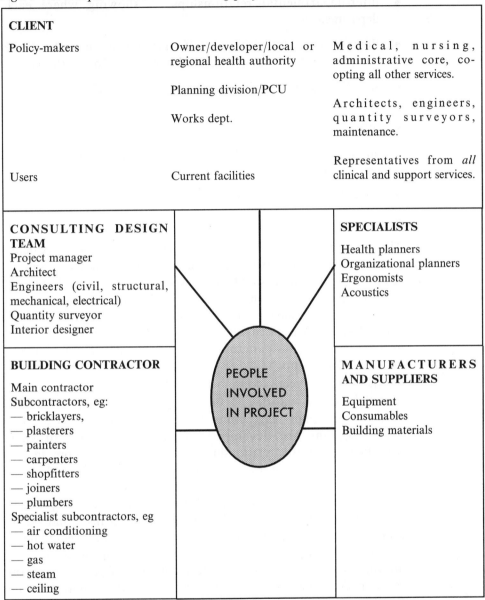

CLIENT		
Policy-makers	Owner/developer/local or regional health authority	Medical, nursing, administrative core, co-opting all other services.
	Planning division/PCU	
	Works dept.	Architects, engineers, quantity surveyors, maintenance.
		Representatives from *all* clinical and support services.
Users	Current facilities	

CONSULTING DESIGN TEAM
Project manager
Architect
Engineers (civil, structural, mechanical, electrical)
Quantity surveyor
Interior designer

SPECIALISTS
Health planners
Organizational planners
Ergonomists
Acoustics

BUILDING CONTRACTOR

Main contractor
Subcontractors, eg:
— bricklayers,
— plasterers
— painters
— carpenters
— shopfitters
— joiners
— plumbers
Specialist subcontractors, eg
— air conditioning
— hot water
— gas
— steam
— ceiling

PEOPLE INVOLVED IN PROJECT

MANUFACTURERS AND SUPPLIERS

Equipment
Consumables
Building materials

should be carried out with great care as changes regarding the layout of the hospital and the layout of individual departments should not be made after approval of the sketch plan stage (Kleczkowski and Nilsson: 22).

The master plan is developed after a careful analysis of the brief provided by the client. The master plan is a proposal for the intended design of the building, illustrated by a set of plans showing various key elements. These elements include:

- inter-departmental relationships — showing where each department is;

- flow of patients, visitors, staff, and goods throughout the complex, ie the major vertical and horizontal flow patterns;

- site development, including parking needs and traffic patterns (see figure 4.7);

- other facilities on the site — for example residence, laundry;

- an assessment of civil, structural, mechanical, and electrical components;

- possibilities for future expansion;

- cost.

The aim is to develop a balanced, functional building for patients and staff alike. The maxim that time one spends walking or waiting reduces working time should always be kept in mind. It would, however, be practically impossible for each department to have its own entrance and have all major services on its doorstep. Decisions about location are based on the operational narrative and other analyses, such as flow patterns and frequency and urgency of access between departments.

Urgent and direct access between the labour ward, theatre, neonatal nursery, and ICU is, for instance, of great importance.

The sketch plan stage follows. Firstly, single line schematic drawings/plans are developed to show the layout of each department and the relationship and size of each room in the department. These line drawings are a reflection of the schedules of accommodation and the operational narrative (see figure 4.8). These are developed in the second phase of the sketch plan stage to produce room layouts (Howie: 14–20). Room layouts are plans of individual rooms which show the internal layout of the room. Built-in equipment, services, wall thicknesses, and door and window openings are now drawn, as shown in figure 4.9. Room layouts/room sheets are based on the room description section of the brief. As shown in figure 4.10, the sketch plan is completed when the room layouts are integrated with the initial line drawings. A realistic cost estimate should be possible from the sketch plan stage (Kleczkowski and Nilsson: 22).

The briefing team should become part of the design team and continue into the design stage as it has to review and approve the requirements specified in the brief. Continuity is, however, often not possible. This increases the demand for a clear brief which conveys the intentions of the original briefing team.

The third design stage is the 'working drawings' stage. The completed sketch plans are further developed into working drawings for the building contractor. Working drawings form part of the contract documents and provide all the necessary information to carry out the project (Kleczkowski and Nilsson: 82). This includes the correct and detailed sizes and specifications of the architectural, mechanical, and electrical services such as building materials, plumbing, or lighting. Schedules which describe the doors, windows, and furniture are also developed.

An understanding of the importance of *ergonomics* is helpful during briefing and it is essential for the evaluation of room layout drawings in particular. Ergonomics refers to the study of the 'fit' between user and machine or tool, and aims to improve productivity and reduce user-fatigue. The main areas of study in ergonomics are shown in table 4.7 (Galer 1987: 6).

Table 4.7: Main areas of study in ergonomics

Area of study	*Examples*
Physical aspects of the user-machine interface	Size, shape, colour, texture, and method of operation of displays and controls for cars, domestic appliances, industrial and commercial equipment.
Cognitive aspects of the user-machine interface.	Understanding of instructions and other information; style of dialogue between computer and user.
Workplace design and workspace layout.	Layout of offices, factories, domestic kitchens, public spaces, etc. Detailed relationships between furniture and equipment, and between different equipment components.
Physical environment	Effects of climate, noise, and vibration, illumination, and chemical/biological contaminants on human performance and health.
Psychological environment	Organizational structure within a group and its effects on satisfaction with the task, productivity, and group membership.
Job design, selection, and training	Effects of shift work on performance; design of instructions, job aids, and training schemes; selection of personnel against criteria of aptitude and personality.

An example of ergonomics applied to a workspace would be the layout of a bathroom for the disabled, which would allow a wheelchair user to reach and use all facilities in an independent manner.

Figure 4.7: Site plan of Crompton Hospital

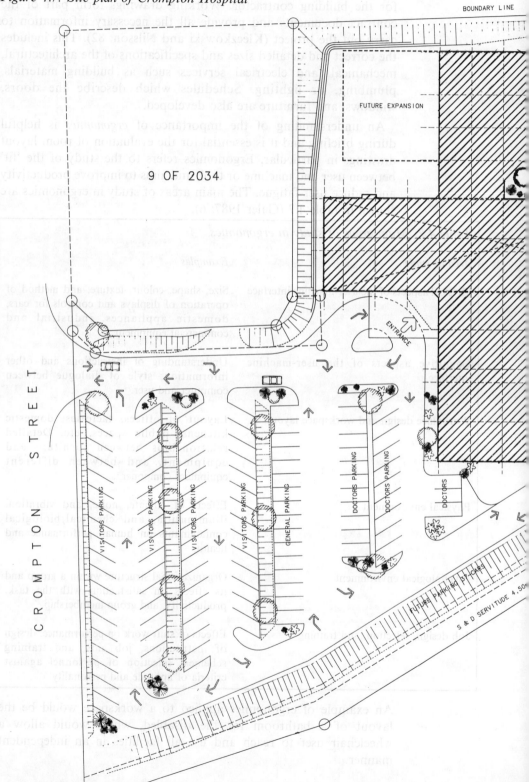

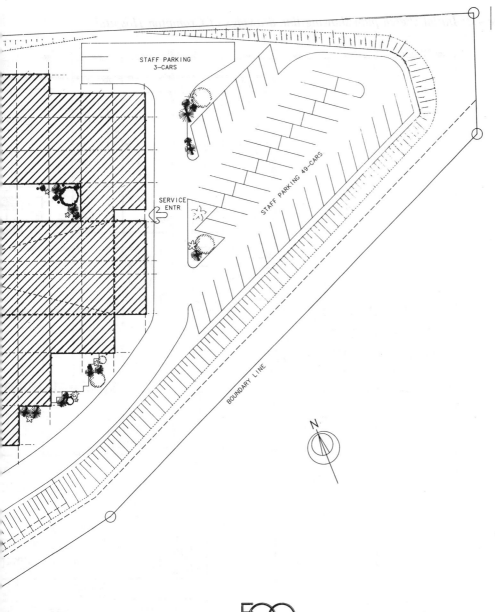

STAFF PARKING
3-CARS

SERVICE
ENTR

STAFF PARKING 49-CARS

BOUNDARY LINE

N

CROMPTON HOSPITAL — SITE PLAN

FGG
ARCHITECTS
FRANKLIN · GARLAND · GIBSON & PARTNERS

5335 — 001

Figure 4.8: Initial sketch plan showing line drawings of Crompton Hospital

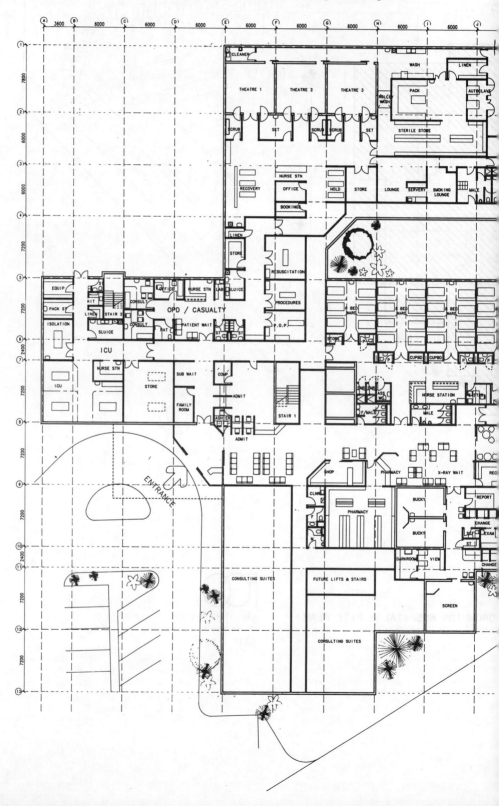

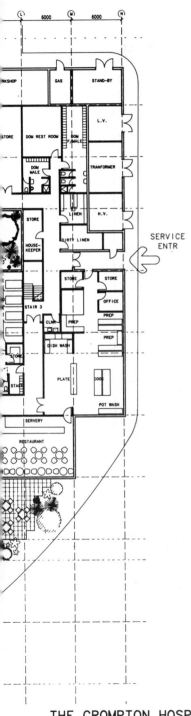

SERVICE
ENTR

THE CROMPTON HOSPITAL — GROUND FLOOR

SCALE 1:200

FGG
ARCHITECTS
FRANKLIN · GARLAND · GIBSON & PARTNERS

5335 — 002

Figure 4.9: Room layout/room data sheet (not to scale)

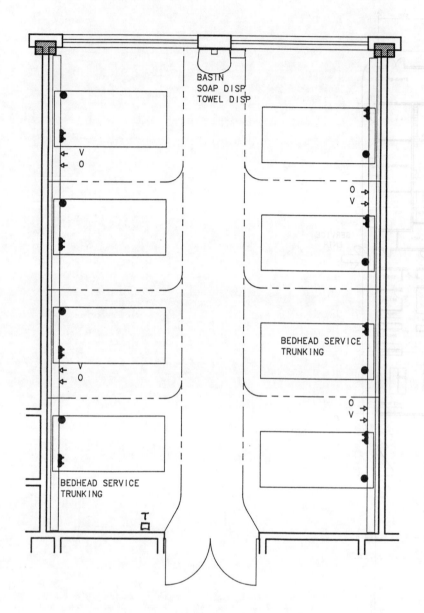

ROOM DATA SHEET   GH5-1

DEPARTMENT	DAY CLINIC
ROOM	WARD 8 BED
ROOM NO.	GH5-1/GI5-1/GJ5-1/GK5-1

	SIGN	DATE
COMPILED	KH	18/3/92
AGREED	I.D./E.S.	27/3/92

FINISHES

WALL	STD	X	SPECIAL		
FLOOR	STD	X	SPECIAL		
DOOR	SIZE	1615	PROTECT	X	VIEW

FITTINGS

WORKTOP	HT		DEPTH				
CUPBS	LOW		FULL HT		WALL		
SHELVES	HT		DEPTH				
	STD		SPECIAL				
X-RAY VIEWER			WRITING BD		PINBD		
SPECIAL							

SANWARE

SURGEONS BASIN	1	BUCKET SINK		WC	
STANDARD BASIN		SLOPHOPPER		BIDET	
SMALL BASIN		BEDPANWASH		BATH	
SS SINK SINGLE		BELFAST S		SHOWER	
SS SINK DOUBLE		DEEP SINK			
SPECIAL					

FIXTURES

SOAP DISP STD	1	GRAB HANDLE	
SOAP DISP ELBOW		GRAB RAILS	
SOAP DISH		EQUIP RAIL	
TOWEL DISP	1	DRIP RAIL	
TOWEL RAIL		DRIP HOOK	
MIRROR STD		CUBICLE TRACK	
MIRROR LONG		COAT HOOKS	
TOILET ROLL HOLD		SPECIAL	

SERVICES

POWER	15AMP	16	EMERGENCY	X	3 PHASE
COMMUN	TEL		INTERCOM		CALL X
COMPUTOR			RADIO	X	TV
LIGHTING	STD	X	DIMMER		EXAM
AIRCON	STD	X	100% FRESH		VENT
MED GAS	O$_2$	4	VAC	4	N$_2$O
	AIR(LP)		AIR(HP)		OTHER
SPECIAL		BEDHEAD SERVICE TRUNKING			

SCALE 1:50

DWG.N . 5335/1286

TEL 3056764   FAX 3056627

FGG
ARCHITECTS

Figure 4.10: Completed sketch plan: day ward

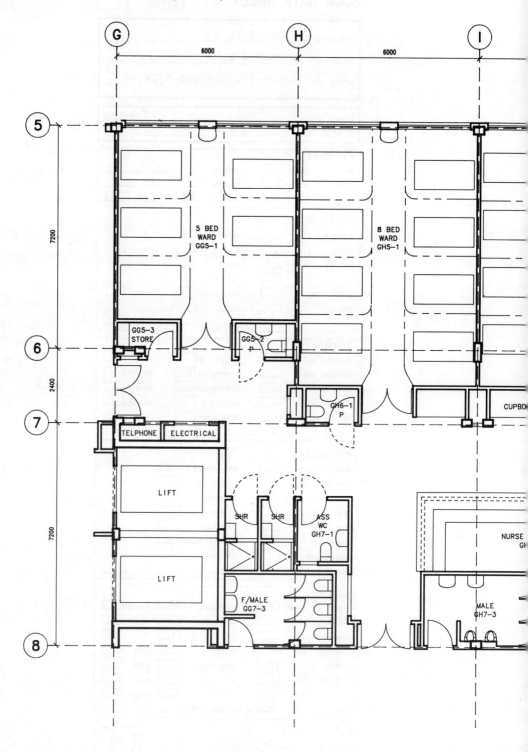

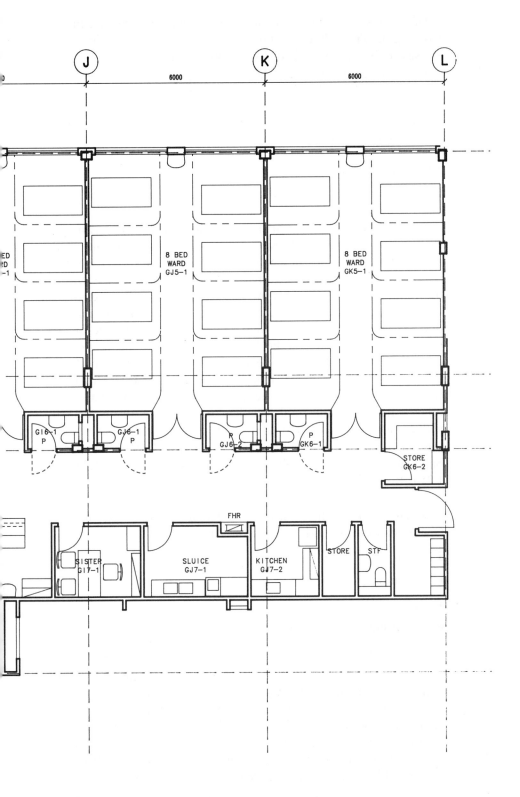

The clients/users have a minor role during the development of working drawings, but they typically interact with the designers in the selection and approval of fixtures and fittings.

The different design stages have to be approved by the client, for example the Provincial Administration, represented by the PCU, Medical Superintendent, heads of departments, the Planning Division of Health Services, the Department of Works, and various management committees or bodies.

Understanding drawings (Abbott 1992)

How do you understand and evaluate what is on a drawing? The starting point is to relate to the scale of the drawing.

The building or department shown on the plan will be drawn to a smaller size but in correct proportion to the proposed facility. The relation between the size of the drawn plan and actual size is called the *scale*. A scale of 1:100 means that one unit of measurement on the drawing represents 100 units in reality — ie 1 cm on the drawing represents 100 cm or 1 metre. At a scale of 1:50, 1 cm on the drawing represents 50 cm or 0.5 m in reality. The scale of the drawing is usually stated in the drawing title block to the right of the drawing or, where more than one scale is used, in the relevant place on the drawing. Where scales of 1:100 are used, an ordinary metric ruler can be used to determine the actual sizes shown on the plans. For other scales an architectural scale has to be used — this is marked with a range of different scales. These are obtainable from stationers.

Building plans are usually drawn at a scale of 1:100, but large buildings may have to be drawn at smaller scales such as 1:200 or 1:250. Room layouts are drawn at 1:50 or 1:20 to show details of equipment, fittings etc.

Different types of drawings depict different aspects of the building. One needs to distinguish between the terms:

- plans;
- elevations;
- sections;
- perspectives; and
- site plans.

Plans are drawn as a horizontal section through the building at about 1 m above floor level. Plans show the internal and external walls, their material and construction, the position of all windows and doors, the position of all fittings (sinks, basins, etc.) and fixtures (built-in cupboards, worktops, etc.), and would preferably also show loose furniture. The drawings shown in figures 4.7–4.10 are therefore all plans. Plans show width and length but not height.

Elevations show the height of walls, the position, size or shape of windows or doors, and the roof or overall profile of the building as seen flat-on — ie not in three-dimensional perspective. They show height and width (as in figure 4.11).

Sections depict vertical slices through the building. Sections show foundations and basements below ground level, the internal height of rooms and ceilings, and roof construction. They show height and length — see the bottom right-hand corner of figure 4.11.

A *perspective* would show the building design in three dimensions — ie height, length, and width. Perspectives are often presented as 'artists' impressions' of the building or room.

The *site plan,* at a scale of 1:200 or 1:500 or smaller, shows the position of the building, in block form, on the site with all roads, paving and external features (see figure 4.7).

Lastly, one has to identify the various objects shown on the drawings — eg windows, doors and fittings. There are various ways to depict an item. Commonly-used items are illustrated in figure 4.12.

A full set of sketch plans usually comprises all plans, including the site plan, elevations, and some sections and perspectives of the building. For a more complete discussion see Abbott (1992) or attend one of the Health Care Facility Workshops presented by the CSIR.

The use of scale rulers, practice and, in particular, the use of simple mock-ups and models all help to understand drawings. Note that it is of vital importance not to fake understanding of drawings. No one likes to admit to not understanding something but, in a meeting, you are usually not the only one who finds them confusing! Ask for references or explanations and make sure that you understand the drawing and the implications of building it before you approve it. By the same token, you and your colleagues may be using clinical terms quite new to the architects and engineers and they, in turn, should ask for clarification of the meanings and implications of procedures or functions. Good communication is as essential in planning as it is in clinical practice. If in doubt — ask!

CONSTRUCTION

The building now has to be constructed within the agreed cost, time, and quality targets. The construction stage must be planned very carefully, as all activities are interrelated and the failure of one can disrupt and lengthen the whole project (Kleczkowski and Nilsson 1984: 22).

The building contractor, along with the subcontractors under him, is responsible for the satisfactory completion of the project in accordance with the documentation. The work is constantly monitored by the professional consulting team.

Figure 4.11: Representations of a building on architectural drawings.

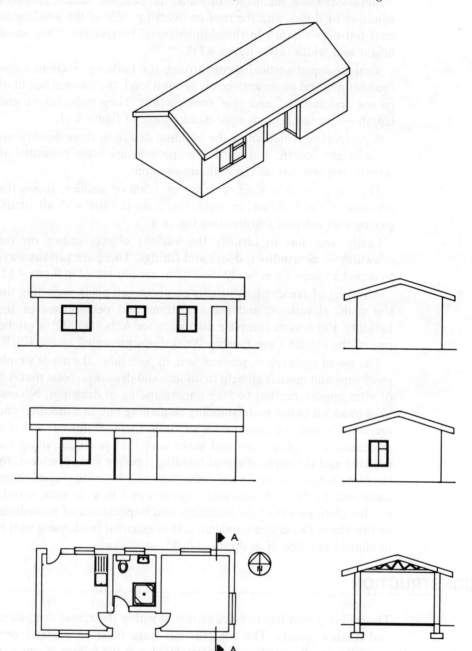

Figure 4.12: Conventional representations of various common building items on architectural drawings

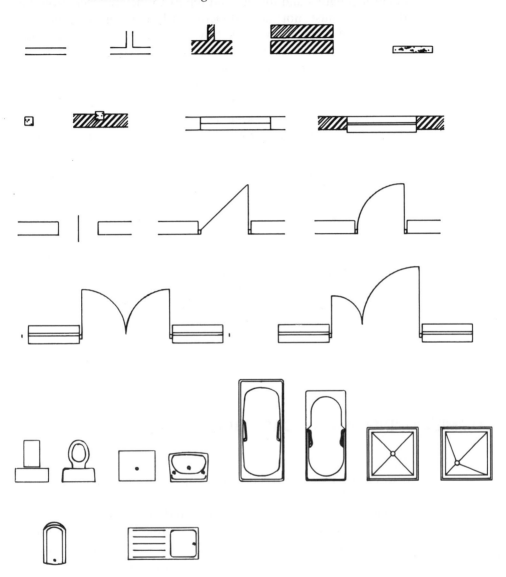

The client may, in big projects, also employ a clerk of works to monitor progress and quality and report to the architect. Note that the client must not deal directly with the contractor(s). The professional team, normally led by the architect, acts as an agent for the client and all instructions must be co-ordinated by the architect. This avoids conflicting instructions and variations which may cause delays and, inevitably, an increase in costs (Howie 1990). Site visits should be managed through the architect. This is definitely not the time to start thinking seriously about the project — that should have been done during the briefing and designing stages.

The main participants in the construction stage are the management team and the construction team. This consists of the main contractor and subcontractors, suppliers of materials and equipment, and designers and specialists (Kleczkowski: 22). If one looks at figure 4.6, it is clear that the main contractor has a full-time job to co-ordinate the many varied sub-contractors and construction staff. He has enough to contend with trying to meet deadlines without having progress halted because some clinical staff have only just taken an interest or begun to understand what they are looking at at a very late stage. It is the responsibility of the planner to assess needs early, to include these in the brief, and to proceed through the design stage carefully. If, however, nurses have been excluded from planning, it is still the nurse manager's responsibility to become involved as soon as she can — briefing being the appropriate place to start.

COMMISSIONING HEALTH CARE BUILDINGS

This concludes the project. The purpose of the commissioning stage is to ensure that construction work is completed according to the approved drawings and specifications and that the buildings can become fully operational on handover to the client (Kleczkowski and Nilsson 1984: 22). It is essential that the project is made operational in terms of the brief (operational narratives) and specifications.

Broadly speaking, commissioning entails staffing and equipping the hospital, so that it is ready for operation.

People involved in commissioning are the management team and the commissioning team. The latter would include the owners or their representative(s), the users or their representative(s), the designers and specialists, contractors, and sub-contractors.

Commissioning begins during construction. It involves so many finely integrated steps that its careful planning and timing is essential. Graphic aids such as the Programme Evaluation Review Technique (PERT) and Critical Path Method (CPM) (Schroeder 1981: 348) and relatively simple bar charts are invaluable tools to ensure that the project is completed on time. Estimates are made of the time which will be needed to complete all activities. These estimates are arranged in chronological order. Programming of phases/activities would usually have been implemented during the early planning stages. If not, it should at least be used during commissioning.

Staff are recruited, appointed, and trained to use the new building and its systems correctly. The ideas expressed in the operational narratives are developed into operational policy manuals to give guidance in the use of the building. Whether staff are being moved from an old facility to a new one, or recruited for a new facility, orientation in the use of the new building and its systems is essential to its success. Refer to chapter 3 for details regarding the staffing function.

Senior staff should be recruited at an early stage in order to have a meaningful input into the design. The key briefing team members may be recruited and appointed specifically so that they are eventually in charge of the various services of the completed facility.

The ordering, receipt, checking, storage and final placement of loose equipment also takes place now. Equipment and services to be installed by the contractor also arrive and should be carefully monitored by the architects and engineer. Note that late changes in the choice of fixed equipment must be avoided. They could be very costly and delay completion as new services and supply systems may have to be installed. Ideally, one should keep abreast of trends and plan for any likely changes in technology.

It is tempting, particularly in private developments, to exclude the installation of major capital items such as kitchen equipment from the brief of the professional team. This is short-sighted and can create major problems as it is essential that such items are properly installed and integrated into the fabric of the building.

Realistic running costs are also calculated during commissioning. Previous estimates, made during briefing, were based on the costs of similar facilities elsewhere. Detailed costs can now be determined for the newly constructed facility.

In due course the building is completed. It is then prepared for handover. The handover process takes place formally, together with a room-by-room inspection of the facility by the designers, owners, and the contractor (or their representatives). Procedures have to be established for the handover and for any follow-up which may be needed. The checking of equipment, both fixed and loose, and of the building and its services, continues for an agreed period, usually six months or as specified in the equipment guarantees.

Moving from an existing facility to a new one is stressful, as is being appointed to a new job. Many staff tend to see a new hospital as merely a new environment in which the methods and procedures they are familiar with can be continued.

It has to be remembered that staff will often have become conditioned to outmoded and inefficient procedures which they had to adapt to. These staff will need considerable sympathy and tact if they are to be persuaded to operate their new department in the way in which it was designed to be used. It should be remembered that when an existing hospital closes down, the process may be likened to the grieving process (Sacewicz 1985: 760). Even though there may be a new facility to replace it, the change process has to be acknowledged and planned for.

Table 4.8: Practical guidelines for a commissioning team (CT), adapted from Steele 1992.

1. Appoint key staff *early* — eg hospital manager/secretary, nursing services manager, hospital engineer.
   - Planning team can evolve into commissioning.
   - Commissioning team often appointed when building tender awarded.
   - Volume of work often underestimated.
   - Dedicated offices essential.

2. Establish timetable.
   - Use CPM or PERT programming.
   - Architect to inform CT of progress, specify delivery time, defect liability period and maintenance in tender.

3. Prepare equipment schedules per room, per category of equipment.
   - Highly technical/expensive equipment — make best choice after consultation with heads and other users, and checking delivery time and latest model.
   - Develop from room descriptions and working drawings.
   - Equipment categories, eg
     — supplied and fixed i.t.o. building contract (eg sterilizers)
     — supplied by Director of Health Services and installed by contractor
     — supplied by hospital/clinic and requiring services (eg gas, water, electricity)
     — supplied by hospital/clinic, nor requiring services, ie losse furniture, equipment, instruments
   - Prepare specifications

4. Ordering equipment	<ul><li>Delivery times often longer than quoted</li><li>Establish procedure for outstanding goods</li><li>Keep good records per policy. Deal with reputable companies who can advise, follow up, and offer *prompt* replacement/ repair service</li><li>Follow up orders well before delivery date</li><li>Ensure that payment terms related to delivery, installation and commissioning dates.</li><li>Negotiate staff training as part of purchase price</li><li>Stipulate warranty period to commence with usage, not delivery date (Fourie 1992)</li><li>Inform professional team if equipment excluded from their brief. Client is responsible for ensuring that details for installation and fitting of excluded equipment are provided timeously and that equipment is available on time.</li></ul>
5. Storage of equipment	<ul><li>Some can be delivered directly *after* handover</li><li>Most would require temporary storage, ie use existing building, build temporary structure, hire warehouse</li><li>Storage area must be well-ventilated and *secured*</li></ul>
6. Receipt of equipment	<ul><li>All goods must be checked on delivery against order and for completeness and damage. Arrange for replacement if needed.</li><li>Ask sales representative to be present</li><li>Keep 'technical equipment' separate until checked and certified correct *by department head*</li><li>On arrival, label items with code, eventual location per floor and department room number, delivery route (eg door of entry/ lift to be used). Colour coding helps</li><li>Store in demarcated areas according to phased move to new building.</li><li>NB — prompt checking of goods for quality and quantity will avoid loss of prompt payment discounts</li><li>Note: existing equipment to be marked for transfer/disposal</li></ul>

7. Prepare operational policies per department and system.

- Use operational narratives and reshape to suit the facility that has been built

8. Staffing

- Establish staffing requirements, perhaps using private firms for cleaning, etc

9. Public relations

- Start early, during planning, to orientate public, suppliers, support groups. volunteers, existing staff. Use public speaking, newspapers, and open days.
- Plan official opening date and ceremony and invite dignitaries early.

10. Cleaning

- Check cleaning responsibilities of contractor
- Arrange cleaning; train cleaners

11. Moving in

- Plan well in advance and inform all of timetable
- Instruct all concerned re. their functions
- Protect corridors, floors, lifts
- Do trial runs of systems, services
- Arrange for security of equipment, staff, and patients during move
- Record the recipt of equipment in deparments
- Support staff emotionally and gastronomically!

12. Defects, liability period, and evaluation

- Hospital staff *not* to effect repairs during this period or the guarantee period — report to architect, etc
- Identify persons responsible for evaluation of each department or service during construction, pre-handover period, and post-occupancy period
- Evaluate building and services according to working drawings
- Formalize 'snag' lists and follow up; exigency budget to be in place

The commissioning stage links the planning and operation stages as shown in figure 4.13.

Figure 4.13: Commissioning links planning and operation

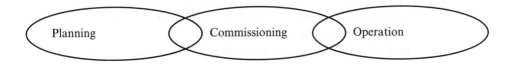

OVERVIEW OF THE PROJECT STAGES

A summary of the products and major functions of each project stage is shown in figure 4.14.

Figure 4.14: Overview of the project stages

STAGE	SUB-STAGE	PRODUCT/FUNCTION
PLANNING	Strategic planning	National health services facilities plan
	Need identification and approval	Service required, cost and space norms, and running cost assessment
	Briefing	Schedule of accommodation Operational narrative Room descriptions
	Designing	Master plan Sketch plan — line drawings / room layouts
		• Cost plan • Working drawings and schedules. • Bill of quantities • Tender procedures
CONSTRUCTION		Building with services Cost monitoring
COMMISSIONING		Staff, equipment, orientation to operational policies, occupy building, evaluation

TRENDS IN HEALTH CARE INFLUENCING HEALTH CARE FACILITY PLANNING

Several trends may influence the planning of health care facilities. These include the restructuring of the health service, an increased emphasis on productivity, a shift towards outpatient care, a tendency to see health care institutions as 'therapeutic environments', an increasing shortage of health care personnel, competition between hospitals, technological development, the concept of 'patient hotels', and changing demographic and epidemiological factors.

Restructuring of the health service

The main objective of restructuring is to provide a cost-effective health service which restores the balance between basic health care and advanced health care. This means that services would be developed so that a patient would receive treatment at the least sophisticated service institution in an area — ie a primary health care clinic — from where he would be referred to a regional or academic hospital if needed. It is hoped that this will prevent the flooding of patients with less serious illness to tertiary centres where primary care is delivered at much higher cost than at a primary care centre.

Whilst this, ostensibly, was the aim of the National Plan and Norms for Health Service Facilities of June 1981, authority for the rendering of services is now being changed to develop a more sophisticated service which includes communities and academic hospitals. From 1 April, 1993, academic hospitals became autonomous bodies.

The main result should be the development of more accessible primary health centres, hopefully open until 22:00. This would enable academic hospitals to use their funds for the true purposes of tertiary institutions, namely training and research, and the rendering of service at tertiary/referral level.

The safety of staff and security of the clinics would be an important consideration, and this would naturally influence the service provided.

Productivity

Any attempt to provide the best possible care within an available budget has to include an in-depth scrutiny of productivity.

With staff salaries commonly forming 60–70% of the running costs, serious analysis is important. The study by Van Tonder (1988) found that registered nurses in public hospitals spent 46.3% of the time that they were observed performing non-nursing duties. A recent study in Britain (Carlisle 1990: 19) found that nurses in outpatient departments spent too long on non-nursing duties and suggested a 70% cut in qualified nurses!

> While this is alarming, our aim for efficiency would be research based and should be 'looking at workloads, how staffing levels match workload, how you get the right staff to the right place at the right time and how all this affects quality'. (Cornwell, in Carlisle 1990)

Computers are used to varying degrees in health care — eg for producing records and in laboratories. Of particular interest is a study of computerized clinical information system in a Wisconsin (USA) ICU: a study before and after the introduction of the system found that indirect care activities decreased from 47.2% to 39.4%. A nearly perfect relationship was also found between the decrease in indirect care activities and an increase in the time spent supporting patients in activities of daily living, including more direct patient care and comfort measures (Lutheran Hospital — 1991). The use of computers should always follow an in-depth cost-benefit analysis.

The layout of departments, departmental relationships, and flow patterns can significantly influence productivity. It would appear that double corridor wards, for example, could decrease productivity as it is difficult to keep contact with staff and patients alike although walking distances are reduced. The development of computer software models can assist designers to evaluate designs and new concepts before they are put into operation. Howard (1992: 7) reports that such models can incorporate a range of nurse management options (such as team and task nursing) and different patient types, so that users can not only test a number of layouts, but can tailor their own management scenarios and simulate different ward functions.

One new concept, developed in the USA by international management and technology consultants Booz-Allen and Hamilton, is the patient-centred approach which involves restructuring the hospital into patient-centred units, with most diagnostic services decentralized and attached to the units, rather than centralized as at present. This model also calls for multi-skilled staff who are able to operate a variety of diagnostic and treatment services. The aim is to prevent the fragmentation of services provided to the patient. This approach has been claimed to result in a 10% reduction in total capital cost compared to a conventional hospital, as well as reduced operational costs (Dix 1990). Studies and articles on ward design and ICUs are listed in appendix 3.

A shift to outpatient care

In America it is expected that, by the year 2000, outpatients will outnumber inpatients by 8:1 and only 15–20% of all surgery will be performed in hospital-based surgery suites. Advances in laser technology and non-invasive procedures, together with advances in MRI and CT diagnostics will move most activities to outpatient facilities (Thomas and Saslow 1992: 33–6). This may be easier to achieve in private hospitals catering for middle income groups. Westville Hospital in Durban, for example, did 60–5% of surgery on a day surgery basis in 1992.

The establishment of day surgery facilities, in association with or separate from hospitals, is also developing in England and locally. Note, however, that a day surgery system requires transport and communications in order to schedule patients.

With 50% of all acute admissions in the UK expected to be for day treatment by the year 2000, rather than for prolonged inpatient stay, the importance of the role of the hospital ward will be lessened (Meara 1992). Whilst Meara questions whether 'patient-focused hospitals' and 'patient hotels' will be around in 10 years time, he suggests that we accept a variety of approaches for the hospital of the future. These approaches will depend on the condition of local hospital facilities, the availability of money, local initiative and innovation, and the willingness of clinicians to adopt new technologies and methods. Figure 4.15 illustrates Meara's model.

Hospitals as therapeutic environments

Beyond efficiency and economy, hospitals have to consider people's needs (De Debuchy 1983: 48–50). De Debuchy reports that the need to move from the view of 'man as an object' to 'man as a person', and to respond to the individual staff member or patient, is becoming increasingly recognized. This would, for example, include community participation in decisions on buildings and the operation of services.

Developing a therapeutic medium means that buildings are designed so that people can relate to them, people will be able to find departments more easily because they are easily recognizable, human rather than technical communications are enhanced, and the design flows toward the outside landscape (De Debuchy 1983).

This approach was highlighted at a recent symposium which featured the creation of 'healing environments' (Malkin 1991: 27–41). Malkin states, however, that one cannot create a healing environment suitable for every person. The most important thing, therefore, is to provide control, so that the patient has options and is able to decide what is best.

The basic components of a healing environment include air quality, thermal comfort, noise control, privacy, light, views of natural surroundings, visual serenity for those who are very ill, and visual stimulation for those who are recuperating. Colour and texture also play an important role, as does accommodation for families.

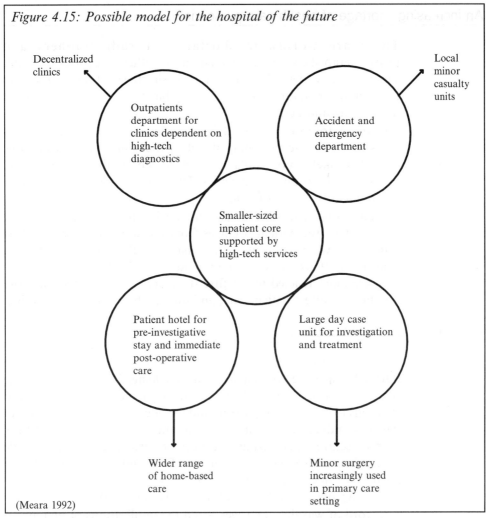

Figure 4.15: Possible model for the hospital of the future

Decentralized clinics

Local minor casualty units

Outpatients department for clinics dependent on high-tech diagnostics

Accident and emergency department

Smaller-sized inpatient core supported by high-tech services

Patient hotel for pre-investigative stay and immediate post-operative care

Large day case unit for investigation and treatment

Wider range of home-based care

Minor surgery increasingly used in primary care setting

(Meara 1992)

Malkin rightly observes that it is still strange to hear a planner say 'I would like you to create a healing environment', because our mind set is such that we do not realize that the physical environment has the potential to support healing. He regards the demand for the creation of healing environments to be the new frontier in health care design.

The health care environment should, of course, also be developed with staff in mind. There are claims that a good working environment attracts staff, and if staff feel that the environment has been created to support them, they feel valued and motivated.

Patients are also asking for more high quality service, convenient locations, quick attention, pleasant surroundings, high-tech equipment, and caring, concerned doctors, nurses and staff (Thomas and Saslow 1992). Provision of rooming-in facilities in paediatrics is now the norm, but patient demands should be balanced against appropriate and cost-effective design.

An increasing shortage of health care personnel

There are worldwide shortages of radiographers and physiotherapists, while the availability of other categories of health care workers varies. There are typically shortages of most categories in the non-urban areas. This obviously has to be taken into account in planning and design.

It would, for example, be advisable to have first stage and delivery areas in very close proximity if not in the same room if only one midwife is likely to be available — which is often the case, especially in small rural hospitals and clinics. Thorough development of a brief would identify such situations.

It has to be remembered that the ideal is to have single delivery rooms which the patient occupies from the start, or a separate first stage area where patients can remain unaffected by patients in delivery. Staff also have different mindsets in the different areas — ie they are more relaxed in the first stage area. Staffing will therefore significantly affect patient care, and this can be influenced by design.

Competition amongst hospitals

In America the reimbursement system (Diagnosis Related Group [DRG] Prospective Price Payment) has challenged hospitals to manage patients at a lower rate than the DRG payment. This has forced hospitals to compete for patients and for doctors who refer and admit patients, and has resulted in the development of 'centres of excellence' such as centres specializing in cancer or cardiology. These provide comprehensive, specialized care in their field, and may be attached to a hospital or free standing, although they have a separate identity for marketing and philanthropic purposes (Thomas and Saslow 1992).

A word of warning, however — all the implications of planning a service have to be identified at a very early stage. A non-medical developer recently proposed the inclusion of a neonatal ICU in a small new private hospital in Durban to act as draw-card. He did not realize, however, that the reason why no hospital in Durban other than King Edward VIII or Addington offered this was that, firstly, one needs to have a reasonable number of potential patients, specialized nurses, and most difficult of all, paediatricians/neonatologists on duty (not merely on call) 24-hours a day.

Hospitals specializing in one field also often offer the use of their expensive equipment to other hospitals for a fee. This is to be encouraged.

One trend in competition, especially noted amongst private hospitals, involves giving the hospital a hotel type atmosphere. Whilst this may originally have been intended to reduce the patients' anxiety when faced with a typically clinical hospital setting, it seems to have become an economic rather than humanitarian consideration. I would, however, urge planners to have a balanced approach — it seems highly inappropriate to spend such a great portion of the budget on marble entrance halls that there are insufficient funds to provide for automatic bedpan washers!

Rapidly evolving technology

As planning is always future-oriented, one has to anticipate changes in technology. These are difficult to predict, but close communication with manufacturers, especially regarding their research and the development of products and equipment, can assist the planner.

It is essential to consider all the implications of new technology. Along with the trend towards developing smaller laboratory equipment (which can also offer more advanced analysis) comes the prediction that mini-labs will be located on wards or in day/ambulatory care settings, with only very specialized tests being sent to clinical labs (Thomas and Saslow 1992). This exemplifies the patient-centred approach. The introduction of any new system must, however, be balanced against the potential frequency of use, the need to care for the equipment, and the need for staff to operate it.

There is much evidence suggesting that advanced technology is inappropriately applied in developing countries. Equipment is often donated or bought with little consideration for its practical installation, operation, maintenance, the use/supply of consumables, or the training of staff (Halbwachs 1992) — ie, a needs assessment is often not carried out. Table 4.9 lists user costs which make up the total cost of an item of equipment. With up to 80% of equipment not working in some centres, the problem is usually not lack of equipment but lack of *functioning* equipment (Halbwachs 1992). Some recommendations include (Schmidt 1992):

1. The establishment of a consulting board for medical equipment. This would consult with donors before donations are made and attend to standardization, budgets for spares, equipment location, operation, and maintenance.

2. The promotion of recognized local training centres for hospital maintenance technicians.

Donors and planners alike have to remember that technology inappropriately applied/placed can be a monster, swallowing scarce financial means for often doubtful ends. Halbwachs also contends that low technology equipment, for example beds, should not be imported, but that local producers should be stimulated to cater for these needs.

> *Table 4.9: Total cost of equipment*
> - Purchase
> - Transport
> - Pre-installation site preparations
> - Installation, calibration
> - User training
> - Personnel (operators)
> - Operating material (consumables)
> - Maintenance and spare parts
> - Energy consumption
> - Disposal of the equipment and/or substances produced
> - Replacement costs   (Halbwachs 1992)

Patient hotels

With the ever increasing costs of health care, the development of the 'patient hotel' is being pursued in an attempt to obtain better value for money. The University Hospital in Lund, Sweden, in 1988 opened a patients' hotel for those patients who:

- required diagnostic examination/treatment at the hospital;

- were unable to stay at home — eg due to geographical factors or because they had no one to support them;

- did not require full ward resources but needed hotel service facilities.

Viterius (1990: 53–5) describes the process of developing a patient hotel and the results. Objectives were reached, running costs were less than half those of running a ward, security of patients was ensured firstly, by having the hotel located inside the hospital and secondly, through staff training. Lastly, the hotel also had improved service.

Accommodating some pre-operative patients in patient hotels would offer patients a less stressful environment, would ensure that patients arrive for their operations on schedule, and may decrease patients' pre-operative exposure to micro-organisms.

Demographics and disease profiles/epidemiology

Demographic and epidemiological trends will obviously play a role in selection and scope of services to be provided. Van Rensburg, Fourie, and Pretorius (1992) give further details.

Environment-friendly facilities

More and more emphasis is being placed on the development of facilities that are built, and operated, to conserve energy, and to promote the efficient use of resources. The increased control of waste materials is also of great importance and efforts are being made to contain and dispose of them in such a way that the environment is not contaminated.

CONCLUSION

No hospital or clinic will ever be perfect. Compromises are always necessary, but if one follows the guidelines for planning, and if one participates in the process in a formal and structured way, the chances of developing a practical and user-friendly building are far greater. In particular, it is critical that nurses at all levels become involved from the outset by participating in the briefing and design stages of hospitals and clinics, irrespective of the size of the project. Once this happens, our hospitals and clinic buildings will enhance excellence in clinical practice.

References

Abbott, G. R. (1992). *A Team Approach to Health-Care Facility Planning and Design.* Health-Care Facility Training Workshop. Division of Building Technology, CSIR: Pretoria.

Allen, D. and Davis, M. (1991). Clinical Information Systems Impact On The Intensive Care Unit, Lutheran Hospital — La Crosse, La Crosse, Wisconsin. March 1991.

Butler, M. (1992). Building the best. *Hospital Development,* volume 23, number 3, pp. 33–5

Carlisle, D. (1990). On the way out. *Nursing Times,* volume 86, number 33, p. 19.

Cowan, D. and Louw, I. J. (1985). *Health Care Facilities — Evaluation of Norms.* Paper read at the third South African Hospital Symposium, Pretoria, 19–20 September, 1985.

De Debuchy, A. B. (1993). Summary of group 2. Design for efficiency, economy and humanity in hospitals. *World Hospitals,* volume 19, number 3, pp. 48–50.

Dix, A. (1990). Patients to the fore. *Hospital Development,* volume 21, number 11, pp. 17–19.

Du Toit, R. (1990). The planning of hospitals part III: planning the New Durban Academic Hospital. *Nursing RSA,* volume 5, number 7, pp. 27–33.

Fourie, C. (1992). *A Team Approach to Health-Care Facility Planning and Design.* Health-Care Facility Training Workshop. Division of Building Technology, CSIR: Pretoria.

Galer, I. (1987). *Applied Ergonomics Handbook.* Butterworths: London.

Halbwachs, H. (1992). *Health Care Equipment for Developing Countries - the Conflict between Needs and Interests.* Paper delivered at the 12th International Congress of Hospital Engineering, Bologna, 25–29 May 1992.

Howard, T. (1992). This year's model. *Hospital Development,* volume 23, number 10, p. 7

Howie, K. (1990). In Du Toit, R. The Planning of Hospitals Part I: Stages of a Project. *Nursing RSA,* volume 5, number 5, pp. 14–20.

Kleczkowski, B. M. and Nilsson, N. O. (1984). *Health Care Facility Projects in Developing Areas: Planning, Implementation and Orientation.* Public Health Papers, number 79, World Health Organization, Geneva.

Langslow, B. (1975). Commissioning New Hospitals and Health Facilities. *World Hospitals,* volume 11, Spring/Summer, pp. 104–7.

Malan, E. (1977). *Die Inwerkingstelling van 'n Nuwe Hospitaal.* Unpublished M.Cur thesis. University of Pretoria.

Malkin, J. (1991). Creating excellence in health care design. Journal of Health Care Interior Design. Proceedings from the Third Symposium on Health Care Interior Design. National Symposium on Health Care Design, Inc. California.

Meara, R. (1992). Millennium agenda. *Hospital Development,* volume 23, number 5, pp. 21–3.

Millard, G. (1986). References for commissioning. In *Commissioning Hospital Buildings.* Third edition. King Edward's Hospital Fund for London: London.

Republic of South Africa (1981). *National Plan and Norms for Health Service Facilities.* Department of Health and Welfare: Pretoria.

Republic of South Africa (1992). *Policy on the South African Hospital Norms (SAHNORMS): Community Health Centres, Maximum Security and Closed Ward Units in Psychiatric Hospitals.* Department of National Health and Population Development: Pretoria.

Sacewicz, L. N. (1985). The death of a hospital. *American Journal of Nursing,* volume 85, number 6, p. 760.

SANC (1984). *The Scope of Practice of Registered Nurses.* R.2589 of 30 November 1984, as amended by R.1469 of 10 July 1987, chapter 2. June 1985. SANC: Pretoria.

Schmidt, R. (1992). *Medical Technology and the 'Fifth Continent'.* Paper delivered at the 12th International Congress of Hospital Engineering, Bologna, 25–29 May, 1992.

Schroeder, R. G. (1981). *Operations Management: Decision Making in the Operations Function.* McGraw-Hill: New York.

Slabber, C. (1991). *Protokol: Primêre Gesondheidsorg In 'n Plakkergemeenskap.* Unpublished.

South African Nursing Council (1984). *The Scope of Practice of Registered Nurses.*

Steele, F. (1992). *Problems and Pitfalls in Commissioning.* Unpublished lecture to nursing management students, Natal University.

Sullivan, E. J. and Decker, P. J. (1988). *Effective Management in Nursing.* Second edition. Addison-Wesley: California.

Thomas, T. E. and Saslow, K. L. (1992). Designing The Next Generation of American Hospitals. *World Hospitals*, volume 28, number 1, pp. 33–6.

Tjam, F. S. (1992). *Concerns in Developing Countries.* International Hospital Federation: London.

Van der Merwe, T. (1993). *Planning Design and Construction of Community Health Facilities.* Unpublished paper delivered at the Southern Africa Federation of Hospital Engineering meeting, Pretoria, 23 March, 1993.

Van Rensburg, H. C. J., Fourie, A. and Pretorius, E. (1992). *Health Care in South Africa: Structure and Dynamics.* Academica: Pretoria.

Van Tonder, S. (1988). Nie-verplegingstake en die Geregistreerde Verpleegkundige. *Curationis,* volume 11, number 1, pp. 6–11.

Viterius, B. (1990). Hotel service. *Hospital Development,* volume 21, number 1, pp. 53–5.

Warner, U. (1990). Trials and tribulations. Community outlook. *Nursing Times,* volume 86, number 28, pp. 29–32.

CHAPTER 5

GENERAL MANAGEMENT APPROACHES

S. W. Booyens

CONTENTS

INTRODUCTION

The nurse manager is faced with the reality of managing or directing a diverse group of health workers. A special brand of eternal vigilance is required in order to lead or direct the different categories of nursing personnel to achieve a good end-product — ie to render a nursing care service which satisfies the patients. This vigilance may take on a variety of forms, but aspects such as controlling the rate of turnover and absenteeism, improving the morale of staff, participating in decision-making, and the formulation of strategies for the improvement of patient care are always debated. It is thus imperative to review a number of managerial approaches in order to supply the nurse manager with the necessary information to handle a diversity of personnel management problems.

MODERN MANAGEMENT THEORIES

There are a number of management theories in common use. We shall examine those of Douglas McGregor, Frederick Herzberg, Chris Argyris, Rensis Likert, and the approach of Robert Blake and Jane Mouton.

Douglas McGregor

McGregor described two types of supervisors. He stated that the type of supervisor who functions according to theory X assumes that people hate work, that they therefore have to be coerced to get something done, and that close control is needed. The supervisory functioning according to theory Y assumes that employees have an intrinsic interest in their work and that they therefore need not be coerced, that they will direct themselves, that they like to be given responsibility, and that they are capable of creative thinking in order to solve problems. McGregor, of course, believed that the second type of manager was the better one and that such a manager could get far better work results than the theory X manager.

Frederick Herzberg

Herzberg enlarged on McGregor's theories and focused on the motivation of workers. According to Herzberg, worker motivation could be accomplished by two 'factors', namely *hygiene factors* and *intrinsic or motivating factors*. The hygiene factors included such things as working conditions, salaries, and fringe benefits, while the motivating factors included the intrinsic worth which the job itself holds for the employee, including responsibility, achievement, and self-actualization.

Chris Argyris

Argyris focused on the effects of organizational life and on individual motivation. He studied the development of organizational structures and control systems in order to obtain a fit between organizational goals and employee goals. He proposed, among other things, such organizational adaptations as job enlargement and participative or employee-centred leadership, and stressed the need for self-actualization of the employee (Argyris 1987). According to Argyris, the employee who finds himself in an organization with rigid controls and an autocratic leadership style will most likely respond by becoming passive, dependent, feeling incompetent, and experiencing job dissatisfaction. On the other hand, when managers take advantage of these people's talents and let them participate in planning, problem-solving, and goal-setting, they become active, independent, and more likely to achieve self-actualization.

Rensis Likert

Likert identified three variables in organizations, namely causal, intervening, and end-result variables. The causal variables include leadership behaviour, organizational structure, policies, and controls. Intervening variables included perceptions, attitudes, and motivations. The end-result variables are measures of profits, costs, and productivity. Likert believed that many managers in organizations only give consideration to the end results without considering what the causes were for poor or good results. He thus developed the Likert scale questionnaire where measures of causal and intervening variables were stated in relation to the end products. This scale measured such aspects as motivation, leadership style, communication, and decision-making processes (Marriner-Tomey 1992: 283).

Likert also described four types of management systems ranging from totally authoritarian to totally democratic: exploitative–authoritative, benevolent-authoritative, consultative, and participative.

In the exploitative–authoritative system the top managers make all the decisions and pass them downwards. The employees are never asked for any ideas, nor are top management aware of any of their problems or needs. Rigid control systems are in place, with punishment meted out often. The employees view top management with suspicion, tend to resist the organization's goals, and form an informal organization system to give them support at work.

In the benevolent–authoritative system the controls are rather less rigid than in the exploitative–authoritative one. Decisions are made by top and middle managers. Employees are sometimes invited to give some input, but they do not feel free to discuss their jobs with managers. Little communication exists between top management and employees, and goals are established through orders, with perhaps a little comment invited. Management have an idea of the employees' situation and occasionally employees are consulted when problems arise. Control is implemented through a system of rewards and punishments. An informal organization is usually in place, and this tends to show resistance to the formal one.

In the consultative system the managers exhibit substantial confidence in their employees. Employees feel free to discuss their work with managers, they give input when goals are set, and they also take responsibility for these goals. A considerable amount of communication flows upwards and downwards, but it is limited in accuracy and, while it is not viewed suspiciously like in the other two systems, it is still only cautiously accepted. Managers are familiar with their staff's working situations, broad policy is set at the top, and decision-making takes place throughout the organization. Control is delegated to the lower levels and is exercised through the use of a reward system and self-guidance. Sometimes an informal organization resists the formal organization's goals.

In participative management systems, managers exhibit complete confidence in their employees. They always seek the ideas of employees with the result that employees freely discuss their jobs with them. Goals are set at all levels. Communication flows freely upwards, downwards, and laterally, is perceived as accurate, and thus is received without trepidation. Managers are well informed about problems faced by their staff, decision-making is well integrated throughout the organization, and control is widely shared through the use of self-guidance and problem-solving. No informal organization operates to resist the goals of the formal organization because the goals are those that were set by the staff themselves (Marriner-Tomey 1992: 284).

Likert strongly supported the use of participative management and supportive relationships and proposed a system where good managers educate poor managers by forming interlinking groups of managers to provide support.

Blake and Mouton

Robert Blake and Jane Mouton proposed a managerial grid which depicted two critical dimensions, namely:

1. a concern for people;

2. a concern for production.

The two dimensions are independent. A manager may thus be high on one and low on the other, or high or low on both. The grid consists of two axes. The vertical axis represents the manager's regard for people. The horizontal axis represents the manager's concern for production. Each axis is on a scale of 1 to 9, representing a minimum to a maximum concern for people or production. There are five basic styles, one in each corner of the grid and one in the middle.

The task manager at 9,1 has the highest regard for production and the lowest concern for people. This manager views employees as tools for production.

The people manager at 1,9 is thoughtful and friendly but production does not really figure in his concerns.

The organization–man manager at 5,5 represents a moderate concern for both people and production but not necessarily at the same time. The emphasis is shifting from time to time.

The team manager at 9,9 is the best manager. This type of manager integrates her concerns for people and production. Problems are confronted directly, and mutual trust and respect prevail (Moorhead and Griffin 1989: 328).

MANAGEMENT TOOLS

A number of so-called management tools were developed during the 1950s and 1960s.

Management by objectives was one such a tool. Management by objectives is still quite popular today because it makes employees and managers more goal-orientated, it stimulates an orientation to the future, and counteracts the tendency to become bogged-down in the everyday problems of managing an organization.

Another management tool which received a lot of attention was the concept of *participative management*. This concept evolved from the idea that the more the individual employee is involved in the decision-making process, the more likely he is to understand and be committed to it.

The idea of job enrichment is related to participative management. Job enrichment is supposed to enlarge the boundaries of a job, thereby increasing the employee's actual decision-making responsibility and allowing for individual achievement (McClure 1984: 17).

The contingency theory

Criticism has been levelled at the different proponents of the above approaches to management because each proponent presented his/ her idea of management as if it was the appropriate style for the management of all the different types of organizations. The different approaches did not make allowance for the fact that there were distinct differences between organizations in relation to the type of work that had to be done, the different managers, the employees, and the organizational settings.

Two researchers, Morse and Lorsch, conducted a study of four organizations, two of which were successful and two unsuccessful. An interesting fact was that the two successful organizations operated on completely different terms; one around McGregor's theory X and the other around theory Y. The researchers concluded that the two organizations were successful because the different managerial styles fitted the task which had to be accomplished and because the employees were able to develop a sense of competence. Morse and Lorsch then developed their contingency theory which emphasized the fit between tasks, organizations, and people. The underlying assumptions of this theory are contained in the following four statements (McClure 1984: 17):

- People bring a variety of needs and motives to the workplace, but one central need is to achieve a sense of competence.

- This competence need may be fulfilled in several ways, depending upon the strength of a person's need for power, independence, structure, achievement and affiliation.

- The need to achieve a sense of competence is most likely to be fulfilled when the individual perceives a fit between the task that he performs and the type of organization he finds himself in.

- This sense of competence keeps motivating one, because if a person feels that he/she has achieved competence in one aspect or task, competence is sought in a higher or more difficult type of task.

According to Morse and Lorsch, individuals tend to gravitate to organizations that meet their needs. Some employees will thus find a theory X organization rewarding and motivating and others will tend to leave such an organization for one with a less rigid control system.

Current management thinking thus favours an eclectic approach towards management. There is no universal theory of management which is useful to all managers in all settings. A manager should become knowledgeable about the different management theories being developed, and will then have to make a careful analysis of the problems inherent in his/her organization and adapt his/her managerial style to fit the circumstances.

When such an analysis or assessment is made, five factors should be examined. These are:

- purpose;
- tasks;

- people;

- technology;

- structure.

The manager must have a good understanding of each of these factors separately, as well as of their action in concert. Added to these internal factors are the external factors which must also be considered such as the economy, political pressures, legal aspects, sociocultural aspects, and the technology involved (McClure 1984: 18).

In order to develop a contingency theory of management in one's own organization, the following four-step methodology is recommended:

- Make a study of the different managerial concepts and techniques which have been developed.

- Analyse these concepts and techniques to develop a crystal clear understanding of the advantages and disadvantages inherent in each one. There is no approach which does not have its own set of negative and positive effects.

- Develop a complete understanding of the situation at hand — ie an understanding of all the internal and external factors involved. It is completely foolish to rush in as a new manager and try to bring about a major reorganization without first taking time to study the situation's weaknesses and strengths.

- When the first three steps are tied together, the new manager is in a position to apply the approach which is fitting for the situation.

MANAGERIAL CONCEPTS

We shall now discuss a number of important concepts that are used in management. These include the issue of centralization versus decentralization, participative management, management by objectives, the span of control, line and staff relationships, and quality circles.

Centralization and decentralization

Health care organizations are among the most complex organizations that exist. Their complexity increases with size, so decisions are better managed at the specific area from where they originate. A decentralized approach to management and decision-making would thus presumably provide better results. This is not, however, always true for all organizations.

During their early years, organizations tend to have centralized authority. If the organization grows from within it tends to stay centralized, in contrast to organizations which grow by merging with others or by acquiring extra smaller units. Organizations with a wide geographical distribution thus tend to be more decentralized.

Functions such as budgeting, accounting, statistical data-processing, and the purchase of capital equipment are usually centralized while functions such as marketing, production, the purchasing of operational facilities, and personnel management are more likely to be decentralized.

In organizations with a centralized concentration of authority, the control is direct. Decisions affecting the majority of the employees are made at the top by a relatively small number of selected managers. They make decisions by virtue of the power which emanates from their positions in the organization. They exert a direct influence on the staff by monitoring the implementation of the organizational decisions (Hein and Nicholson 1986: 353). Centralization of authority and decision-making usually occurs where the top managers do not wish to weaken their positional authority by empowering managers in the middle and lower levels. It is also practised where top managers fear that the overall goals of the organization may not be achieved because the self-contained divisions, with their relatively greater powers of authority, may work against the best interests of the organization.

An organization that operates in a relatively stable environment, is well organized, and does not need to change its operations frequently, is usually effective if it is run by a centralized authority.

Decisions made at the top, however, need to be communicated through more intermediate levels to reach the operational personnel than those which originate at or near the functional level, with the result that centralized organizations are slow in adapting to change. The rank-and-file workers in such organizations are not used to critical thinking and problem solving, with the result that they become passive and unenthusiastic workers. In such an organization, the nurse manager acts as a liaison officer between top management and care-givers.

Decentralization of authority increases morale and promotes interpersonal relationships. There is a greater feeling of individuality and informality in a decentralized system and the employees become more creative in, and enthusiastic about, their jobs. Decisions may be more effective because the people who make them know the situation and have to implement the decisions. Communication is swift, co-ordination is improved, and the organization can adapt better to changes in the environment. The main goal of decentralization is to push responsibility and authority downwards. The effect is often better-informed decisions.

In such an approach middle managers become more accountable and so it is difficult for them to engage in buck-passing behaviour. The middle manager is thus developed and this makes the principle of promotion from within the organization more realistic. Top management is released from the burdens of daily administration, and this allows them time for their prime functions of long-range planning, goal and policy development, and the integration of the variety of systems in the organization.

In the nursing department, decentralization means that, in practice, nurses will provide the major input in the development and interpretation of patient care norms, standards, and criteria for excellence. This leads to increased personal and professional satisfaction in the nursing process.

Decentralization also involves a great change in the role of the unit manager in that she will usually become responsible for the budget of her unit — sometimes even for the staffing of the unit. It may not always be wise to give such managerial responsibility to a unit manager on the basis of seniority or clinical expertise without considering her educational preparation and managerial aptitude.

Many proponents of decentralization claim that it increases the power of nurses because it increases the number of voices that speak for, and have control over, nursing. This expansion of power through the greater involvement of the individual nurse in decision-making and the implementation of goals and objectives at the operational level is the key to improvement in patient care (Wellington 1986: 39).

Some managerial functions may be decentralized while others are best controlled at a centralized level. When deciding to use a decentralized approach, careful consideration must be given to the following: who controls the budget; who has the power over hiring and firing; who handles disciplinary matters, promotions, and transfers, and who handles disputes between staff and management.

There are, however, a number of disadvantages in a decentralized approach. If there are not enough qualified managers to take responsibility for decentralized units, it is difficult to implement decentralization. Decentralization is costlier than centralization because more managers are needed. Sometimes there may be an underutilization of managers, or specialists at headquarters may not be adequately consulted. There may be a lack of standardization. Because decentralization develops managers, they are still novice managers and will most probably make mistakes. Divisions might not inform top management of their problems and might not implement policies correctly. The most obvious disadvantage of a decentralized system is loss of co-ordination. When each unit or department independently runs its own affairs, duplication of effort, unnecessary problems in effecting change, and mismanagement by unqualified personnel can occur. The management process can also be very time-consuming when large numbers of people take an active part in the system. Decentralization also opens the door to interdepartmental power struggles (Wellington 1986: 39).

Participative management

Participative management takes place in flat organizational structures where there is increased association between employees and managers and where there are decreased numbers of policy manuals, managerial titles, and executive offices.

During participative management, subordinates are actively involved in problem-solving and decision-making. The subordinates are thus allowed some measure of influence in the manager's decisions. This is done in a decentralized organizational structure. The process of participative management involves training and changed roles for supervisors, and changes in organizational communication. There is a complementary relationship between managers and practitioners rather than a hierarchical one.

Management training of supervisors will include such aspects as group dynamics, problem-solving, planning and decision-making. It will also develop supervisors' abilities for frankness and openness with employees, and will encourage contributions from them.

In participatory management, the supervisor facilitates rather than directs the workforce. Increased interpersonal skills and conceptual abilities will be demanded of supervisors. When supervisors have mastered the above skills, and when the employees become committed to taking an active role in problem-solving and decision-making, the facilitator or supervisor will find herself freed of the everyday running problems of her division and will have more time to organize the work and to be creative. Management by objectives, group brainstorming, and quality circles are often used in the participative management style.

The advantages of participatory management include:

- increased feeling of responsibility among employees toward organizational goals and objectives;

- better working relationships because of increased trust and mutual support among employees;

- better attitudes towards work among employees;

- increased productivity;

- fresh ideas for managerial decisions and problem-solving;

- identification of potential leaders;

- decreased turnover and increased stability of the workforce;
- the development of mature, healthy, self-directed personalities among employees.

Some of the disadvantages of participative management include:

- staff may misinterpret the concept as meaning that they make all the decisions;
- organizational policies and procedures will have to be changed;
- the initiation of programmes takes time and money;
- employees who are only used to an autocratic management style may not appreciate this style and may view it as insincere, patronizing, and manipulative at the beginning;
- employees may feel threatened by the use of self-evaluation.

Implementation of participative management

Full participation by employees is neither realistic nor desirable for all decisions. Even in an organization with participatory management, it is the top managers' responsibility to determine the appropriate direction the organization must take and then to structure it for the accomplishment of the strategic goals that have been decided upon.

There are a number of prerequisites for the effective use of participation in an organization (Yukl, as referred to by Callahan 1987: 10). These are:

- the leader of a group has the authority to make important decisions;
- decisions are made without strong time pressures imposed on the team;
- subordinates must be in possession of relevant knowledge;
- subordinates must be willing to participate;
- the leader has confidence in participative techniques;
- the leader is skilled in the use of participative techniques.

The leader must have authority to make decisions, otherwise she will not be in a position to encourage or seek participation from subordinates. Participation is, however, feasible only for problems over which she has jurisdiction. There are decisions in which even the leaders have no participation, for example decisions about medical practice which influence nursing practice (Callahan 1987: 11).

The three critical elements which have been identified for the effective implementation of the participative management concept are decentralization, group decision-making, and management by objectives.

If an organization wishes to implement participatory management, it is recommended that the following guidelines should be followed:

- Top management should write out guidelines for participation, for example stating the types of decisions to be delegated to participatory groups, methods for assessing the quality of decisions, and top managements' responsibilities in developing and monitoring such a style in the organization.

- All staff should be taught about the relationship between responsibility, accountability, and authority inherent in the system, about the types of decision participation procedures, and about the expected level of participation for planning how the decisions should be implemented.

- The group's leader must take on the final responsibility and accountability for the group's decisions. She must clearly describe to the group the level of input which is needed from it as well as the nature of the assignment.

- The best decisions are worthless if they are not implemented. Activities to implement decisions must be defined and described in chronological order. The leader or manager must estimate the resources needed for their implementation.

- Formal guidelines must exist regarding the flow of communication regarding decisions from top to bottom, from bottom to top, and laterally.

- Staff development programmes will have to be arranged to teach personnel about effective communication skills, group processes, and negotiation skills.

- The participative process must be monitored and its relative success or failure must be evaluated by the groups themselves. If changes are necessary, the groups must decide which changes should be made.

When the employees know the limits within which they participate, and are committed to the process, they will experience increased job satisfaction (Callahan 1987: 11–3).

Management by objectives

Management by objectives is a system for setting organizational objectives for a given period, devising plans to implement the objectives, and carrying out periodic evaluation of progress towards the attainment of the objectives.

It is a process whereby the manager and subordinate jointly identify the common goals of an organization, define each individual's major areas of responsibility in terms of the results expected, and utilize these measures as guides for evaluating the contribution of each worker. It is a system which stresses an individual's ability and achievement rather than personality. Management by objectives assures the protection of individual idiosyncrasies and does not require personality changes; it is indifferent to activities, but deeply concerned with output.

Before engaging in management by objectives, the major responsibilities of the incumbent of a job must be identified. Once the major responsibilities of a job are listed, the expected levels of accomplishment can be determined. The setting of job performance standards and criteria is done by determining the objectives to be attained.

The objectives set must conform to the following criteria (Bell 1980: 25):

1. They must be specific, personal, and risky.

2. The time period in which they must be accomplished must be realistic.

3. They must be measurable.

4. The objectives must be determined through dialogue between manager and subordinate and must be confirmed in writing.

5. The employee should be guided by the manager to remain within her limitations when setting objectives.

6. The objectives should be used as a tool for coaching, developing, and improving the employee, and for rewarding good results.

7. They should be stated in a way that will affect behaviour and results.

8. The objectives should be realistic and flexible, but should not include routine activities which will be performed anyway.

9. They should be stated in a format which will enable one to do an evaluation of the results later and to provide feedback regarding attainment of the objectives. This type of format will also guide the employee when assessing her individual progress.

10. Once the objectives have been set and target dates for completion have been determined, the plan should be adhered to. Results should be published in the newsletter of the hospital or health-care organization.

11. Not more than three or four objectives should be set at any one time. Once they have been attained, new ones can be set.

12. It must be possible to count, measure, or describe an objective, otherwise it should not be used.

13. Four types of objectives have been identified by Odiorne — routine, problem-solving, creative or innovative, and personal development objectives.

14. The expected standard of performance for each objective — for example, whether it is unsatisfactory, satisfactory, or outstanding — should also be determined. A concrete plan must be devised to accomplish each objective.

Some advantages of management by objectives are the following (Marriner-Tomey 1992: 381):

- improvement of the relationship between managers and staff;

- clarity of goals;

- the nurse feels that she has some input and control over her future;

- there is a better basis for evaluation of performance — personality traits do not play a role;

- management by objectives is future-orientated, and the future can be changed;

- it stimulates better individual performance and morale.

A number of disadvantages are also encountered (Marriner-Tomey 1992: 381). These include:

- a manager's development may be hampered, because if she is only concentrating on the staff's attainment of the objectives which they have set, she does not develop abilities to handle improbable, unforeseen, uncertain situations, where an ingenuity for problem-solving is needed;

- if there is too much emphasis placed on objectives and their achievement, it might lead to neglecting the normal necessary routine and repetitive tasks such as budgetary control, writing procedures, and updating policies, with the result that the workplace is not maintained properly (Gillies 1989: 69–70);

- it is not an easy system to implement and to maintain;

- some managers may be assessing activities that seem to indicate results rather than the results themselves;

- not all staff members are willing to be involved in goal- and objective-setting;

- nurses can become frustrated if they believe that they will have to conform to increasingly higher goals;

- management by objectives lends itself to quantitative assessment, with the result that qualitative facts may be overlooked;

- it does not provide comparative data on which to base merit rating for promotions or salary increases.

Management by objectives is necessary for the development of the organization. Interpersonal competence among staff members should be aimed at, the individual goals of employees should influence the organizational goals once such a system operates well, organizational structures and systems should be adopted and adapted by the employees for goal attainment, and individual self-actualization should be achieved (Swansburg 1990: 346).

Span of control

The span of control, or span of management, refers to the number of people reporting to a manager. It thus defines the size of the organization's work groups.

The optimal unit size for supervision depends on a number of variables such as the requirements for consideration within the unit, the degree of job specialization within the unit, the similarity of tasks in the unit, the type of information available or needed by unit members, differences in the need for autonomy by unit members, and how much direct access to the supervisor is needed by the members (Moorhead and Griffin 1989: 405).

The span of control is also affected by the patient profile in a unit, the type of nursing care delivery system(s) used (patient-nurse assignment), the geographical dispersion of subordinates, the managerial and supervisory skills that the manager possesses, the educational level(s) of the employees, the number of support systems available (eg unit clerks and other administrative assistants) the organization's management philosophy (eg decentralized or centralized structure) and the prevailing environmental factors (for example an organization functioning in a fast changing environment will have to adapt to many novel problems regarding changing disease patterns and will need more supervisory support, thus necessitating narrowing the span of control) (Shehnaz 1988: 35–9).

It has been shown by research that the executive at the top of the bureaucratic pyramid can effectively supervise three subordinates and at the bottom the common ratio is 1:6.

When the span of control is too broad, the supervisor does not have enough contact with the staff to observe a representative sample of their work, with the result that the quality of work performance cannot be accurately assessed. This again leads to insufficient encouragement of staff or to a failure to institute remedial measures as soon as they become necessary.

A span of control which is too narrow is equally problematic because there are only a few subordinates to monitor, with the result that the supervision becomes stultifying. This inhibits the development of skills for problem-solving, individual judgement, and creative thinking in employees. According to Drucker (1976) worker productivity is higher when close supervision is impossible.

Line and staff relationships

Line authority is depicted in the chain-of-command system. The chief nurse manager delegates authority to the senior nurse manager who in turn delegates authority to a senior professional nurse and so on. The command relationship is a direct line from the one to the other and is shown by a solid line on organizational charts. The line positions are related to the direct achievement of the goals of the organization.

A staff function is one that has been separated from the chain of command to permit specialization and increased effectiveness. A staff officer does the work that an executive is too busy to do. A staff officer's specialization gives her the status of an expert in a narrow sphere of management.

If a nursing department with a pure line structure becomes so large that the chief nurse manager cannot effectively execute all her managerial responsibilities, she may appoint staff officers to share her workload. The manager thus assigns certain management tasks — staff development, for instance — to a staff officer who is not in a position to supervise activities in the line structure.

The staff officer is expected to improve the functioning of the organization through her analyses and proposals. She must try to get voluntary acceptance of her ideas by the line officers, or she must persuade the chief nurse manager to order the line workers to carry out her suggestions (Gillies 1989: 154).

A staff officer usually has a service, advisory, or control function. An example of a staff officer with a service function is the staff development specialist who orientates newcomers and develops existing line employees to function more effectively in their line function capabilities. An example of a staff officer with an advisory function is a research specialist who assists line staff members to plan and carry out research projects. An example of a staff officer with a control function is a quality control officer who evaluates the care given in units on a regular basis, or who, with her staff, conducts regular audits and then not only advises on remedial measures to be implemented regarding shortcomings but actually oversee their implementation.

When a staff organization's function is too large for one person to handle, and grows to the extent that a corps of staff members are appointed or seconded to this staffing function — eg the staff development section — there again appears a line organization within this staff authority in order to distribute responsibilities among the staff members.

The staff organization is there to serve the line organization. It often happens that the staff organization must stand quietly in the background, while the line officers are praised for the good ideas which were actually originated by the staff specialists. Sometimes staff personnel may attempt to enlarge their sphere of authority by usurping the authority of the line managers. Conflict thus arises between the two types of officers. Staff officers should not be allowed to take over responsibilities which are the domain of the line managers, but the line managers (who are often older, but less well educated than the staff specialists) should not be free to ignore the advice of the staff specialists.

In a third type of formal organization structure, the staff officers no longer fill a purely advisory capacity but are utilized in a command authority over line staff members. An example is where the manager responsible for in-service education has the power to decide what the programme of in-service education will consist of and when the sessions will be presented, and where she controls the attendance of the sessions by keeping registers of names of the staff members attending. This type of organization is called a *functionalized line and staff organization*. In this type of organization, the morale of staff specialists is higher than in the line and staff organization and their talents are used more effectively. It is, however, possible that the communication network in this type of organization can become tangled and that confusion may develop.

Quality circles

The idea of using small groups of workers to solve work-related problems was advocated by management consultants in the United States of America and adopted by the Japanese after the Second World War. The quality circle concept has become widespread in Japan, raising the quality of Japanese products to world class standards, with the result that companies in the United States are now in turn borrowing back the idea from the Japanese.

A quality circle is composed of a group of five to ten people who are trained especially for this process. They meet for an hour once a week to spot problems in their work area and to solve them. The group members use statistical analyses to make improvements in the quality. Group members must share common interests and common problems, and they are usually people who work together to produce a specific component or service.

There are four steps in establishing and leading a quality circle (Dessler 1984: 444):

- planning;

- training;

- initiation;

- operation of the circle.

During the planning phase, the top level management decides to implement such a system, and a facilitator and a quality circle steering committee are selected. The steering committee directs the quality circle activities in the organization. This committee is also responsible for establishing circle objectives which should be worked upon, such as bottom-line improvements (eg more effective teamwork), increased motivation, and increased job involvement.

There must be an initial training session, which usually takes four days, where the facilitator and the pilot project leaders learn the leadership techniques which must be applied in quality circle sessions.

During the initiation phase, the concept is introduced to the employees. Managers of sections, quality circle leaders, the facilitator, and someone from top management explain the concept to the employees at meetings and ask them to consider joining the circle. The circle is then formed and can turn to its real job, namely the analysis and solving of problems.

First the problem must be identified. The problems are typically mundane ones which would not interest someone outside the circle's work area, such as how to speed up the packing or, in a health care unit, how to speed up the administration of medicines. Big interdepartmental problems, such as reducing the turnover rate, are not within the realm of quality circles and are none of their concern.

When the circle considers the problems it wants to focus on, it will select the number one problem inhibiting the work of its members. Only when a solution has been produced for this can they move on to another one.

During problem analysis, members of the quality circle collect data regarding a problem, analyse them, and try to solve the problem using the problem-solving techniques for which they were specially trained. During this phase the quality circle members derive a real sense of satisfaction from the process, and so quality circles become just as much a morale-booster and teamwork-promoter as an output improvement tool.

The group now recommends a number of solutions during an official oral presentation to management. The group must thus sell its ideas to management.

This presentation is not made to top management but to the immediate supervisor in the group's chain of command. It is found that 85–100% of the suggestions of the circle are usually approved during the presentation meeting. In those unusual instances where a manager must turn down a recommendation, he or she should be trained to explain the reason for not accepting it, so that the enthusiasm of the circle members is not dampened (Dessler 1984: 445–6).

Problems encountered by quality circles

1. *'It's just another programme.'* When workers view quality circles as just another programme to entice them to get more out of them, they will view them with scepticism. It is thus essential that management must stress to them that they are first and foremost a people-building exercise and only secondly a cost-reduction programme.

2. *'Management does not heed our ideas.'* When management does not pay attention to the quality circle's suggestions, the concept will not be successful. The employees must, however, be made aware of the fact that they will not be allowed to generate a list of problems and then turn this over to management to solve. They will have to understand that they must solve the problems they identify themselves.

3. *Selecting problems outside the area of the circle's expertise.* The leader of each group should keep the group on track so that only problems within their own immediate area of work are identified and selected for problem-solving.

4. *Problems are too difficult to handle.* When the group cannot solve a problem, outsiders might be called in. This might involve the organization's quality circle facilitator.

5. *There is no time for quality circle meetings.* This approach from supervisors and managers will definitely inhibit progress. Their attitude can be overcome by showing them the results of achievements of quality circles and/or inviting them to attend a circle meeting. Quality circles require planning, patience, and long-term commitment from health care managers. They must believe in their employees' ability to contribute to the institution

and be willing to invest the necessary time and resources in the activities of the different circles (McKinney 1984: 86).

6. *Labour unions' fears of interference.* Often labour unions oppose the idea of quality circles because they erroneously think that matters such as wages, salaries, and grievances are being discussed during meetings. Union leaders should be involved right from the start in the steering committee and that union stewards be involved as members of quality circles (Dessler 1984: 446–8).

Benefits of quality circles

Research indicates that productivity and morale improve when employees participate regularly in decision-making and the implementation of changes. In a hospital in the United Kingdom 15 quality circles were set up and their achievements include:

1. Quality of care improvements
   - Reducing the number of accidents in toilets by changing nursing practices and fitting new handrails.
   - Involving families in the treatment of elderly patients.
2. Working environment
   - Research was being carried out into the use of special equipment, such as the mechanical bed.
   - The roles of staff were being clarified.
3. Service provision
   - The quality and presentation of patients' meals have been improved.
   - New health education programmes were initiated (Hyde 1984: 50).

In another hospital in the United Kingdom, quality circle efforts in the radiology department resulted in zero waiting time for patients. Previously, patients had to spend an excessive amount of time waiting to be x-rayed and the x-ray department also had trouble with 50% of its patients not being on time for x-rays. A scheduling system was introduced and waiting time on both sides was effectively eliminated (Cornell 1984: 91).

MANAGEMENT OF STRESS AND BURNOUT

Nursing is a stressful occupation. Anyone will find constant interaction with people who are sick to be stressful. Hospitals are furthermore seen as extremely stressful environments to work in.

Sources of stress in nursing

There are many variables that contribute to the stress and burnout syndrome.

1. Stress resulting from job tasks and the organizational environment.

2. Stress developing from such conditions as conflicting tasks, task assignments for which the nurse feels herself inadequately prepared or experienced, and unclear or insufficient information regarding what is expected of a task assignment.

3. The behaviour of the supervisor who has an authoritarian, punitive, and closely controlling style of supervision creates much stress.

4. Organizational factors which cause stress are: major or frequent changes in instructions, policies and procedures; when the institution is undergoing a major reorganization; when a sudden, significant change in the nature of a person's work is experienced, and when the requests of different supervisors conflict with one another.

5. The rapidly changing environment of health care institutions (which include technological changes and advancements, liability issues, and increased pressure for efficiency due to competition among institutions) is making the role of nurses more difficult and stressful.

6. Chronic work-related stresses include having too much to do in too little time, and experiencing decisions or changes that affect one's work without having any knowledge about them and without being involved in them.

7. Stress resulting from interpersonal factors. Interdisciplinary conflicts and conflicts with supporting services are a common source of discontent.

8. Nurses frequently encounter difficulty in making the system work for the patients, for example when the nurse has difficulty in persuading the doctor to take the patient's symptoms seriously; when convincing the radiology technician that the patient's chest x-rays must be taken immediately; trying to get the kitchen or dietary department to deliver a late tray of food. Such routine frustrations can become rather overwhelming over time (McClure 1984: 15).

9. The multiple roles of the married nurse are a severe source of stress. The nurse experiences conflict when she has to make the quick role-shift from working as a professional in the hospital

and then coming home and playing the roles of mother, housekeeper, lover, spouse, and parent. Added to this is the strain of working rotating shifts which is exhausting because an individual's biorhythm takes several weeks to adjust to changes in shifts.

10. A number of factors or changes which commonly occur in the life of most individuals contribute to stress. These include divorce, death of a spouse, pregnancy, death of a close friend, marriage, personal injuries or illness, vacations, family get-togethers, revision of personal habits, children leaving home, changing homes, and the birth of children. Stress is also experienced when one does not feel in control of one's life, when an individual's low self-esteem makes it difficult to cope with ambiguous and conflicting roles, and when an individual's expectations or ideals are so high that they can never be satisfied in either the work situation or the home situation.

11. Stress resulting from role conflict and role ambiguity. Role ambiguity occurs when there is a lack of clear, consistent information about the activities which must be performed or goals that must be pursued in a given position in the organization (Sullivan and Decker 1992: 205). Role conflict is often experienced by new nurse managers when they find that staff members expect them to view their needs as the first priority, while management expects that their primary loyalty must be to the organization and its goals. The two sets of loyalties can conflict.

Consequences/symptoms of stress and burnout

Burnout is defined as 'an evolutionary process of growing emotional exhaustion, occurring in a nurse as a consequence of being exposed to chronic work-related stress factors' (Bailey, Burnard and Smith 1987: 17). Three degrees of burnout have been identified (Bailey et al. 1987). Characteristics of *first degree burnout* included:

- short-lived bouts of irritability;

- fatigue and worry;

- work situations and colleague relationships are viewed negatively (Bailey et al. 1987: 17).

Characteristics of *second degree burnout* included:

- feelings of failure;

- lack of interest in the work;

- a sense of powerlessness and inadequacy.

Characteristics of *third degree burnout* resulted in:

- development of psychosomatic illnesses, such as ulcers, migraine and chronic backache;
- excessive use of sick leave;
- overuse of alcohol and tranquilizers;
- sarcasm and cynicism in interpersonal dealings;
- displaying judgmental and overcritical attitudes towards others.

Apart from symptoms of burnout, the symptoms of experiencing too much stress are also evident from the following:

- frustration
- bewilderment
- inadequacy
- unhappiness
- feelings of insecurity
- worry
- lack of assertiveness
- foolishness
- fatigue
- nervousness
- incoherence
- apprehension
- lack of confidence
- fearfulness
- anger
- feeling deserted
- anxiety
- wanting to run away
- forgetfulness
- self-criticism
- tearfulness
- restlessness
- depression

- withdrawal or sudden gregariousness
- decrease in self-care
- disorganization
- inability to relax

(Bailey et al. 1987: 17)

- absenteeism
- increased turnover
- job dissatisfaction
- decline in productivity
- occurrences of pilfering and theft
- impaired job performance

(Patrick 1984: 16–17).

Methodologies that are currently available for assessing individuals at risk from burnout, as well assessing actual levels of burnout, are (Patrick 1984: 17–18):

- the Maslach Burnout Inventory
- Health Hazard Appraisal
- the Jones Staff Burnout Scale for Health Professionals, and
- the Wellness Workbook.

Control of stress

Several measures can be used by managers and employees themselves to lessen the effect of stressors in the workplace and in one's own life situation. Managers can lessen their own levels of stress by:

1. Increasing self-awareness. The nurse manager should take time to evaluate herself, her way of performing her job, and her career advancement possibilities as objectively as possible.

2. Developing outside interests, such as hobbies, recreational activities, and being a member of a social group.

3. Maintaining a programme of regular physical exercise, because tension is reduced by physical exercise.

4. Taking regular vacations, because a change of scene is essential to take one's mind off some problems.

5. Learning how to relax, for example listening to music, doing yoga exercises, meditating (Sullivan and Decker 1992: 208).

Managers can lessen the stress levels of subordinates by the following measures:

1. Developing systems for effective two-way communication. It is necessary to make time to hear what the lower level employees think and what they have to say about top-level management's organizational measures. It is also necessary to supply personnel with sufficient up-to-date information about what is going on in the organization.

2. Clarifying role and performance expectations. Expectations of participatory management decision-making and what is expected of each employee in her job should be spelt out as clearly as possible.

3. Promoting prompt, constructive resolution of conflicts. Nurse managers should receive training in handling conflicts and should apply their knowledge to resolve conflicts before they become too complex and emotive to be handled by one manager.

4. Managers should become familiar with staff and their work — eg by learning names, being more visible, doing more rounds and visits (Wadsworth 1986: 26–7).

5. Psychological counselling and therapy should be easily accessible and available for troubled staff members. It is essential, however, that absolute confidentiality must be guaranteed by the psychologist and nursing manager.

6. The nursing manager should demonstrate good listening skills and empathy by not interrupting people, by allowing them time to lead up to an important point, by acknowledging the feelings behind the words, and by not joking about important matters (Firth et al. 1987: 56).

7. Continuing education and staff development should be promoted. Increased skills training, even for those personnel who are more experienced, pays by leading to reduced levels of stress, less turnover, and better performance. Career development and growth should also be actively promoted. A programme of job enrichment that is matched to the individual's goals and desires could also promote development of self-worth.

8. Assertion should be encouraged in all staff, and sessions could be conducted to teach staff essential assertive skills.

9. Clear procedures should be followed regarding discipline and the handling of grievances.

10. Greater participation in decision-making should be aimed at, especially in decisions affecting work increases, job involvement, and commitment.

11. Personal respect must be shown to staff members by passing information promptly to staff, giving time for staff, encouraging discussion before giving one's own views, consulting staff before taking action, being encouraging in difficult times, and by thanking people for their contributions (Firth et al. 1987: 56).

12. Showing openness, or an absence of defensiveness, in discussions with others by giving direct answers to questions, by being straightforward, by being open about one's doubts, uncertainties, faults and mistakes, and by avoiding a defensive response when one feels that one is being criticized (Firth et al. 1987: 56).

13. The manager should endeavour to increase her observational skills in order to detect increased stress levels or signs of burnout among her personnel in the early stages and in order to identify the sources of stress and to reduce or eliminate them.

14. Policies which reduce stress from shift work should be developed. These could include reducing the number of hours of the night shift, increasing rest time between shifts, providing adequate meal times, and providing a fair distribution of weekend and holiday work.

15. A support group for nursing personnel is recommended. Such a support group, which should consist of a group of non-judgmental nurses and nurses who have handled a difficult period of stress and burnout in their own lives, can be helpful to nurses who are experiencing distress. The group should have a particular approach to the way in which frustrations and problems are ventilated; it should emphasize the solutions to the problems presented, it should provide support for lifestyle changes, and it should provide emotional support to enable nurses to cope with stress.

16. A health care support programme for individual employees suffering from problems with substance abuse, weight, diabetes, or hypertension could be helpful. It is, however, essential that confidentiality is maintained (Peterson 1986: 20).

17. Nutritional support should also be considered for employees, including weight control classes with group support and follow-up, and information regarding the calorie, sodium, and cholesterol content of foods.

18. Health fitness programmes comprising screening for health risk factors such as cardiovascular problems could be provided, as well as fitness classes (Peterson 1986: 20).

Personal strategies for coping with stress could include, among other things, the following:

1. The goals one sets oneself must be consistent with one's values.

2. Stress regulation should be practised in that routine habits should be maintained during periods of high stress. It would, for instance, be unwise to try to stop smoking at the same time as starting a new job.

3. Setting aside specific time to adapt to stress is important. When one is promoted to a managerial position, for example, setting aside specific periods to read about management might reduce anxiety about the new work expectations.

4. Time management reduces stress.

5. Assertive people reduce their own stress levels as they can say 'no' to demands which they know they cannot meet, they can request help from others when needed, and they can set limits on other attempts to block their achievement of their goals.

6. Deliberate stopping and compartmentalization of one's thinking pattern helps a person to set aside an allotted time for negative thoughts and worries and then to switch over deliberately to positive thoughts such as 'I am an intelligent person who is completely capable of handling my own life successfully'. (Thoughts lead to feelings and feelings lead to behaviour.)

7. Humour is developed through a flexible attitude towards life, trying to look at a situation from several different viewpoints, and actively employing some playfulness in one's life.

8. Getting sufficient sleep is one of the best ways to combat stress. The different remedies and sources of advice for getting a good night's sleep should be heeded (Marriner-Tomey 1992: 420–2).

The effect of burnout on the budget, on organizational functioning, and on personal effectiveness in the health care setting is such that the nurse manager cannot afford to leave this important aspect of the managerial function to chance.

EXCELLENCE IN NURSING MANAGEMENT

The eight concepts of excellence as identified by Peters and Waterman in their classic book *In Search of Excellence* can be applied to nursing management in the following ways:

1. *Bias for action.* It is important to delegate certain tasks to a task force or an ad hoc group to avoid being caught up in endless meetings and discussions. These can analyse problems, make decisions, and make plans for implementing changes. The group is given a problem to address and the authority to solve it, and it is expected that the group should have the solution to the problem implemented after a few weeks when the group is dissolved.

2. *Staying close to the customer.* Staying close to the customer in nursing means that:

   - the process of quality assurance must be enhanced by research, in-service education, and the promotion of innovative ideas for practice;

   - a strong sense of personal commitment of nurses to patient care must be fostered;

   - supporting the nursing staff at ground level (the staff who deliver nursing care), and showing respect for their contributions (Loveridge 1991: 46).

3. *Support and encouragement of autonomy and entrepreneurship.* Nurse managers must be flexible enough to allow the innovative individual in the nursing workforce to try out new practices and new methods. They must be willing to allow failures, for failures are a part of innovative endeavour.

4. *Productivity through people.* Dedicated nursing staff are entitled to all the support and appreciation that management can provide. They should receive recognition and rewards for excellent service apart from their normal salary increments or merit increases, and management should display a philosophy that the staff are the most important asset of the organization (Loveridge 1991: 47).

5. *Value-driven organizations.* The leader's responsibility is to provide a suitable environment for the expression of the identified values of the nursing personnel and the organization, such as ongoing research, quality patient care, and quality assurance.

6. *'Stick to the knitting.'* The organization should stick to what it knows best, and in health care what is known best is clinical nursing care. It is thus necessary for the manager to exercise exceptional management skills in addition to sound clinical judgement.

7. *Lean organizational structure.* Matrix organizational structures, bureaucratic structures, or decentralized structures are recommended for different health care settings, but none of

them really addresses all the managerial problems of managers. It is thus immaterial what type of structure is used as long as it results in authority for unit and departmental nurse managers in terms of budgetary accountability, personnel management, and inter-unit co-operation (Loveridge 1991: 47).

8. *Tight control.* Tight control should be maintained through strict adherence to an explicit set of values and painstaking attention to detail. This gives employees confidence to be innovative, as they know what is expected of them (Loveridge 1991: 47).

The following conditions in the work setting also promote excellence:

- the presence of a congenial work atmosphere where there is a positive inclination and job satisfaction among subordinates, and where sure signs of empathy are displayed;

- strong levels of risk-taking, initiative, and perseverance, with encouragement is given to these behaviours within the limits of the existing policy, procedures, and acceptable practice;

- staff are uninhibited in approaching supervisors and managers, do not ignore channels of authority, and acknowledge achievements — in other words, good mutual utilization of manpower is achieved coupled with loyalty and respect;

- solid and clear structuring of tasks which leads to high productivity and acceptable standards;

- an analytical working climate where sound judgements, realistic flexibility, and well-considered firmness are applied;

- the promotion of innovation and creativity by encouraging healthy interactional debating and reasoning;

- a move towards the limiting of crisis management through adequate planning and organization;

- the expectation of a high degree of self-discipline and organizational discipline;

- establishing effective leadership which has vision and can clearly indicate the path to be followed. The leaders should bring out the best in their employees, should communicate with them continuously, and motivate them to work together as a team.

CRISIS MANAGEMENT

A number of general points to consider when faced with a crisis in management are coming forth from business management literature, namely:

1. When faced with a crisis, consider what is the worst possible scenario and then act according to this scenario.

2. Develop a crisis management plan.

3. Demonstrate human concern for what has happened by visiting the scene of the disaster.

4. It is essential to communicate effectively in a time of crisis in order to acknowledge that you are aware that something is wrong and to inform the employees or the outside world of your plans to combat the crisis.

5. In a time of crisis it is important to remember that the routine activities of the organization must be continued. The crisis must be managed in addition to organizing the smooth running of everyday activities (Regester 1987: 21).

6. Extra telephone lines should be set up and manned by senior trained personnel to handle incoming calls from outside.

7. Maintain a continuous dialogue with the staff members or members of the public who are disrupting the service, and listen to their grievances.

8. Try to get your opponents on your side by getting them involved in solving the problem.

9. Inviting unbiased, objective, authoritative outside bodies to help end crises, can take the 'sting' out of many crisis situations.

10. When communicating about a crisis, use clear language which shows that you care about what has happened and which clearly demonstrates that you are trying to remedy the situation (Regester 1987: 31).

11. It is an integral part of crisis preparedness to investigate what specialized training programmes are available and to train a senior group of people for the handling of external communications in times of crisis (Regester 1987: 40).

CONCLUSION

The nurse manager is faced with numerous managerial and personnel management problems in her everyday experiences in an organizational setting. A variety of modern management theories have been presented to aid her in her approach to managerial problems. Managerial concepts have been explained at length, some strategies to manage stress and burnout among staff members have been discussed, and a few general points to remember when a crisis has to be managed were presented.

References

Argyris, C. (1987). *Personality and Organization*. Garland: London.

Bailey, C., Burnard, P., Smith, R. (1987). Signs of stress. *Nursing Journal,* January 1987, pp. 16–18.

Bell, M. L. (1980). Management by objectives. *JONA,* May 1980, pp. 19–26.

Callahan, C. B. (1987) Participative management: a contingency approach. *JONA,* September 1987, volume 17, number 9.

Cornell, L. (1984). Quality circles: a new cure for hospital dysfunctions? *Hospital and Health Services Administration,* September/October 1984, pp. 88–93.

Dessler, G. (1984). *Personnel Management*. Reston: Virginia.

Firth, H., McKeown, P., McIntee, J., Britton, P. (1987). Burn-out, personality and support in long-stay nursing. *Nursing Times,* August 1987, volume 83, number 32, pp. 55–7.

Gillies, D. A. (1989). *Nursing Management: a Systems Approach*. W. B. Saunders: Philadelphia.

Hein, E. C. and Nicholson, M. J. (1986). *Contemporary Leadership Behaviour*. Scott, Foresman: Illinois..

Hyde, P. (1984). Quality circles: something for everyone. *Nursing Times,* volume 80, number 48, 1984, pp. 49–50.

Loveridge, C. E. (1991). Lessons in excellence for nurse administrators. *Nursing Management,* volume 22, number 5, pp. 46–7.

Marriner-Tomey, A. (1992). *A Guide to Nursing Management*. Mosby: Philadelphia.

McClure, M. L. (1984). Managing the professional nurse. Part 1. *JONA,* 10 February 1984, pp. 15–20.

McKinney, M. M. (1984). The newest miracle drug: quality circles in hospitals. *Hospital and Health Services Administration,* September/October 1984, pp. 74–85.

Moorhead, G. and Griffin, R. W. (1989). *Organizational Behaviour*. Houghton Miffin Company: Boston.

Patrick, P. K. S. (1984). Organizational burnout programs. *JONA,* volume 14, number 6, pp. 16–20.

Peterson, M. E. (1986). Shared governance: a strategy for transforming organizations. Part 2. *JONA,* volume 16, number 2, pp. 11–21.

Regester, M. (1987). *Crisis Management*. Hutchinson Business: London.

Shehnaz, A. and Funke-Furber, J. (1988) First line nurse managers: optimizing the span of control. *JONA,* volume 18, number 5, pp. 34–9.

Sullivan, E. J. and Decker, P. J. (1992). *Effective Management in Nursing.* Addison-Wesley: California.

Swansburg, R. C. (1990). *Management and Leadership for Nurse Managers.* Jones and Bartlett Publishers: Boston.

Wadsworth. N. S. (1986). Managing organizational stress in nursing. *JONA,* volume 16, number 12, pp. 21–7.

Wellington, M. (1986). Decentralization: how it affects nurses. *Nursing Outlook,* volume 34, number 1, p. 36.

CHAPTER 6

FINANCIAL MANAGEMENT

S. Koch

CONTENTS

INTRODUCTION

Ever-shrinking health service budgets mean that nursing managers must possess essential financial skills. According to Strasen (1987: v), nursing managers need business skills if they are to function effectively in a rapidly changing health service environment.

The change of emphasis towards more business-orientated hospital management has, therefore, led to a need for additional skills and expertise in order for organizations to function effectively within an affordable financial framework. Nursing managers' knowledge of financial management, marketing of services, economics, affordable strategic planning, and budgeting procedures will probably have to be extended before they can function effectively in the work situation.

What, therefore, should successful nursing managers be doing to protect, maintain, and manage resources? Del Bueno argues that nursing managers will have to learn the terms and expressions used in the financial world. It is also important that nursing managers are aware of the difference between managing a personal budget and the management of an organizational budget.

With a personal budget, only one individual is responsible for the success or failure of the budget. In an organization, on the other hand, errors, mismanagement, or bad decisions are shared. With a personal budget, the individual is directly responsible and easily identified when failure or success occurs. Bad financial management in an organization has a far greater impact and much wider implications. Another difference between a personal budget and an organizational budget lies in *control*. While a personal budget is controlled by the individual, an organizational budget is subject to control by internal bodies such as budget review committees, and external bodies such as auditors. An organization's budget also exceeds that of an individual by far. Personal budgets are more flexible than organizational budgets, the latter being subject to established rules and regulations.

The task of nursing managers involves providing nursing services as an income-generating service, rather than merely as a service that uses resources without contributing to the organization's income. Nursing professionals have to prove that, without their services, the provision of a health care service would not be possible.

COST-EFFECTIVENESS IN NURSING MANAGEMENT

The nursing manager is the key figure in the planning, organizing, leading, and controlling of cost-effectiveness in nursing management. In order for her to ensure the provision of a cost-effective service, she must examine motivation, job satisfaction, on-the-job training, management participation, optimum employment of human resources, and productivity.

According to Dunn and Bradstreet, poor management is responsible for more than 90% of business failures (Resnik 1988: 2). The nursing manager must be capable of running the nursing services according to business principles. This is the only way to achieve cost-effectiveness.

Resnik (1988: 2) states that effective management can be learned. He maintains that effective management is the factor that determines the continued existence and success of a business. It involves the ability to understand, to give guidance, and to control the business. Resnik's comments are applicable to nursing management. Nursing managers must have the ability to understand business principles, give nursing staff guidance in this respect, and exercise control over the financial aspects of the nursing service.

Effective management is a goal-oriented, directive activity (Resnik 1988: 3). Nursing managers can play a crucial role in goal-oriented and directive financial activities.

According to Resnik (1988: 5) an effective manager is an expert at overcoming restrictions and limitations. In the history of nursing in South Africa, professional nurses have always faced up to situations where restrictions were at issue. If a nursing manager possesses sufficient knowledge of financial and management aspects, she can contribute considerably towards overcoming the financial restrictions imposed on nursing care.

In the light of her knowledge of nursing practice, the nursing manager could make a considerable contribution towards cost-effectiveness.

In order to gain a better understanding of cost-effectiveness, two concepts, namely *cost-benefit analysis* and *cost-effectiveness analysis* should be examined.

In both of these two concepts three elements are important, namely:

- costs;

- benefits; and

- effectiveness.

Cost-benefit analysis

This technique is used frequently in the planning of health services in order to establish priorities. In this method the costs and the benefits of one health project are weighed against those of another. For example, the costs of immunizing all health workers against hepatitis can be weighed up against the benefits which the organization will reap if fewer of their health workers contract this disease, reducing the costs of the treatment of such cases and possible liabilities that may flow from claims against the health organization. Cost-benefit analysis thus provides an estimate of the inherent value of a programme through a consideration of whether the benefits exceed the costs, as well as a consideration of competing alternatives (Warner and Luce 1982: 49). *In a cost-benefit analysis, all the outcomes and advantages are assessed in monetary terms.*

Analysis of cost-effectiveness

In the case of a cost-effectiveness analysis, *the results of programmes can be measured in non-monetary units.* In a health service, cost-effectiveness can be measured in terms of general measures such as years of life that can be saved, or days of sickness, or disability that can be prevented (Warner and Luce 1982: 48).

The reason for measuring the effectiveness of a health service programme in non-monetary terms is that it is sometimes impossible or undesirable to evaluate important results in monetary units (Warner and Luce 1982: 48). Cost-effectiveness may be expressed in units such as rands saved per annum, or life-years saved, or life-years added. Cost-effectiveness analysis does, however, allow a comparison of costs per unit of effectiveness between competing alternatives designed to serve the same purpose (Warner and Luce 1982: 48).

Cost control

Nurse managers have a high degree of sensitivity to the need for cost-effectiveness and cost-control. They are usually inundated with requests, policies, and programmes designed to hold down the ever-escalating costs. As in business organizations, each health service organization will view cost-control measures somewhat differently in the sense that there will be shifts in emphasis regarding different strategies and priorities for cost-control. According to Blaney and Hobson (1988), there are, however, a number of approaches in health service management which will promote cost-effectiveness, for example:

- the effective management of time;

- improving the productivity of staff by establishing a regular physical fitness programme for staff members;

- monitoring and controlling the use of supplies in order to detect misuse immediately, and implementing stricter controlling measures where necessary;

- establishing and maintaining a sound performance appraisal system in order to promote the productivity of staff;

- promoting a positive attitude among all staff members regarding cost-control;

- improving the scheduling of prescribed tests on patients, in order for them to undergo tests without delay, which would in many cases lead to fewer patient days spent in hospital.

A cost-effectiveness strategy described by Turban (1980) consists of four stages (McBrien 1986: 21):

- cost-awareness;

- monitoring costs;

- managing costs; and

- incentives for cost-saving.

Each one of these stages of development could lead to considerable cost savings, but for long-term results it is important that all these stages should occur in the correct sequence.

McBrien (1986: 21) suggests that hospitals should:

- set up cost-effectiveness committees;

- initiate strategies for cost-effectiveness;

- monitor productivity;

- evaluate terms of reference, aims, and objectives by concentrating on cost-effectiveness;

- train all staff members in cost-awareness.

McBrien's (1986: 21) recommendations should be implemented by hospitals to promote cost-effectiveness. Various authors emphasize the importance of management expertise and management training. Resnik (1988: 3) maintains that management expertise consists of attitudes, perceptions, ideas, and knowledge that motivate and direct key management activities. The nursing manager, being the leader of the nursing corps, can apply management expertise to promote cost-effectiveness. Demanding information about cost-effectiveness from providers of health services helps promote efficiency in the provision of health services (Warner and Luce 1982: 54).

Those who finance health services — ie the taxpayers who bear the brunt of financing — clearly have an interest in ensuring that the care provided is cost-effective. Those who receive health care would also like to see value for money (Warner and Luce 1982: 185).

The potential for creating awareness of cost-effectiveness in medical and health care services is considerable. Such an awareness could contribute to the creation of an environment in which both attitudes and behaviour could change constructively (Warner and Luce 1985: 205). In this way, cost-effectiveness in hospitals could be promoted.

TERMINOLOGY IN FINANCIAL MANAGEMENT

For nursing managers to function efficiently and credibly in the business milieu they will have to acquire a basic knowledge of financial terminology. This knowledge of financial terminology will enable them to negotiate the financial interests of the institution/ organization in which they work on an equal footing with other managers. Knowledge, understanding, and use of financial terminology will give nursing managers the necessary confidence to state their views on financial matters in management meetings and other fields.

Strasen (1987: 85–117) has set out the basic terminology which she regards as important in financial management:

1. *Direct costs* are costs that are directly associated with providing patient care services. Examples are:
   - the costs of nursing staff salaries; and
   - the costs of medical supplies for patients.

2. *Indirect costs* are costs that are necessary, but are not directly associated with providing patient care services. Examples are:
   - the costs of the engineering department;
   - the costs of the medical records department; and
   - the costs of administration.

   These indirect costs relate to the support services that are required for the functioning of the health service as a whole.

3. *Fixed costs* are the costs of health services, not taking into account fluctuations in the numbers of patients using those services. These costs are incurred regardless of the number of patients using the service. Examples of fixed costs for a nursing unit include:
   - the salary of the professional nurse in charge;
   - the minimum staff provision requirements of a department;
   - the costs of the infection control nursing professional.

   Examples of fixed costs for the whole hospital include:
   - the expenditure of the medical records department;
   - the costs of the administration staff;
   - the costs of depreciation;
   - the costs of insurance;
   - the costs of financing capital projects.

4. *Variable costs* are a function of the volume of patients using the service. They are costs that are incurred over and above the fixed costs. Examples of variable costs in a nursing unit include:
   - medical supplies for specific patients;
   - the costs of linen;
   - the costs of food.

5. *Total costs* are the sum of the fixed and the variable costs.

6. *Unit costs,* or *costs per unit of service,* are the costs of producing a single product or unit of service. The unit of service for inpatients is the patient day.

There are two basic methods of calculating costs: *direct costing* and *full costing*. Direct costing is a method of calculating all costs directly incurred by a specific department. Full costing is a method of calculating costs which includes direct departmental costs, as well as the indirect costs allocated to the department. The strength of the full costing method is that it accounts for all the hospital's costs. The weakness of the full costing method is that some of the indirect costs allocated to a department may be irrelevant to the real income obtained by the patient care service provided by the department.

INTERPRETATION OF FINANCIAL STATEMENTS

Finances are based on accounting principles. To understand financial statements, knowledge of terminology is essential. Important concepts in the interpretation of financial statements include the following:

1. An *asset* is any tangible or intangible property owned by an institution or an individual. Examples are cash, equipment, and supplies.

2. *Liquidity* is the term used to give an indication of the time it takes to convert an asset into cash in order to purchase something else.

3. *Accounts receivable* refers to money that will be received by an institution at some stage in the future. In the case of a health service, accounts receivable are usually accounts for the services provided to patients on a continuous basis.

4. An *inventory* describes the actual supplies on hand which an institution owns and which will be used for providing health services in the future — eg drugs, food, linen.

5. A *liability* is a debt (short-term or long-term); ie it refers to the money that an institution owes to other businesses. Examples are: accounts payable, notes payable, bonds payable, and mortgages payable. *Accounts payable* are records of the short-term debt that

the organization owes. A credit card account is an example of an account payable. *Notes payable* are records of money an institution owes for a loan over a period of one to ten years. *Bonds payable* are records of loans for a period of more than ten years. *Mortgages payable* are records of money owed for the mortgage taken out on an institution's property. *Wages payable* refers to the cash owed to employees for services rendered to an institution. Wages payable are often recorded under the heading 'accrued liabilities'.

6. *Owner's share capital* is a term used in the private sector. It is the money that would be divided among shareholders should the firm be sold and should assets exceed liabilities. If a profitable hospital were to decide to close its operations, for example, it would pay off all its liabilities with its assets. The remaining assets, or owners' share capital, would be divided among the shareholders.

$$Assets = R\ 1\ 000\ 000$$
$$Liabilities = R\ \ \ 800\ 000$$
$$\overline{Owner's\ share\ capital = R\ \ \ 200\ 000}$$

After liabilities have been paid, the institution will have R200 000.00 worth of assets or owners' share capital. If there are 100 000 shares, this money is divided among the shareholders by paying them R2 for each share they own. A non-profit business has no shareholders.

ACCOUNTING RECORDS

The accounting records of a business or institution are kept in a general journal, in the general ledger, and in various other special journals/ledgers. A general journal is the book in which raw information is recorded, including the dates of transactions, the relevant accounts, and the size and the direction of changes in the accounts.

The *fundamental accounting equation* is the following:

$Assets = liabilities + owner's\ equity\ (owner's\ share\ capital)$

Because the equation has to be balanced at all times, any transaction has to maintain the balance. For this reason each transaction should have at least two entries. This is called the double-entry principle. The double-entry system of accounting was designed to always retain the balance of the ratio between assets and liabilities. Accounts receivable are always entered in the left column. Accounts payable are entered in the right column.

Figure 6.1: Example of a page from a general journal

Date	Account	Debits	Credits
1993-02-26	Creditor's ledger	R20 000	
	Cash		R20 000

A balance sheet

A balance sheet is a financial document that shows the financial position of an organization on a specific day — ie what it owes and what is owed to it.

A balance sheet is divided into two parts, either horizontally or vertically. Assets are shown on the left-hand side or towards the top of the sheet. Liabilities and owner's share capital (owner's equity) are shown on the right-hand side or at the bottom of the sheet. Both components of the balance sheet are always balanced, or the one is equal to the other. Terms used on the balance sheet include the following:

1. *Current assets.* These are defined as assets that can be converted into cash within one year after the date shown on the balance sheet.

2. *Fixed assets.* These are long-term assets, generally referring to property, buildings, and equipment. Fixed assets have value that can be converted into cash in the long term. Examples of fixed assets are land, buildings, equipment, and constructions. Constructions refer to the part of a construction project completed when an institution is undergoing building improvements.

3. *Depreciation.* This is a decrease in the value of fixed assets such as buildings and equipment, based on the fact that their value or usefulness or suitability will decrease over a period as a result of wear and tear.

4. *Liabilities* and nett worth. Specific current liabilities shown on a hospital's balance sheet are accounts payable, notes payable, and accrued liabilities.

5. *Long-term liabilities.* Long-term liabilities are debts of the institution due more than a year from the date shown on the balance sheet. Examples are: bonds payable, interest expenses, and bond costs.

6. *Nett worth* is assets minus liabilities. Nett worth is sometimes referred to as a balance of funds that appears on the balance sheet of a non-profit making institution. In the balance sheet of a profit-making institution it is referred to as the *proprietor's share*

capital or the shareholder's share capital. The proprietor's share capital or the shareholder's share capital (nett worth) is equal to the value of the institution after all debts and liabilities have been subtracted.

7. *Own capital* is sometimes referred to as the *balance of funds* (surplus) on a non-profit institution's balance sheet. On a profit-making institution's balance sheet it is referred to as *owner's share capital or shareholder's interest*. Owner's share capital/ shareholder's interest is the value of the institution after debts and liabilities have been deducted.

Figure 6.2: A balance sheet (adapted from Strasen 1987)

CURRENT ASSETS			CURRENT LIABILITIES	
cash receivable		R200 000	accounts payable	R1 000 000
accounts receivable			notes payable	50 000
patient revenues		2 200 000	accrued liabilities	100 000
			current portion of	
Less			long term	300 000
bad debts		200 000		
charitable allowances		50 000		
contractual allowances		200 000		
Inventory		100 000		
TOTAL CURRENT ASSETS		2 050 000	TOTAL CURRENT LIABILITIES	1 450 000
FIXED ASSETS				
land		4 200 000	LONG-TERM LIABILITIES	
buildings		20 000 000	bonds payable	4 000 000
equipment		5 500 000	mortgage payable	600 000
		29 700 000	nett worth	21 000 000
Less: depreciation		4 700 000		
NETT FIXED ASSETS		R25 000 000		
TOTAL ASSETS		R27 050 000	TOTAL LIABILITIES &	
			NETT WORTH	R27 050 000

An income statement

An income statement is a record of the money or income that an institution receives for services rendered and of the money the institution loses as a result of expenses.

Income can be divided into *operational income* and *non-operational income*. The former is income from the institutions normal business. Non-operational income is the income derived from sources other than the institution's main business. Interest derived from an institution's investments is an example of non-operational income.

Expenditure is also divided into *operational expenditure* and *non-operational expenditure*. Operational expenditure includes salaries, rent, equipment, and depreciation. Non-operational expenditure includes interest expenses and income tax for non-profit making institutions.

Income for profit-making institutions comes from services rendered to patients. Non-profit institutions derive income from public authorities. Factors that can decrease income include the writing-off of bad debts, and welfare allowances. Welfare or charitable allowances are the amount that the institution budgets for the provision of free or charitable care.

Figure 6.3: An income statement (adapted from Strasen 1987)

GROSS PATIENT REVENUE		OPERATING EXPENSES	
routine patient services	R20 000 000	salaries	R17 000 000
ancilliary services	30 000 000	employee benefits	2 000 000
total gross patient revenue	R50 000 000	medical supplies	4 000 000
		non medical supplies	5 000 000
DEDUCTIONS FROM REVENUE		maintenance	5 000 000
provision for bad debt	R5 000 000	depreciation	4 000 000
contractual allowances	3 000 000	total operating expenses	R37 000 000
charitable allowances	2 000 000		
total deductions	R10 000 000		
nett revenue from patients	R40 000 000	NETT INCOME FROM OPERATIONS	R3 000 000

THE BUDGETING PROCESS

An understanding of the budgeting process can have a positive influence on nursing managers' financial control performance as well as on the performance of their nursing staff.

The budget and cost-effectiveness

Planning is an important component in drawing up a budget. Finkler (1984: 3) states that a budget is a written plan, stated in financial terms. This plan represents the management's expectations. Budgeting is the process during which plans are made, after which an effort is made to achieve or exceed the stated objectives.

Finkler (1984: 3) is of the opinion that a budget without a formal controlling mechanism to ensure that the actual results are as close as possible to the requirements of the plan loses most of its value for management, and that a budget can be used to motivate and evaluate the performance of managers and departments. The different elements of an organization can be co-ordinated through the budget. A budget also serves as a means of conveying the objectives and expectations of an organization (Finkler 1984: 17).

Finkler's (1984: 3) statements about budgets could be borne in mind by nursing managers in their efforts to contribute towards cost-effectiveness. If nursing professionals in control of units were to handle unit budgets in the same way as managers handle department budgets it would be easier to motivate nursing staff and to evaluate their approach towards the functioning of the budget. If a hospital strives for cost-effectiveness, the budget could serve as a means for conveying these expectations.

Nackel, Kis, and Fenaroli (1987: 231) concur with these opinions and state that once the aims and objectives of the hospital have been documented within the strategic plan, these aims and objectives become the basis for the organization's annual budget. The authors also state that a budget converts the strategic plan into a defined set of departmental activities, expectations, income levels, expenditure targets, and eventually into financial statements that can be forecast.

Stevens (1985: 297) indicates that, once a budget is approved and implemented, it becomes a controlling system. Scott and Rochester (1987: 153) maintain that a budget should be used to give a better understanding of the funds for which the management is responsible.

According to McClure (1989: 3), nursing managers are currently responsible for the largest staff component and for more than half of the operational budget in most health service institutions. McClure's statement emphasizes the importance of the role that nursing managers have to play in contributing towards a cost-effective budget. DiVincenti (1986: 113) regards the budget as a guide for the financial year for which it is prepared; it specifies a framework in which the nursing department can function, evaluate results, and modify organizational tasks. The author maintains that the main purpose of a budget, however, is to prevent expenses from exceeding what is reasonably required for the organization to function. A budget is a method of controlling the progress made by keeping costs and expenses within the limits of the organization's financial plans and allowances. A review of a nursing unit's financial statements allows nursing managers an opportunity to control expenses involved in the nursing service as a whole, as well as those involved in individual units.

Herkimer (1986: 144) defines an effective budget as a systematic documentation of one or more carefully-developed plans for all individual supervisory activities, programmes, or sections. Herkimer maintains that a budget is an instrument that can help decision-makers in the evaluation of operational performance and in the projection of what future actions may bring forth.

In order to be an effective planning instrument, a budget should contain sufficient, reasonable, achievable, and reliable information inputs, on which suitable decisions can be based. Herkimer emphasizes that a budgeting procedure by itself is not a management tool — it only becomes one if it is put into practice during performance. All information contained in a budget should be objective, consistent, reliable, and realistic.

The functions of a budget

A budgeting system which reflects the objectives of the organization can do several things (Lambrechts 1990: 162–3).

1. It can be a term of reference for subordinates and an authorization to act. It helps subordinates know what is expected of them. If the budget is used correctly it motivates subordinates to contribute towards achieving the overall objectives of the organization.

2. A budget is a means for communicating with those subordinates who are responsible for realizing the objectives of the budget. When subordinates understand precisely what is expected of them, the organization can put its planning into action more easily.

3. A budget is a co-ordinating instrument. It helps to make the various activities function together. It also helps integrate the ideas of various management levels.

4. A budget estimates those external influences that are beyond the control of management. The calculation of a short-term budget almost always leads to a refinement of plans. A budget makes management aware of the fact that circumstances may change and that steps might need to be taken to adjust to the changing situation. The future is thus projected and the direction of action is determined.

5. A budget performs an indispensable task as a controlling measure. It serves as a norm against which actual performance can be measured. When differences between budgeted results and actual results are analysed, crucial areas for improvement, as well as unexpected opportunities that can be exploited, are usually indicated. Such an analysis could also indicate whether a budget was unrealistic.

6. Budgets contribute towards the task of educating managers regarding their responsibilities towards their own departments and other departments in the organization. Newly-appointed managers, in particular, find this very valuable.

Conditions for successful budgeting

According to Lambrechts (1990: 160–1) conditions for a successful budget include:

1. A sound organization. An advantage of an integrated budgeting system is that it strengthens the organizational framework. The

responsibilities of each department should be clearly defined. It would be impossible to determine who is responsible for the application and control of the budget if these two conditions were not met. There should always be someone in overall control of the budget. The name of this person should be made known in writing.

2. A satisfactory accounting system. Planning is based chiefly on information and data concerning past events. The accounting system should be of such a nature that all the required data can be obtained. It should be possible to draw conclusions, based on information from the past, which show the exact relationship between costs and results, as well as the effectiveness of, for example, departments, products, and individuals. Important trends in current financial ratios should be observable. In a nutshell, the financial information system should be able to present information in such a way that it can help the management to draw up a budget.

3. Analysis of achievements. Management must be informed not only of what has been achieved, but also of what was not achieved. This approach is based on the fact that there is always something more to be achieved, as well as different methods or better ways to achieve objectives.

4. The support of management. The success of a budgeting programme depends on the enthusiasm and support of top and middle management in an organization.

5. Responsible staff, at every level of management, should participate in the development of the budget. The staff involved should understand the ideals of the service and the financial objectives of the hospital.

6. An effective system should exist to provide reliable financial and statistical information to the person responsible for the budget.

7. The budget should allow sufficient freedom to achieve departmental objectives.

8. The budget should be sufficiently flexible to make provision for unforeseen circumstances.

Advantages of a budget

- It enables a complete and detailed programme of activities to be planned.

- The analysis required for drawing up a detailed budget helps to explain and promote the task of supervision and administration.

- The co-operation and support of all the departmental heads can be obtained in achieving mutual objectives.

- The orderly handling of financial matters can be assured.

- The budget has a balancing effect on the organization as a whole.

- Monthly trends can be defined and exploited.

- Drawing up a budget encourages an exchange of information; ideas are conveyed and expressed, so that staff stimulate each other. The budgeting process promotes teamwork.

- The budgeting process gives the hospital administration an opportunity to evaluate the thoughts of the heads of departments. Is the budgeting plan realistic? Are standards too high or too low? The budget can help to evaluate quality and initiative in performance.

- Once budgeting standards have been set, they can be compared with actual expenditures (DiVincenti 1986: 114).

ORGANIZING AN EFFECTIVE BUDGETING SYSTEM

In the absence of an effective organizational framework it would be extremely difficult to draw up and control a budget. A budget cannot be controlled solely by accounting activities; it is a management tool that affects all levels of an organization. Co-operation from all the participating parties is essential. Lambrechts (1990: 164–6) suggests that the following steps could inspire trust in an organization's budgeting system:

1. The establishing of a budgeting department and an effective accounting system.

2. Training in budgeting techniques. All the staff members involved in the budget should be trained in budgeting techniques. When these staff members know what is supposed to be achieved through the budget, and how it fits into the overall objectives of the organization, this will inspire confidence in the employees — it will give them a feeling of active participation, and it will make them feel that they are capable of handling the budgeting programme.

3. Drawing up an organogram. Successful implementation of a budgeting programme can only be achieved if each member of the management team knows precisely what her responsibilities entail. Each member's position relative to other members of the management team should be known. An organogram is the best way of setting out these relationships.

4. The establishment of a budgeting committee. The smaller an organization, the easier it is to combine and co-ordinate the activities associated with a budgeting system. In larger organizations it is customary to establish a budgeting committee consisting of heads of departments. The general manager of an organization draws up guidelines for carrying out procedures, but he usually delegates the responsibility for executing these procedures to those who are responsible for the various budgets. The financial manager of the organization is usually the secretary for this budgeting committee.

5. Drawing up a budgeting manual. A budgeting manual contains instructions concerning the responsibilities of staff members, procedures, forms, and other relevant information about the presentation and use of a budget. Such information may include:

- the objectives, principles, and benefits of a budget;

- classification and division of the budgeting system;

- an organizational matrix in which budgeting responsibilities are set out;

- the composition and duties of the budgeting committee and an explanation of the interdependent relationships between the various budgets;

- a description of available information sources;

- time schedules setting out the course the budget is to follow, as well as due dates;

- accounting guidelines to be followed;

- cost calculation practices to be followed;

- guidelines on problem areas and control points;

- methods setting out budgeting control;

- budgeting periods. There are no fixed budgeting periods which are universally applicable. Periods will depend on the type of organization and its internal requirements. The most effective practice is to have a range of budgeting periods for a large enterprise. The sales budget may, for example, be organized according to a five-year plan, and the production and cost budgets may, for example, be on a one-year basis. The annual budget may also be divided into three-month or monthly periods, and in certain cases the cash budget may be divided into days.

6. Priorities must be set for each budget in the budgeting system.

Attitudes towards budgeting and cost-effectiveness

A budgeting system in any organization can only be successful if the underlying budgeting philosophy is right. This philosophy is based on a positive attitude towards planning and controlling the budgets. When attitudes are right, the staff responsible for carrying out the requirements of the budget accept that a budget suggests definite boundaries and limitations which must be taken into account in the best interests of the organization. When no objectives, or very 'light' objectives are set out, the staff soon realize this and find it unacceptable. Unrealistic objectives, on the other hand, lead to all kinds of loopholes and malpractice.

Over-budgeting expenditure leaves room for manoeuvring, which means that it requires little or no effort by the staff to achieve the objectives of the budget. This could lead to dissatisfaction or criticism from the public sector.

Attitudes towards a budget are influenced by characteristics of human behaviour. Lambrechts (1990: 163) describes this as follows:

- Authority begins with the top structure of an organization. The line of authority always runs from top to bottom.

- Relationships between higher and lower levels of an organization are only meaningful when described in terms of responsibilities.

- The setting of objectives leads to an improvement in human performance.

- Management participation improves performance in an organization.

- When there is a deviation from standards that have been set, staff react immediately.

- An effective manager manages by means of the principles of exception — ie only exceptional problems, which cannot be handled by routine work and control measures, are brought to the attention of the manager.

- People react to control systems if their own interests are at stake.

Stumbling blocks on the way to a successful budget

Lambrechts (1990: 163–4) states that certain stumbling blocks may occur on the way to a successful budgeting process:

- A conflict of interests. For example, a nursing manager may wish to keep supplies as low as possible, while the nursing professionals may wish to keep supplies as high as possible.

- Demands made on nursing staff may be too high. There is a mistaken belief that unrealistic demands encourage staff. When nursing staff participate at all levels in establishing objectives, they make high demands on themselves and are more motivated to achieve the objectives they have established themselves.

- The control functions of budgets are overemphasized. This could result in staff being disheartened and it may deter them from giving adequate feedback since they perceive the control elements as a method of spying on them. Much time is wasted thinking up excuses. This wasted time could be used much more effectively in planning better future performance.

- Too many control mechanisms allow no room for discretion or judgement. Sometimes budgets are taken so seriously that large amounts of money are left over at the end of the budget cycle. Sometimes ill-considered purchases are made in order to 'use up' the amount budgeted for because it is feared that a smaller amount will be allocated to the relevant department or section in the next budgeting period.

The stages of the budgeting process

The preparation of a budget is done through a series of steps or stages.

Stage 1: planning

During this stage the operational goals and policies for the entire organization are reviewed. In order to have operational goals, the organization's long-term (three-to-five-year) goals must be reviewed, taking into account the community's future health care needs. A careful review of how the current budget performed, in terms of objectives set and achieved, must also be made.

Management must then decide on the approach which will be used for the next fiscal period's budget preparation — eg an incremental approach, where incremental adjustments are made to the current year's budget, or a zero-based approach, where the cost of each activity to be performed and budgeted for must be analysed as if it is a new activity in the organization. A timetable must be prepared that stipulates the due dates for submission of each department's budget, the individuals responsible for preparing and submitting proposals as well as guidelines that must be followed in the preparation of the budgetary proposals.

Stage 2: preparation

During this stage, each unit or department prepares its budget by translating the objectives set in the planning stage into projected costs and revenues. Calculations regarding projected personnel numbers and their salaries are made, as well as projected average length of stay for patients, total number of outpatient visits, and expected changes in the level of demand for particular services or products (Dieneman 1990: 285).

Stage 3: modification and approval

The requests of each unit or department are compared with the revenue which could be reasonably expected to be earned during the next financial year. This usually results in the elimination of the lowest priority items until the budget is balanced. Then the operating, payroll, capital, and cash budgets are incorporated into the master budget. The final budget is then communicated to all departments (Tappen 1989: 179).

Stage 4: monitoring

Monthly summaries of expenses and incomes are usually distributed to each unit or departmental manager by the accounting department. Variances of more than 5% must be carefully checked. Sometimes the variance is the result of a new purchase, for example a new incubator, but when averaged over the year, the expenses for the unit should equal the budgeted amount. Sometimes, if expenses for additional staff members and/or supplies exceed the amount that has been budgeted for them on a regular basis, the situation will need to be brought under control, or otherwise the budget will have to be adjusted, depending on the situation (Tappen 1989: 182).

The monthly variances are depicted on a monthly variance report. This report usually depicts the budgeted amount, the actual amount spent during the month, and the variance between the two amounts, expressed as a percentage. The variance percentage is calculated as follows:

$$\frac{actual\ expenditure}{budgeted\ expenditure} \times \frac{100}{1} = \%\ variance$$

When the variance is less than 100% it means that less was spent than was budgeted for, and when the variance is more than 100% it means that more was spent than was budgeted for.

Another important aspect of monitoring is the in-depth analysis which could be made regarding different factors in nursing services — for example, one could analyse the cost of using disposable versus reusable supplies, using different mixes of personnel categories, or the costs of home visits versus clinic visits in a community service.

Budgetary control

Apart from the controlling functions which are inherent in the planning, modification, and approval stages (where budgetary proposals are often pruned) and in the monitoring stage (where administrative control is exercised by monitoring the monthly variances), final control is carried out by auditing. The auditor examines the expenditure on each activity/purchase in relation to the amount budgeted for it. The auditor's report usually states the amounts spent on particular items in the service — eg provisions and salaries — but it does not indicate how much is spent in terms of a particular unit of service, such as cost per patient per day.

The measure of control used to assess such service unit costs are termed cost-accounting.

A cost-accounting system matches all revenues to costs. This uses time periods, but it is not always complete. While monthly reports of revenues and costs are provided to managers, there are many indirect costs which are only incurred once a year — eg costs for doing accounting, data processing, and administration. These costs are usually hidden in the operational budget in the form of room costs. These costs are accumulated and averaged as unit costs within a cost centre. Costs are thus expressed in units — eg cost per patient per day in a particular cost centre or department. When there is a rise in the unit costs, eg in cost per patient day from R30.00 to R33.00, the factors responsible for the rise must be examined closely and accounted for.

Cost containment

Cost containment is geared at keeping costs within acceptable limits. It involves a number of strategies, described by Mariner-Tomey (1992: 82–3).

Cost awareness

By orientating and educating each manager and nursing staff member on how the budget is drawn up and how it is controlled, an awareness of the need to keep costs within limits can be developed.

Cost monitoring

By monitoring such costs as turnover, absenteeism, sick time, and inventories, the staff and managers become aware of where, when, and why expenses are incurred.

Cost avoidance

This means not buying certain supplies, technology, or services. For example, disposable items are not bought because reusable items are utilized, or a new monitor is not bought because the older, less-sophisticated one is still working properly. It also means that the least expensive supplies, equipment, and technology are identified and utilized.

Cost reduction

This means that less is spent for goods and services. Significant reduction in costs can often be brought about by reducing waste of supplies and by reducing absenteeism costs.

Cost control

Costs can be controlled by using resources effectively, careful forecasting, planning, budget preparation, and monitoring.

Other cost-cutting actions

According to Swansburg et al. (1988: 211) cost-cutting actions by nurse managers which have proved worthwhile include the following:

- giving more autonomy to unit managers;
- increasing unit managers' management training;
- reducing overtime work;
- utilization of flexible staffing patterns;
- utilization of centralized staffing;
- expanding the use of computers;
- expanding the monthly distribution of financial information to all units.

Types of budget

A well organized institution's master budget usually consists of an operating budget, a cash budget, a capital budget, a manpower budget, and a programme budget.

The operating budget

The operating budget is defined by Finkler (1984: 6) as 'the plan for day-in and day-out operating expenses for a period of one year.' This budget deals with the routine operating costs of each department in the organization.

Data describing the revenue and expenses of a cost centre (the unit of operation, ie ward or department) are contained in activity reports. The activity report describes the workload of a given unit or cost centre. The report gives an account of the total number of times a particular service was charged to patients within a given period of time — eg number of patients occupying beds at midnight, number of clinic visits, and number of laboratory procedures (Finkler 1984: 65).

The preparation of the operating budget sometimes includes the personnel budget for the cost centre if the organization does not have a separate manpower budget for personnel requirements.

The ongoing budgetary requirements for equipment and supplies are usually the main components of an operating budget.

When planning the operating budget, the cost centre's activities during the last fiscal period must be reviewed and projected increases, decreases, or alterations must be calculated. Costs which must, among others, be taken into account during budgeting include (Stevens 1980: 242–3):

- ongoing supply costs;
- inflation;
- anticipated price increases;
- travel expenses;
- educational expenses;
- administrative overheads such as heat, light, housekeeping, general administration, supplies, equipment servicing costs, repairs, and renovation costs.

The cash budget

A cash budget is an important issue in an organization's budgeting process. A cash budget ensures that an organization has an adequate cash flow to meet its obligations and to take advantage of important opportunities which may arise. These obligations include the payment of accounts and the pay roll.

The format of the cash budget is fairly standard. At the beginning of each month there is an initial cash balance. The expected cash receipts for the month are then added to this balance. These expected cash receipts may come from inpatient and outpatient payments, from medical aid payments, from donations, and from sales such as cafeteria sales if the cafeteria is owned by the health service.

The payments which it is expected will have to be made during the month — eg salaries, payments to suppliers of provisions, and loan repayments — are then determined and subtracted from the initial cash balance. The result is called a *tentative cash balance*.

This tentative cash balance may be more or less than the minimum cash balance. The minimum cash balance is the amount that an organization considers to be necessary to have at the end of each month after all cash payments are made. This is a safety measure, because unexpected expenditure should be provided for.

If the tentative or projected balance exceeds the minimum desired balance, the excess can be invested, but if the tentative cash balance is less than the minimum desired balance, the organization will have to borrow some money to meet its expected expenses (Finkler 1984: 180).

Some months there may be a surplus, and other months there may be a cash shortfall. Managers should plan their cash flow carefully so that surpluses are invested skillfully to cover shortfalls, thus preventing the need to resort to emergency measures.

The cash budget may be drawn up on a monthly, weekly, or daily basis. Cash is not a direct nursing responsibility, but nursing managers must be capable of providing the finance department with sufficient information about when expenses are to be paid or when additional cash may be required.

The capital budget

According to Finkler (1984: 60) a capital budget refers to budgeting expenses for resources (capital assets) with a lifespan of more than one year.

Sullivan and Decker (1992: 416) believe that a capital budget is established to finance the purchase of large equipment or architectural alterations. Lambrechts (1990: 174) refers to a capital budget as:

> . . . those planning actions dealing with the acquisition and utilization in the longer term of funds for purchasing new machines and equipment, the introduction of new product lines, the upgrading of existing installations or parts thereof, or any other investing opportunity that offers the required return.

Each organization, however, has its own description of what will qualify as a capital expense. Commonly the criteria set for what constitutes a capital expense are that the item must cost more than a certain amount and that the expected lifespan of the item must be longer than a set time limit — often not less than three to five years.

Sullivan and Decker (1992) state that when a purchase is considered in line with a capital budget, certain questions should be answered:

- How will it affect the volume of work or workload?
- How will it affect patient days/revenue?
- How will it affect the supplies budget?
- Will additional space be required?
- Will other departments be affected?

Capital budget items should be requisitioned on forms especially designed for this purpose. Motivations for each item should be well prepared. Included in the capital requisition are installation, delivery, and the estimates for expenses which will be incurred for the servicing of the item/piece of equipment.

The purchase and accounting departments can help nursing managers by providing information about items — for example, the lifespan of the items.

It is also necessary to take cognizance of other aspects associated with the purchase of an item. Aspects to be considered include whether the organization has staff who are capable of using the item, or whether training will be necessary. Any additional requirements for operating the item should be determined, recorded, and included in the operating budget.

Rapidly changing technology may make it difficult to compose a capital budget. If good co-operation exists between the medical staff and the nursing staff, and if they keep abreast of internal changes and external trends, nursing managers will be in a position to contribute to an effective capital budget.

The manpower budget

The manpower budget for nursing personnel can account for as much as 90% of the total nursing service budget. Included in this personnel budget are salaries for the nursing staff, as well as the compensation for sick leave, overtime payments, merit increases, orientation, and education time — eg in-service education, and college education time. When calculating the manpower budget per unit, the following steps are usually followed:

1. The bed capacity — eg the number of beds in the unit (ward or clinic) — is defined.

2. The average bed-occupancy rate is determined. The lower the bed-occupancy rate, the greater is the possibility of daily variation in the rate. If the rate is in the lower range — eg 65% or lower — it is necessary to determine patterns of patient distribution because this will significantly affect the staffing patterns and personnel budget. If, for example, the pattern of patient distribution shows a high census during weekdays and a low census over weekends, staffing will be affected in the sense that a fairly large number of personnel will be needed over weekdays, but these numbers cannot all be given their off-duty days during weekends because there are still a number of patients to be cared for. It follows that more personnel will be required than when the distribution of patients would be more equally divided over the seven days of the week.

3. The acuity levels of the patients must be established. A classification system is necessary where the nursing care needs are expressed in nursing care hours to be provided per unit per week and per month (see *patient classification systems* in chapter 14).

4. Other variable factors affecting staffing needs in a health service must also be considered. These are technological advancements, changes in medical practice, statutory staffing norms, and future projects.

   - Technological changes, such as the addition of more monitoring equipment in an intensive care unit, may increase the need for nursing staff, whereas the addition of equipment which eases the handling of heavy patients, such as patient-lifting devices, may decrease staffing needs.

   - Statutory staffing norms must be taken into account. They often provide a baseline which the manager can adjust according to existing needs.

   - New plans for the future, eg new projects planned, or the planned opening of new or added facilities and health care services must be taken into account when staffing needs are budgeted for.

5. Staffing patterns — eg the distribution of the required nursing care hours over all the shifts — and the staffing mix must now be determined. Factors affecting staffing patterns and staff mixes are the patient care modalities used in a service and the policy regarding distribution of staff over day and night shifts — eg 60% of staff to be allocated for day-service and 30% of staff for night duty.

6. Benefits and differentials. Benefits usually budgeted for in the calculation of the personnel budget are leave pay, sick leave, pension contributions, and indirect labour costs such as travel expenses or transport services provided. If night staff are paid more per shift than day staff, the extra amounts must be determined, as well as the extra allowances paid for work in intensive care units, rural clinics, and other high-stress units — eg cancer wards.

Programme budgeting

According to Finkler (1984: 8) programme budgets are special budgets for specific programmes. Such a programme may be an existing one or it may be a new programme — for example the addition of open-heart surgery facilities.

Programme budgeting examines feasible alternatives for any given programme — for example maintaining the use of outside laboratory services or opening up a fully-equipped laboratory for the institution. Programme budgets often include the labour and equipment of the various departments.

Programme budgeting differs from other kinds of budgeting in the sense that programme budgets are long-term in nature. The revenue and expenses of a programme or programmes, and how they will effect the entire organization over a period of years, must be determined. Programme or long-range budgets thus examine the organization in general terms over a number of years. Capital, operating, and cash budgets examine all programmes in detail, but only for the following year. Programme budgets combine a large volume of detailed information and long-term planning, but only for specific programmes. While most budgets concentrate on departmental income and costs, programme budgets compare income and costs for the total programme.

Programme budgeting methods focus on the identification of costs and benefits of different programmes or of different approaches to one programme. Programme budgeting often focuses on trade-offs. Thus the qualitative benefits of one programme might have to be relinquished in order to achieve the qualitative results of another programme.

Programme budgeting techniques are normally used to examine suggestions for new programmes but they may be used to review an existing programme where, for example, technological changes and demographic shifts may have changed the patient profile.

Sometimes the cost of undertaking a certain programme, or providing a certain service, increases gradually over time. During programme budgeting a careful review of the programme will elicit whether the increased costs are justifiable. Sometimes a total review of all the components of the programme is called for in order to remove unnecessary, unproductive costs.

It is wise to use the programme budgeting approach — ie looking at the costs of all components of a service well beyond the initial year — when a department's discretionary costs are high. Discretionary costs refer to those costs where the 'consumption of resources cannot be directly tied to the varying levels of output measures, such as patient days' (Finkler 1984: 26).

The main advantage of programme budgeting lies in its multi-period orientation. One is forced to look at all the costs of initiating a programme well beyond the initial year. This forces one to pay attention to the hidden future costs which may offset the initial savings.

Zero-based budgeting

Zero-based budgeting is a budgeting approach which analyses the alternative ways of offering any one programme or service within an institution. The analyses which have to be performed in order to justify the inclusion, institution, or maintenance of a programme include the following (Finkler 1984: 28–9):

- statement of the purpose of the programme and the consequences of not performing it;

- the ways that the costs and benefits of the programme may be measured;

- alternative ways of providing the same service;

- alternative outcomes which will be achieved with the various approaches.

The rationale of zero-based budgeting is that the objectives to be achieved, methods of achieving them, and the revenue and expenses of each programme must be reviewed regularly. Such reviewing is necessary because the traditional way of budgeting allows managers to add to the previous year's budget in order to allow for inflation without analysing whether the service or programmes budgeted for are still necessary or whether they can be rendered in an alternative way which might yield the same results but with lower costs. In zero-based budgeting, managers are required to justify all costs of the different programmes/services they intend performing during the coming year, as though they were instituted for the first time. No cost is simply allowed continuing into the future without being examined (Sullivan and Decker 1992: 414).

In large organizations, zero-based budgeting is very valuable because this kind of budgeting enables top management to quickly identify key areas in the organization. The advantage is that resources can be adjusted rapidly, according to priorities. Another advantage is that nursing managers are forced to consider a wide range of alternatives between different programmes or within any individual programme.

The analysis of alternative, and often more economical, ways of rendering a service, or of maintaining or instituting a programme, provides a greater measure of sophistication regarding budgetary justifications.

The greatest disadvantage of zero-based budgeting is that the preparation of zero-based budgets is a rather time-consuming activity.

THE FINANCIAL STRUCTURE

The financial structure of a health organization is based on cost centres. A cost centre is a functional unit that generates costs within an organization. A cost centre may generate income (for example a laboratory and pharmacy) or it might not generate income (for example household services and the administrative department of a health organization). A department may be a single cost centre. Nursing departments, however, include multiple cost centres. Examples are individual patient care units, operation wards, recovery rooms, emergency rooms, outpatient clinics, and nursing administration. Nursing services are usually included in the costs of the accommodation of, procedures for, and treatment of patients.

All nursing units are usually seen as cost centres. It is increasingly expected of nursing professionals in charge of units to deal with the budgets of their departments. The nursing manager is responsible for co-ordinating these budgets in order to be able to submit a nursing department budget to the organization.

CONCLUSION

Ever-increasing demands are being made on nursing managers to utilize the funds available to health services cost-effectively. This requires additional skills in nursing management, which include a knowledge of business principles. Nursing managers should understand the budgeting process. Drawing up an effective nursing services budget is essential, and knowledge of the different kinds of budgeting is essential in order to promote cost-effectiveness in nursing management.

References

Bennett, A. C. (1980). *Managing Hospital Costs Effectively as a System*. American Hospital Association: Chicago.

Blaney, D. R. and Hobson, C. J. (1988). *Cost-Effective Nursing Practice: Guidelines for Nurse Managers*. Lippincott: Philadelphia.

Booyens, S. (1991). The future nursing service manager. *Nursing RSA*, volume 6, number 8, pp. 39-41.

Cronje, G. J. de J., Neuland, E. W., Hugo, W. M. J. and Van Reenew, N. H. (1989). *Inleiding tot die Bestuurswese*. Second edition. Southern: Johannesburg.

De Klerk, F. W. (1991a). Openingstoespraak deur die Staatspresident by die Suid-Afrikaanse Verpleegstersvereniging Eeufeeskonferensie 'Excellence in clinical nursing', 19 September, Bloemfontein.

De Klerk, F. W. (1991b). Toespraak deur die Staatspresident by Groote Schuur hospitaal, 26 September, Kaapstad.

Dienemann, J. A. (1990). *Nursing Administration: Strategic Perspectives and Applications*. Appleton and Lange: Norwalk.

DiVincenti, M. (1986). *Administering Nursing Service*. Little Brown: Boston.

Douglass, L. M. (1988). *The Effective Nurse Leader/Manager*. Third edition. Mosby: St Louis.

Faul, M. A., Pistorius, C. W. and Van Vuuren, L.M. (1988). *Rekeningkunde — 'n Inleiding*. Third edition. Butterworths: Durban.

Financial Management Series (1971). *Budgeting Procedures for Hospitals*. American Hospital Association: Chicago.

Finkler, S. A. (1984). *Budgeting Concepts for Nurse Managers*. Orlando: Grune Stratton.

Gillies, D. A. (1989). *Nursing management — A Systems Approach*. First edition. Saunders: Philadelphia.

Haley, R. W. (1986). *Managing Hospital Infection Control for Cost-Effectiveness*. USA: American Hospital Association.

Herkimer, A. G. (1986). *Understanding Hospital Financial Management*. Second edition. Aspen: Rockville.

Hobson, C. J. and Blaney, D. R. (1987). Techniques that cut costs, not care. *American Journal of Nursing*, February 1987, pp. 185–7.

Hobson, C. J. and Blaney, D. R. (1988). *Cost-Effective Nursing Practice: Guidelines for Nurse Managers*. Lippincott: Philadelphia.

Hoffman, F. M. (1984). *Financial Management for Nurse Managers*. Appleton-Century-Croft: Norwalk.

Hoffman, F. M. (1986). The capital budget: developing a capital expenditure proposal. *American Association of Operating Room Nurses Journal*, volume 44, number 4, pp. 604–10.

Johnson, R. and Varroll, P. E. (1987). Hospitals must start budgeting like a business. *Health Care Financial Management*, volume 41, number 2, p. 18.

Kish, L. (1965). *Survey Sampling*. John Wiley: New York.

Koch, S. 1992. *Die Bydrae van die Verpleegdiensbestuurder tot Koste-effektiewiteit in Geselekteerde Hospitale in die Republiek van Suid-Afrika*. Ongepubliseerde D.Litt et Phil. proefskrif. Pretoria: Universiteit van Suid-Afrika.

Lambrechts, I. J. (ed.) (1990). *Finansiële Bestuur*. Van Schaik: Pretoria.

Lock, M. V. L. H. (1989). *The Role of the Nurse Administrator in Rural Hospitals in the Republic of South Africa*. Unpublished D.Litt. et Phil. thesis, University of South Africa, Pretoria.

Mark, B. A. and Smith, H. L. (1987). *Essentials of Finance in Nursing*. Aspen: Rockville.

Mariner-Tomey, A. (1992). *Guide to Nursing Management.* Fourth edition. Mosby: St Louis.

McBrien, M. (1986). Cost containment. Who's job is it? *Nursing Success Today,* volume 3, number 4, 20–1.

McClure, M. L. (1989). The nurse executive role: a leadership opportunity. *Nursing Administration Quarterly,* volume 13, number 3, pp. 1–8.

Minnaar, A. (1990). Wat vra die toekoms van verpleegadministrateurs in privaathospitale? *Nursing RSA,* volume 5, number 10, 40–1.

Nackel, J. G., Kis, G. M. J. and Fenaroli P. J. (1987). *Cost Management for Hospitals.* Aspen: Rockville.

Nel, C. (1986). Realistiese beplanning binne 'n verpleegdiens. *Nursing RSA,* volume 1, number 4, pp. 33–4.

Olenick, A. J. (1989). *Managing to have Profits.* McGraw-Hill: New York.

Porter-O'Grady, T. (1987). *Nursing Finance Budgeting Strategies for a New Age.* Aspen: Rockville.

Resnik, P. (1988). *The Small Business Bible — the Make-or-Break Factors for Survival and Success.* John Wiley: New York.

Scott, J. and Rochester, A. (1987). *Effective Management Skills. Managing Money.* Cox and Wyman: Reading.

Searle, C. (1966). *Die Geskiedenis van Ontwikkeling van Verpleging in Suid-Afrika 1652-1960.* Suid-Afrikaanse Verpleegstersvereniging: Pretoria.

Shaw, S. (1989). Nurses in management: new challenges, new opportunities. *International Nursing Review,* volume 36, number 6, pp. 179–84.

Sonberg, V. and Vestal, K. W. (1983). Nursing as a business. *Nursing Clinics of North America,* volume 18, number 3, pp. 491–9.

Spitzer, R. B. and Davivier, M. (1987). Nursing in the 1990s: expanding opportunities. *Nursing Administration Quarterly,* volume 11, number 2, pp. 55–61.

Steenkamp, W. F. J. (ed.) (1986). *Ekonomiewoordeboek.* Butterworths: Durban.

Stevens, B. J. (1980). *The Nurse as Executive.* Second edition. Nursing Resources: Wakefield, Massachussetts.

Stevens, B. J. (1985). *The Nurse as Executive.* Third edition. Nursing Resources: Wakefield, Massachussetts.

Strasen, L. (1987). *Key Business Skills for Nurse Managers.* Lippincott: Philadelphia.

Sullivan, E. J. and Decker, P. J. (1992). *Effective Management in Nursing.* Third edition. Addison-Wesley: New York.

Swansburg, R. C., Swansburg, P. W., and Swansburg, R. J. (1988). *A Nurse Manager's Guide to Financial Management*. Aspen: Rockville.

Tappen, R. M. (1989). *Nursing Leadership and Management*. F. A. Davis: Philadelphia.

Warner, K. E. and Luce, B. R. (1982). *Cost-Benefit and Cost-Effectiveness Analysis in Health Care – Principles, Practice and Potential*. Health Administration: Michigan.

PART TWO:

ORGANIZING

CHAPTER 7

ORGANIZATIONAL STRUCTURE, CULTURE, AND CLIMATE

S. W. Booyens

CONTENTS

INTRODUCTION

When the planning function has been completed, it is necessary to organize resources and manpower to accomplish the goals which were set during the planning phase. The nurse manager must thus ensure that the organization of her nursing service is such that the philosophy and mission of the institution — ie to provide quality patient care cost-effectively — can be realized. This will, among other things, require the correct utilization of the abilities and skills of personnel, the effective co-ordination of support services, and the skilful utilization of resources.

DEFINITION OF ORGANIZATION

Organization may be defined as follows:

Organization is the grouping of activities for the purpose of achieving objectives or goals, the assignment of such groupings to a manager with authority for supervising each group, and the defined means of co-ordinating appropriate activities with other units, horizontally and vertically, which are responsible for accomplishing organizational objectives. (Swansburg 1990: 264)

PRINCIPLES OF ORGANIZATION

There are several important principles which need to be taken into account. These include the chain of command, the principle of unity of command, the span of control, the principle of requisite authority, the principle of continuing responsibility, the organizational centrality principle, and the principle of management by exceptions.

Chain of command or scalar chain

The chain of command is the chain of reporting ranging from the ultimate authority at the top to the worker with the least authority at the bottom. In practice, communication usually flows in a downward direction. It is wrong not to follow the line of authority without a good reason, but it is an even greater error to follow it when, in doing so, you are not supporting the organization's objectives. In modern nursing organizations the chain of command is flat with more professionals working on a collegial basis than before.

Unity of command

Unity of command means that an employee should receive orders from one superior only. This principle is not always followed in nursing services, especially when a nurse in a unit may receive orders from the professional nurse in charge as well as from doctors and/or other professionals — for example the physiotherapist.

Span of control

This principle states that a person should only be in charge of a group which he or she can effectively supervise in terms of numbers, functions, and geography. Implementation of the principle, however, needs to be flexible because the more highly trained an individual is, the less supervision she needs, while employees in training need more then the usual amount of supervision in order to prevent serious mistakes (Swansburg 1990: 264).

The choice of span of control for the nursing division in an organization is important because it determines the number of managers within the division, and this directly influences the total cost for salaries of nursing personnel. Narrow spans of control result in tall organizational structures with many supervisory levels between the nurse executive and the first line nurse manager. Wide spans of control, on the other hand, result in flat organizational structures with fewer levels of management (Shehnaz and Funke-Furber 1988: 34).

Requisite authority

This principle states that when an employee is assigned the responsibility of executing a certain task, the authority which the employee may need in order to obtain and use the resources necessary for the accomplishment of the task must also be granted to her.

Continuing responsibility

This principle means that the supervisor who delegated the responsibility for the execution of a task to a specific employee or number of employees is not absolved from taking the final responsibility for the successful completion of the task.

Organizational centrality

This principle refers to the fact that the more people an employee interacts with directly, the more information she receives and the more powerful she becomes in the total organizational structure (Gillies 1989: 146).

Management by exceptions

This principle is followed in some organizations. The employees are expected only to report exceptions or departures from the normal routine functioning to higher authority. Managerial efforts are thus only channelled to the management of unusual or exceptional cases which cannot be controlled by the routine organizational mechanisms.

ORGANIZATIONAL STRUCTURE IN HEALTH CARE INSTITUTIONS

There are several different ways of structuring health care institutions. These include the bureaucratic structure, the collegial structure, the open systems structure, the adhocracy, and the administrative adhocracy.

The bureaucratic structure

The word 'bureaucracy' is often used pejoratively to indicate an institution where excessive enforcement of rules leads to inefficiency. However, some degree of bureaucracy is found in the formal operation of virtually every organization. Even informal working groups often take on some of the characteristics of this organizational structure because bureaucracy is designed to promote smooth operations within a large and complex group of people.

Max Weber, the father of the bureaucratic organizational structure, outlined the following four basic characteristics of this structure:

- Division of labour: specific parts of the job which must be done (eg the provision of quality patient care) are assigned to different individuals or groups. For example, nurses, dietitians, laboratory workers, doctors, all provide a part of the care which the patient needs.

- Hierarchy: employees are organized and ranked according to their degree of authority within the organization. For example, the superintendent and the chief nurse manager are at the top of most hospital hierarchies, while nursing aids and cleaning personnel are at the bottom.

- Rules and regulations: acceptable and unacceptable behaviour, and the correct way to perform predictable tasks, are usually specifically set out in writing. For example, procedure and policy manuals prescribe many types of behaviour from the correct method of performing aseptic procedures to policies for the transfer of patients, to guidelines which must be followed when an employee must be disciplined.

- Emphasis on technical competence: people with certain skills and knowledge are employed to carry out specific parts of the total service of the organization. For example, in a comprehensive health care centre in the community, there are, among others, professional nurses who do deliveries, a pharmacist who dispenses medicines, doctors who examine and treat patients, a social worker who organizes grants and community support, and clerical staff who do the typing and filing.

In the traditional bureaucracy, the emphasis is on vertical relationships or the vertical chain of command. In this chain of command, the superintendent or chief nurse manager delegates authority to the middle managers, and the middle managers delegate to the unit charge nurses, and so on (see figure 7.1). Employees in the technical and support staff compartments have relatively limited power and authority compared with those in the centre who have line authority (Tappen 1989: 195–7).

The bureaucratic organization consists of sets of positions arranged in a hierarchical order. Each occupant of a position has formal duties with a high degree of specialization, and there is a formally established system of rules and regulations that governs her decisions and actions. Individuals are employed on the basis of professional or other qualifications rather than political, family, or other connections. In this idealized type of organization, bureaucratic officers hold their positions because of their expertise; they apply the rules and regulations in an impersonal manner, without favouritism; they make rational decisions, and they achieve administrative efficiency (Sullivan and Decker 1992: 42).

Varying degrees of bureaucracy are found in different organizations. A highly controlled and bureaucratized approach is based on the belief that employees must be told what to do, that they must be closely supervised to ensure that they will do it, and that some employees are more skilled and responsible than others and should therefore have authority over the others. Organizations where these beliefs reign would have many detailed rules and regulations, close supervision of employees, little autonomy delegated to individual employees in general or even to professional employees, although this last mentioned group of people is perfectly capable of functioning independently.

Disadvantages of the bureaucratic approach

1. The long lines of delegated authority and decision-making which are often found in bureaucratic organizations make it impossible for an employee or outsider to identify exactly who is responsible for having made a certain decision or who created a certain unpopular rule. No one person in the organization takes full responsibility for the results of decisions and nobody seems to know where the rules and decisions originated from. A 'rule by nobody' thus prevails, and in some of these organizations

Figure 7.1: Chain of command

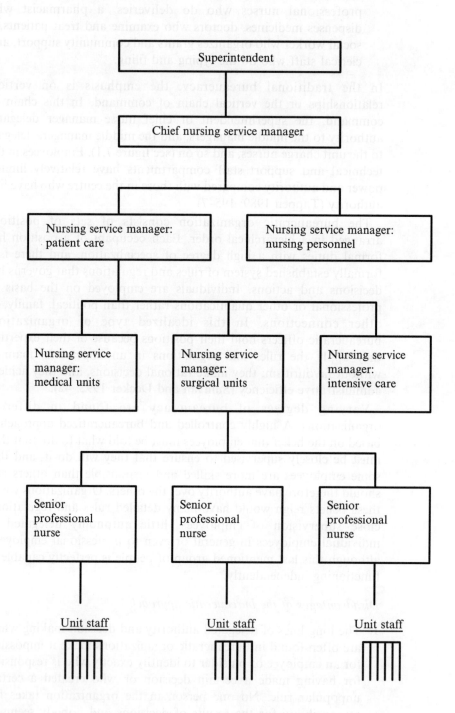

employees believe that they are controlled by impersonal rules and regulations. Having no influence on decisions within an organization creates a feeling of powerlessness and alienation among the employees.

2. One of the greatest frustrations experienced by both employees and clients of bureaucratic organizations is the diffusion of responsibility and the subsequent refusal to make a decision. For example, to get something done in some organizations, you need the approval of six different people on six different forms, and each of the six people refuses to give approval until the other five have given theirs. This is known as 'bureaucratic red tape' (Tappen 1989: 197).

3. The typical bureaucratic structure which contains rules, divisions of labour, hierarchies, specialists, line and staff positions, and records, contributes to stability. This stability, however, leads to paralysis because the structure's response to changes in the environment is sometimes non-existent, and when there is a response it is too slow. The structure is too inflexible to effect meaningful and necessary changes quickly and efficiently.

4. The extreme division of labour also makes it impossible to identify who is really responsible for the successful or unsuccessful results of care. The result is that people do not derive the necessary satisfaction from, or pride in, their work because it is too difficult to determine their specific contribution to the end result. When an employee does not get the necessary recognition for his or her contribution to successful patient care outcome, self-actualization is also not readily achieved and it is difficult to sustain motivation to deliver a high quality of work.

5. In a bureaucratic structure it is the top management which makes the important decisions. In the current climate, with its rapidly-changing health care technology and complex organizations, it has become impossible for the management team to maintain the level of knowledge required for sound decision-making. The employees who are most knowledgeable in the different areas of speciality are the specialized lower-level workers who are carrying out their functions on a daily basis. These specialists should use their expert knowledge to make the necessary decisions for their field of speciality. In most bureaucracies, though, this is not done (Fuszard 1983: 14).

The collegial structure

A collegial structure or 'professional model' of organization, which is sometimes found in hospitals, is more sensitive to the changing environment than the bureaucratic structure, yet it retains enough components of the bureaucratic model to provide organizational stability.

The unique characteristic of the collegial model is the group of professional specialists who function completely independently of the bureaucratic structure and who are responsible for decisions affecting patients. The housekeeping and other support personnel are arranged hierarchically as in the typical bureaucracy and are directed and controlled by the administrative staff.

The decisions regarding patient care are made by the specialists. These specialists are the physicians working in the hospital. Change in patient care decisions can be effected relatively easily for it affects only the work of the specialists, not the structure of the administrative hierarchy (Fuszard 1983: 15).

In this model, the hospital administrator's main functions are to maintain the facilities of the institution and to ensure that the decisions of the professional specialists — the doctors — are implemented. The specialist group of professionals would make decisions regarding their own patients, but also decisions regarding the purchase of equipment, the use of ancillary departments, and the determination of policies affecting various departments of the institution.

The nurses and other health care professionals are categorized as 'support' personnel. Their role is merely to carry out the physicians' decisions. The model thus seems to make an erroneous assumption that physicians (not the top administrators) possess all the knowledge needed for decision-making in the health care institution (Fuszard 1983: 15).

The open systems structure

While bureaucracies are seen as closed systems, the open system concept is usually seen as one that readily interacts with the environment on a continuous basis. When the open system interacts with the environment, it trades materials or energies with the surroundings. The inputs for such a system are likely to be raw materials, human labour, and work-related information which is transformed during throughput into output in the form of products and services. An open system is goal-directed, its components are dynamically related, and its boundaries are open to influence from the environment (Gillies 1989: 83). An open system has the flexibility to meet the constantly changing health care needs of society.

A large organization, however, cannot fully adapt to the rapid changes in its environment. It requires some form of stable structure together with flexibility. The open system structure creates too much uncertainty and complexity, and too little predictability, to be effective for large organizations.

Adhocracy

The term 'adhocracy', originated by Alvin Toffler, refers to the use of ad hoc committees or ad hoc project teams. These teams, or committees, or task forces, are used to carry out special assignments.

A project team is a group of diverse specialists who have been called together to unite on a temporary basis to carry out a non-routine task of a complex nature which is of critical importance to the organization. The members of the project team come from different parts of the organization, they work together until the assignment is completed or until a specific problem given to them has been solved, and they stay together as a group to implement their ideas. Once this has all been achieved, the team is dissolved.

Most project team members come from several different hierarchical levels. Team members are usually relative strangers to each other, coming from different professional backgrounds. The group works against a strict deadline, with the result that little group cohesiveness develops, but a great need is nonetheless felt for free- · flowing communication and interaction between team members. There is a tendency to develop temporary, intense relationships and to ignore differences in status between group members in order to achieve the goal of the project. The project leader gives commands and provides direction to the team members but there is no clear structure binding the team together. Each specialist works independently for part of the time and serves as a consultant to the other members when the need arises (Gillies 1989: 159).

The nurse manager who wishes to incorporate adhocracy as a structure in the nursing division must take the following guidelines into consideration:

1. *Group decision-making.* In an adhocracy, decisions are made by the team or group of persons who are most appropriate because of their expertise. If the people who are responsible for the planning, implementation, evaluation, and follow-up care of an individual patient are regarded as a project team, the nurse manager must place the full responsibility for decision-making regarding a specific patient's care on the members of the patient care team. All the members of the patient care team — ie the doctor, the professional nurse(s), the physiotherapist, and the dietitian — must be regarded as equal contributors to decision-making.

   The nurse manager must allow the membership of patient care teams to be fluid. For example, when a patient needs the care of a clinical nurse specialist, the clinical nurse specialist must be included in addition to the existing members of the project team.

2. *Use of experts.* In an adhocracy it is the experts in the field who make up project teams and who are responsible for decision-

making. This would imply that the patient care team would include registered nurses, physicians, dietitians, and physiotherapists. An all-registered nursing staff should thus be needed if ad hoc project teams are to be formed for individual patient care assignments.

3. *Communication and co-ordination.* In an adhocracy every team member shares responsibility for communication and co-ordination. When the work of an ad hoc project team is accomplished, the team dissolves. Because of the constantly changing membership of committees and project teams, each team member becomes aware of the functioning of the entire institution. In this way each member can become a link-pin of communication and co-ordination in the organization.

4. *Fluid organizational structure.* A feature of an adhocracy is its fluid organizational structure. It is not possible to represent this type of structure on a diagram like the organizational chart of the bureaucratic structure. Rapid and continual change eliminates the predetermined positions common to the typical administrative organizational chart.

5. *Decentralization.* A final component of adhocracy is decentralization of the organization. Three different types of managers exist in the operating adhocracy: they are functional, integrating, and project managers. Managers do not supervise — they liaise, negotiate, and co-ordinate the work laterally among the different project teams and between the project and the concerned functional units. The system needs a large number of managers because of the small size and the large number of the project teams. The project managers are the most numerous of the three types of managers.

Managers responsible for integration or liaison promote co-ordination among different project teams, represent their own teams in meetings of various project teams, and keep the project teams aware of each other's activities.

Functional managers maintain communication and co-ordination with the functional units (nursing, physical therapy, purchasing, etc.), representing the project team in meetings of a single functional unit or in a group of such units (Fuszard 1983: 17).

Advantages of adhocracy

1. The increased participation in decision-making by each employee reduces the feelings of powerlessness and alienation which can arise in bureaucracies. Increased motivation to render a high quality of service should thus take root among employees.

2. The members of a project team are given much more authority than in a bureaucratic structure. A project team is responsible for much of its own self-correction and self-control.

3. The structure provides for many opportunities to pool needed talents and skills, and thus establishes a climate that fosters innovation and creativity.

4. An advantage of ad hoc groups is the greatly increased flexibility to respond to the changing needs of the organization.

5. The professional nurses, as team members in different project teams, have a chance to seize some of the free-flowing power which exists in the modern adhocracy.

Disadvantages of adhocracy

1. The frequent use of ad hoc project teams tends to decrease the formal chain of command. Many teams find themselves reporting to two or more managers. Two or more managers may also complete evaluation forms and make recommendations for salary adjustments and promotions. The chain of command becomes confusing which can result in conflicts over territory, power struggles, and duplication of effort (Tappen 1989: 198).

2. Those highly-skilled specialists who are appointed to one project team after another move back and forth so frequently between different project assignments that they have no time to develop close relationships with co-workers or a strong commitment to any single working group in the organization (Gillies 1989: 159).

3. The uncontrolled autonomy of project teams weakens the strong superior–subordinate link that stabilizes the line organization (Gillies 1989: 159).

4. The rapid movement of personnel from one role to another throughout an adhocracy upsets existing power relationships. The development of these imbalances in the power structure makes it possible for employees in key positions to seize additional power (Gillies 1989: 159).

5. There is a disruption of the departments or areas from which people are taken to form a team.

6. The creation of temporary task forces or project teams may threaten some employees' feelings of security.

7. The large number of managers, the small size of project teams, and the large number of specialists, make the adhocracy system appear to be an expensive one (Fuszard 1983: 17).

8. It can be expected that the top administrators and physicians in an organization will resist any attempt to reduce their authority for making decisions, as would occur in an adhocracy (Fuszard 1983: 18).

9. A high degree of sophistication in conflict management is required in such a system.

Administrative adhocracy

According to Fuszard (1983) there are a number of health care administrators who have been attracted to the concept of administrative adhocracy. They see it as a way to increase creativity in their organizations, to effect changes, and, at the same time, maintain their bureaucratic administrative authority and accountability. In this structure, the administrative/managerial staff divide themselves into different project teams to investigate and plan for institutional innovations and to take charge of the implementation of the developed changes. Physicians have also sometimes been involved in these project teams (Fuszard 1983: 19).

ORGANIZATIONAL CULTURE

Organizational culture is different from ethnic or national culture in that it focuses only on organizational life. Culture is the combination of the symbols, language, and behaviours that are openly manifested in the values and norms of an organization. It is a pattern of basic assumptions or behaviours that have worked in the past and are taught to new members as the correct way to perceive, to think, to feel, and to act (Del Bueno 1986: 15).

Objective aspects of culture exist outside the minds of the members of an organization and include such artifacts as pictures of leaders, monuments, stories, ceremonies, and rituals. Subjective aspects are related assumptions and mind-sets such as shared beliefs, values, meanings, and a shared understanding of how things will be done (Marriner-Tomey 1992: 144). The cultural values and norms of the organization are reflected in policies and practices related to dress, personal appearance, social behaviour, the physical environment, communication, and status symbols (Del Bueno 1986: 16).

The cultural network is the primary informal means of communication within the organization and it carries the corporate values and heroic mythology. The manager should use this network to understand what is going on beneath the surface and to get things done (Deal and Kennedy 1982, referred to by Marriner-Tomey 1992: 144).

The leaders in an organization help shape the culture by their demonstration of what the organization's philosophy entails, by their projection of a vision for the future, by setting policies, professing values, creating systems, and supporting organizational reward systems (Marriner-Tomey 1992: 144).

Culture and the manager

The first thing that one encounters in an organization's culture is its visible artifacts — how members behave, and how things look and feel. Initially it is difficult to decipher why individuals behave in the way they do or what their behaviour really means. The real culture is not easily revealed. To be accepted, and to manage successfully, it is important to discover the assumptions and values that lie beneath the surface. The new manager needs to discriminate between what people say they value and what is, in fact, valued (Del Bueno 1986: 18).

To be a successful manager it is important to recognize the cultural indicators and to make a conscious decision to commit or not commit oneself to norms and values of the culture. The nurse manager must also consider the following facts regarding an organization's culture:

1. Managers and personnel who survive in a culture are those who have learned to support the values and norms of that culture.

2. There is potential for conflict if the cultural norms of the organization differ markedly from the personal values and norms of employees.

3. To change an organizational culture is very difficult. It often involves revolution and severe conflict and may only be achieved by installing a new leader.

4. When the manager is considering a change in the organizational culture, sacred cows and taboos are discovered.

5. A strong culture that encourages participation and the involvement of employees in decision-making affects an organization's output positively.

6. The chief executive officer of an organization has a prominent influence on the culture of an organization (Swansburg 1990: 269).

The nurse manager who wants to find out what is really going on in the organization's cultural set-up may examine the following indicators of culture (Del Bueno 1986: 17):

1. Image. How does the organization wish to be perceived? Which words, slogans, or phrases are used to describe the organization — eg friendly, caring, safe? Is money being spent on creating this image?

2. How do people dress: formally or informally? Is there a code for dressing? May people let themselves go at parties? Is sexist behaviour tolerated?

3. Status symbols and reward systems. Are there any acknowledged status symbols, such as private dining rooms? Which are the committees, events, or projects which are only shared by elite members? Do titles mean anything?

4. Rites, rituals, ceremonies. What are the established rituals and how do you learn about them? Is orientation planned and is it the same for every newcomer? Does the organization recognize length of service, outstanding performance, marriage, or other important personal events in the lives of its employees?

5. Sacred cows. These are persons, things, places, or beliefs which cannot be discussed, attacked, or ignored. Are there heroes, dead or alive, who must be honoured? Are there myths which must be perpetuated? What rules and policies may not be changed or challenged even when they are illogical? What subjects are taboo?

6. Environment. Are there places for employees to relax? Where are they, and what do they look like? May employees decorate their areas of work with plants, pictures, etc? Are there conference rooms? Who may use them? Who eats with whom, and where?

7. Communication. How does one conduct important communication in this organization — by writing a memo or letter, or by seeing a person face-to-face? How many documents are marked 'confidential' or 'restricted information'? Where does important communication take place — in meetings, at the golf course, or in the chief executive's office?

8. Meetings. What meetings can be missed without reprisal? Is discussion at meetings allowed, encouraged or limited, or does it depend on the type of meeting? Is smoking permitted?

The manager may also assess the culture in her organization by measuring it with an instrument solely designed for this purpose — the organizational cultural inventory. This inventory is designed to assess quantitatively the ways in which members of an organization are expected to think and behave in relation to their tasks and to other people. Participants answer a set of 120 questions which describe the behaviours or personal styles which might be expected of members in their organization. The questions produce twelve scales corresponding to the following cultural styles:

1. Constructive styles. These styles emphasize members' higher order needs for achievement and affiliation.

- Achievement culture. Members are expected to set challenging yet realistic goals and to pursue them with enthusiasm.

- Self-actualizing culture. Creativity and individual growth are valued by encouraging members to develop themselves, to gain enjoyment from their work, and to take on new and interesting activities.

- Humanistic–encouraging culture. The organization is managed in a participative and person-centred way. Members are expected to be supportive and constructive in their dealings with one another.

- Affiliative culture. Constructive interpersonal relationships are emphasized. Members should be open and sensitive to each other's needs (Thomas et al. 1990: 20).

2. Passive/defensive styles. The security needs of members are promoted — eg the lower-order needs for acceptance and for the avoidance of failure.

- Approval culture. Conflicts are avoided and members feel that they should agree with, gain the approval of, and be liked by others.

- Conventional culture. Conservative, traditional, and bureaucratic controls are in place. Members should conform, follow rules, and make a good impression.

- Dependent culture. The non-participative, hierarchically-controlled organization values centralized decision-making and members only doing what they are told to do.

- Avoidance culture. In these organizations success is not rewarded but mistakes are punished. This leads to the shifting of responsibilities among members to avoid the possibility of being blamed for a mistake (Thomas et al. 1990: 20).

3. Aggressive/defensive styles. The security needs of members are promoted — eg their need for power. This requires them to approach tasks forcefully to protect their status and position.

- Oppositional culture. Confrontation prevails and negativism is rewarded because members gain status by being critical and in this way they are encouraged to oppose the ideas of others.

- Power culture. The authority inherent in the position of individual members is valued. This leads to members believing that they will be rewarded for taking charge, controlling others, and being responsive to demands from their superiors.

- Competitive culture. Winning is valued, and members want to outperform each other with the result that they work against each other in order to be noticed.

- Perfectionist culture. In these organizations, persistence and hard work are valued. Members feel that any mistakes must be avoided, that they must keep track of everything, and that they must work long hours to attain narrowly defined objectives (Thomas et al. 1990: 20).

Philosophy, mission, and vision

Studies have shown that organizations with a strong vision and a strong sense of values and beliefs outperform those that do not.

Written philosophies of nursing have existed in many health care organizations for a number of years. They often include philosophical beliefs about man, the environment, health, and nursing. It is not clear to what extent these philosophies have contributed to the development of a common belief system within the nursing service (Barker 1990: 88).

Most health care organizations also have mission statements which describe, in broad terms, the reason for the organization's existence. They usually describe the patient population and the services provided, and they are orientated to the present rather than the future (Barker 1990: 88).

A similar, but somewhat different, approach for organizations is to write a vision statement. This statement describes what the organization is working towards and where energies should be focused. The vision statement generally includes information about patients, nursing staff, management systems, and the relationship of the department to the organization, community, and society. According to Britton and Stallings as referred to by Barker, a vision statement should include, at a minimum, the following elements:

- Statements of excellence or success. These statements may include financial objectives, such as cost-effective care, but the statements must address the quality of patient care.

- A transcending purpose focusing on the long term, not the short term.

- Statements about tapping the talents and enthusiasm of all the levels of employees.

- Statements which reflect the organization's attitude towards fairness and humanity.

- Statements which show the value placed on creativity and innovation.

- Words which reflects the organization's acceptance of an informal structure.

- Statements about the organizational structure (Barker 1990: 89).

Policies and procedures

Policies and procedures are means for accomplishing organizational goals and objectives. Policies explain the steps to be followed in achieving goals: they serve as the basis for future decisions and actions, help co-ordinate plans, control performance, and increase consistency of action by increasing the probability that different managers will make similar decisions when faced by similar situations. Policies also serve as a means by which authority can be delegated (Marriner-Tomey 1992: 144–5).

Policies should be comprehensive in scope, stable, and flexible so that they can be applied to different conditions which are not so diverse that they require a different set of policies. Policies should be consistent to reduce feelings of uncertainty and unfairness. They should be written and should be understandable.

Policies may be implied or expressed. Implied policies are not directly voiced or written but are established by patterns of decisions. Sometimes policies are implied simply because no one has ever bothered to express them. At other times they may be deliberately implied because they reflect questionable ethics (Marriner-Tomey 1992: 145).

Written policies must be reviewed and revised periodically. They originate at the top level of management, or sometimes come from the first line managers. At times policies are generated at the functional level when there are insufficient guidelines regarding a particular service aspect from top management, eg rules to be followed regarding the admission of visitors to an intensive care unit.

The expected areas which should at least be addressed in policy formulation in health care institutions are patient care modalities, physicians' orders, administration of medications, safety precautions for patients, charting, and infection control. Labour policies are often directed by contracts with labour unions or by collective bargaining principles (Marriner-Tomey 1992: 140).

It is advisable to have the policy statements reviewed and approved by superiors and by the managers who will be affected by them before the policy is finally written down. New policies should be introduced and explained to personnel members as soon as they have been formulated because policies are useless when they are not known by all.

Policies should be written following a specific, concise, and complete format, and should be stored in a policy manual which is easily accessible by all personnel to whom the policies apply. The manual should be organized by classifying policies into different categories, or by indexing them by topic, and by summarizing them in a table of contents (Marriner-Tomey 1992: 150).

Procedures provide a specific guide for actions. They help achieve regularity by setting out the steps which must be followed in a chronological sequence.

Procedure manuals can serve as a basis for orientation and staff development, and are a ready reference source for all personnel. They standardize procedures and equipment with the result that they can provide a basis for evaluation. Good procedures will save time and effort.

Productivity is increased by improving work procedures. It is therefore imperative to simplify each part of a procedure so that productivity is enhanced maximally. The first step in work simplification is to identify the procedures which are problematic. These identified procedures are then carefully analysed. It is often useful to make use of specific charts which shows the different components of the work and their flow in order for the procedure to be executed. It is, however, necessary to ask a number of relevant questions in order to really get down to the 'nitty gritty' of the selected procedures. These questions are:

- What is the purpose of the work?
- Is it necessary to do it?
- Can it be eliminated?
- Who does the work?
- Can someone else do it better?
- Can it be delegated to someone with less skill?
- Is there a duplication of effort?
- Can two or more activities be combined?
- Will changing the chronological order improve the outcome?

When these questions have been answered satisfactorily, the work should be simplified by rearranging, combining, or eliminating components. The improved methods must then be made known to all the personnel members for implementation (Marriner-Tomey 1992: 153).

The procedure manual should also be easily accessible and well organized (with a table of contents), and indexed. It is recommended to have this manual in a ring file so that old procedures may be revised and replaced with the updated versions. It stands to reason that the procedure manual, like the policy manual, should be reviewed and revised periodically. Changes to procedures should be dated. Before writing out procedures one must consider whether they are not already written out in textbooks for bedside nursing, or whether they are contained in the literature which accompanies the many disposable products on the market. It seems important that the procedure manual should contain information which may vary from institution to institution — in other words information which is only specific to one's own organization.

ORGANIZATIONAL CLIMATE

The organizational climate serves as a measure of individual perceptions or feelings about an organization. The working climate is often described in general terms such as 'formal', 'relaxed', 'defensive', 'cautious', 'accepting', or 'trusting'. It is the employee's subjective impression or perception of her organization.

The work climate is determined to a large extent by the management and leadership style adopted in an organization. The practising nurse in an organization contributes to a large extent to the creation of the climate as perceived by the patients. The work climate set by the nurse manager determines the behaviour of the nurses.

When the climate is being assessed, the following aspects are usually measured:

- the understanding which exists among employees regarding the organization's goals;

- the effectiveness of its decision-making processes;

- integration, co-operation and vitality;

- the effectiveness of its leaders;

- openness and trust;

- job satisfaction;

- opportunities for growth and development;

- level of job performance;

- orientation;

- effectiveness of teamwork and problem-solving;

- the overall confidence in management which exists among the employees.

According to Sullivan and Decker (1992) the organizational climate centres around whether the beliefs and expectations of employees are being met. They give the example where in one institution the nurse manager adopted an autocratic leadership style and in another one the nurse manager displayed a more democratic leadership style. The employees in both institutions were satisfied with their leaders' behaviour simply because the expectations of the employees in the two institutions were different.

Nurses like to work in a climate where they can achieve satisfaction from their jobs. They derive satisfaction from their jobs when the jobs are perceived as challenging, when patients and managers recognize their achievements, when they can participate in decision-making on a collegial basis with other health professionals. The nurse manager should thus make the jobs of nurses challenging by seeing to it that nurses are not working at piecemeal sections of a job but that they complete a whole piece of work. They will then be able to see the result of their specific inputs.

In an ideal climate the nurse should have to use a variety of skills and talents to achieve the patient health improvement set out as her goal. The nurse should also be provided with sufficient autonomy for her task and receive adequate feedback on the satisfactory completion of a task (Swansburg 1990: 273).

The use of disciplinary measures in nursing management influences the climate as well. Discipline must be applied fairly and in a uniform manner. It is thus necessary to have a disciplinary code in an institution, and this should be followed. A uniform grievance procedure should also be in place, as well as an open door policy that really works.

The rights of employees should be protected. It is the nurse manager's responsibility to stay informed of the salaries, fringe benefits, and personnel policies of other health care institutions, and to act to promote her own staff's rights if they are not in line with those of the other institutions.

The climate can further be enhanced by creating suitable career ladders for clinical nurses, by actively seeking the input of clinical nurses in patient care and unit-management decisions, by reducing boredom and frustration, by instituting positive programmes of job enrichment and personal health promotion, and by giving awards for special achievements and seniority (Conway-Rutkowski 1984: 16).

Nurse managers who fail are not different from other managers. They fail when they go about their daily work as usual, make no special effort to learn the culture, ignore organizational problems, treat all their responsibilities with equal interest and effort, take on too many conflicting priorities, promise without keeping their promises, try to take over the jobs of line managers, do not respond adequately to higher concerns of the organization (eg strategic planning), represent only the interests which they themselves are enthusiastic about, do not evaluate or anticipate the influence of their actions on other people and projects, have poor timing, do not criticize themselves, and are insensitive to the needs of the clients.

Activities to promote a positive organizational climate

These include the following (Swansburg 1990: 274; Conway-Rutkowski 1984: 15–16):

1. Develop the organization's vision, mission statements, goals, and objectives by making full use of the input from practising nurses.

2. Avoid managing by surprises. When you are contemplating the introduction of major changes which will affect everyone, ensure that employees are informed in understandable terms of precisely what can be expected.

3. Tune in to the your employees' needs for recognition and for improvement in self-esteem.

4. Keep morale high by establishing trust and openness through communication, including prompt and frequent feedback.

5. Provide opportunities for growth and development by establishing career development programmes and continuing education programmes.

6. Apply a disciplinary code which is fair and consistent.

7. Provide your employees with clear statements of what is expected in terms of appropriate behaviour and adequate job performance.

8. See that employees who do unsatisfactory work or continually drag others down with a chronic negative attitude are disciplined.

9. Analyse the compensation system for the entire nursing organization and try to get it structured so that productivity, longevity, and competence are rewarded.

10. Provide an open-door policy and employee complaint system that really works.

11. Provide an environment where communication is promoted upwards, downwards, and laterally. This can only be achieved by encouraging the free expression of ideas, criticism, and opinions. Employees should be able to speak their minds without fear of reprisal, threats, or confrontation.

12. Encourage and support loyalty, friendliness, and civic consciousness.

13. Provide opportunities for employees to give input in managerial decisions and in the formulation of policies. See that they are informed about the ideas which you implemented in decisions and policies.

14. Provide a workable career ladder.

15. Evaluate yourself by rating yourself on the following:

    • Creative and equitable staffing patterns.

    • Incentives for the staffing of difficult periods such as holidays, weekends, night shifts.

    • Specific policies for seniority and promotion.

    • Provisions for continuing education.

    • Provisions for accessible child care services.

    • Establishment of guidelines for staffing policies and patterns, especially where use is being made of 'float' nurses.

TEAM BUILDING

The employees in an organization commonly relate their feelings about the organization using words such as 'this organization really cares about its employees' or 'this organization does not care about its employees'. The first statement reveals a high morale or *esprit de corps* among employees and the second one a low morale.

When morale among employees is high, they tend to work enthusiastically, courageously, confidently, productively, and in a disciplined manner. When morale is low, employees are timid, rebellious, and unruly, and display an indifferent attitude towards their job with the result that their productivity is low (Swansburg 1990: 275).

To promote motivation among her nurses, and to create high morale, the nurse manager should find out what the values are which the personnel would regard as 'caring for the worker' and she should try to match these values in her management. Some of these values are as follows:

1. Some nurses want to work fewer hours per day or per week; some want to work longer shifts. The nurse manager should try to accommodate as many of these requests as possible. She should be flexible about shifts and working hours and try out as many schedules as possible while still staying within the organization's policies.

2. Child care services are often needed not just when employees are on duty but also at other times.

3. People want to be involved in decision-making. The nurse manager must thus try to involve her staff in decision-making at unit level, departmental level, and at the organizational level.

4. People want inside knowledge about the organization. The manager should thus ensure that information is flowing from the top on a continuous basis and in language which is easily understood (Swansburg 1990: 275).

Apart from satisfying the wishes of personnel using the methods discussed above, the nurse manager can enhance motivation or good morale by building teams in her service which are effective in problem-solving.

To be able to be an effective team-builder the nurse manager should, however, be a good collaborator who is effective in the establishment of networks and relationships. She should display the following qualities (Jacobsen-Webb 1985: 17):

- self-esteem (by recognizing the contribution she has to make and by identifying the value of the contributions of others);

- co-operation;

- trustworthiness (by interacting with others in a warm and open manner);

- open relationships (by identifying with the values of other people);

- an ability for independent decision-making when appropriate.

The nurse manager who wishes to build teams throughout her nursing service would do well to structure her teams so that they are made up of individuals who possess contrasting styles of thinking. There are four distinctive behavioural types into which individuals can be divided. These types are the self-reliant individual, the loyal one, the factual one, and the enthusiast. Here is a short description of each type (Jacobson-Webb 1985: 18):

1. *Self-reliant*. These individuals appear cool and distant, tend to be precise about their timing, and are willing to take interpersonal risks. They prefer telling others what to do. They combine competitiveness with self-control and are task orientated.

2. *Enthusiast*. These individuals, who are verbal and fast-acting, show their feelings and concerns. They are extroverts, take risks, and easily become interested in several things, only to lose their interest quickly. They prefer to tell others how they are feeling.

They combine competitiveness with self-expression and are people-orientated.

3. *Loyal*. These people are more concerned with feelings than facts and are flexible about the use of time. They are orientated to people rather than tasks, and prefer low-risk, non-threatening situations. They prefer to ask others how they are feeling, combine self-expression with co-operation, and appear warm and close in their relationships.

4. *Factual*. These people are co-operative and non-verbal, and dislike taking risks. They seem cool and distant because they try to remain precise about the use of time, preferring to work with facts and figures. They like to study the facts before making a decision. They combine co-operation and self-control in their interpersonal relationships and tend to ask others what they are doing.

The purposeful utilization of this profile brings out the best in the individual and it provides the talent needed to deal with a variety of problems. The leadership in the group may also be shifted from one individual to the next as the problem-solving task evolves. When completing a task or solving a problem, the team is well served by the self-reliant individual who sets the timetable to meet the goals and who concludes the discussions, by the enthusiast who initiates new and creative ways of thinking about the problem, by the loyal individual who does her best to reduce conflicts and to make encounters as pleasant as possible, and the factual individual who supplies the necessary data so that final decisions can be reached after a thorough review of all the relevant information (Jacobson-Webb 1985: 18).

ORGANIZATIONAL STRUCTURES: CONCEPTS

We now discuss formal and informal structures, the organizational chart, hierarchical and matrix structures, and tall and flat structures.

Formal and informal structures

The formal structure consists of the officially-agreed graphic table of the organization which shows how each position in the department is related to every other and how the entire nursing department is related to other parts of the institution. On the formal level, communication flows along established lines (the proper channels of communication). The formal level of operation would also include the way in which the employees are divided into groups, the work which each group does, and who acts as the supervisor of each group.

The informal structure includes all the unwritten, unofficial relationships which are found in an organization but are not displayed anywhere. Traditions and norms about how people work together are included in the informal structure. This structure is closely intertwined with the official one, but the two are not always in harmony with each other.

The informal level of operation exists in every organization, even the best-controlled ones. On close inspection one may find that some rules and regulations are circumvented, that the hierarchy is sometimes ignored, that an official high up in the hierarchy does not have the authority which normally would be inherent in such a position, that messages are sent across and around the so-called proper channels of communication, and that requests are sometimes approved without going through the prescribed number of officials (Tappen 1989: 204). The informal network also provides for the informal communication network, known as the grapevine.

The organizational chart (organogram)

It is the normal custom to display the formal organizational structure in a diagram. When drawing up such a diagram, one usually considers the following rules:

- Each position is given a title that broadly describes the responsibility of the job (eg nursing service manager — patient care).

- Each job title is enclosed in a box

- The distance of the job title from the top of the chart indicates the relative status of that position within the organization as a whole.

- The lines which connect the different job titles show the direction in which communication should take place and in which authority is delegated.

- A solid line (————) between two positions indicates a direct command-flowing relationship.

- A dotted line (. . . . . .) between positions may indicate a communication channel which is used frequently, but not for the purpose of delegating orders.

- A dashed line (- - - - -) may indicate a co-ordinating relationship which enables people in widely separate parts of an organization to co-operate during complex planning, control, or problem-solving activities.

The organizational chart is often used to orientate new employees, to provide the necessary overview of the functioning of the organization for interested visitors and inspection officials, and sometimes (together with flow charts of nursing procedures) to analyse the origin of departmental inefficiency.

Hierarchical structure

In any complex organization one finds many levels of systems and subsystems. These systems and subsystems are identified as areas, divisions, departments, units, etc. These different levels are arranged in a hierarchy within the organization. This is also sometimes called the *bureaucratic structure*.

In most organizations, people are ranked according to their function and the amount of authority which they have. This hierarchy can best be viewed as a pyramid, where the top is formed by the smallest number of people (possessing the greatest amount of authority) and the bottom of the pyramid is formed by the largest number of people (with the smallest amount of authority). People in a hierarchy are also ranked according to their status and salary (Tappen 1989: 192).

The flow of communication up and down the hierarchy varies in different organizations, depending on the organizational culture and climate.

Matrix structure

When an organization is making use of the adhocracy style as well as the hierarchical style, the result is called a *matrix organizational structure*. In a matrix type of organization, the skills and efforts of numerous specialists are co-ordinated both vertically and horizontally.

The difference between a line and staff organization and a matrix type of organization lies in the fact that the latter contains fewer levels of hierarchy, greater decentralization of decision-making, and a less rigid adherence to formal rules and procedures (Rabich et al. 1985, as referred to by Gillies 1989: 160).

Employees' skills in lateral relations are increased in a matrix structure because the emphasis on the large number of short-term, single-objective project groups develops the communication skills of employees in relation to the other professionals with whom that employee is forced to interact frequently on an in-depth level while serving on a project team.

The nurse manager's role is more complex in a matrix organization than a vertical one. The managers are expected to co-ordinate different project efforts laterally, and these lateral relationships are more time-consuming and difficult than the vertical relationships. The manager's responsibility in a matrix-type organization is to provide the conditions that are required for the optimum functioning of the different project teams. They are expected to ensure that the support, the information, the funds, and the materials which are needed in order for the different project teams to function effectively are all available. They are also expected to co-ordinate the efforts of the different project teams so as to ensure that those teams are all working to achieve the organization's goals and are not working against each other (Tappen 1989: 199).

Tall and flat structures

A tall structure in an organization — that is a structure with many intermediate levels from the top to the bottom — paves the way for an autocratic leadership style. This type of structure is the preferred one in situations requiring rapid minor changes and precise co-ordination. In a tall structure, communication from managers is given more attention than that from colleagues, with the result that messages pass quickly from top to bottom. This narrow range of management allows the staff members the time and opportunity to evaluate the managers' decisions on a frequent basis. The many levels in such a structure are rather expensive because many managers are needed, each earning a relatively high salary.

Apart from the advantage that communication passes relatively quickly from the top to the bottom in tall structures, there are a number of disadvantages concerning communication in such a structure:

1. Each additional level makes communication more cumbersome.

2. The more levels that the message must pass through, the more it becomes distorted.

3. The taller the structure, the less understanding is found between the top level and lower levels.

4. The taller the structure, the more impersonal the organization becomes.

The flat structure is flat because a number of organizational functions are identified separately and are then placed on a structural diagram which is more horizontally- than vertically-organized. It is thus obvious that the flat structure shortens the administrative distance between the top and the bottom levels in the organization. Communication is thus made easier because it is direct, fast-flowing, and does not get distorted through many organizational levels.

Another advantage of the flat organizational structure is that the large groups that are responsible for each horizontally-placed organizational function have a greater variety of skills between them and they are thus capable of solving a greater variety of problems. It is commonly believed that this type of structure improves morale among employees and that it assists in the development of confident and capable staff members, mainly as a result of the democratic type of management style which is an integral part of this kind of structure.

In a large organization, however, a flat structure may prove to be impractical because large groups require more co-ordination and have more difficulty in reaching consensus. The nurse manager, in a flat structure, can easily become overburdened because her span of control is wide (Marriner-Tomey 1992: 132–3).

ASSESSMENT OF THE ORGANIZATIONAL STRUCTURE

The degree to which nurses are able to function successfully in an organization will depend on the extent to which they understand the system, its structure, and its daily operations. In order to understand the health care institution fully it is advisable to analyse both its formal and informal structure. Some of the questions which one needs to ask in order to do such an analysis are the following (Hein and Nicholson 1986: 354; Shehnaz and Funke-Furber 1988):

1. Authority

   - Is the authority centralized or decentralized?

   - How long does it take to change a policy or a procedure?

   - Is the chain of command to the superintendent and nurse manager in charge followed or circumvented?

   - What kinds of decisions are made by nurses who are in positions of authority?

   - How are conflicts resolved and by whom?

   - How do nurses contribute to the decision-making process?

   - Who holds legitimate power?

   - How does the informal structure function?

   - How much influence is exerted by the informal structure?

2. Physical environment

   - How much energy must be expended to obtain equipment and supplies?

   - Is there a place where nurses can relax?

   - Is the ward duty room designed to promote functional efficiency?

- What is the overall noise level in the institution?
- For whose comfort are the patient rooms designed?

3. Role expectations

- What functions or specifications are included in job descriptions?
- Are performance standards included in job descriptions?
- Does the job description duplicate another title or function?
- To what extent are non-nursing duties performed by nursing staff?

4. Types of communication

- What are the formal channels of communication?
- How are rules, policies, and procedures made known?
- Does communication flow freely upwards?
- Is important information withheld from the people in the formal chain of command?
- How does lateral communication occur?
- Which subgroups interact with each other and which avoid each other?
- How accurately does the grapevine function?
- Who seems to have all the 'latest news'?

5. Leadership behaviours

- What pattern of behaviour do most of the nurses and other health workers exhibit daily?
- What is the main leadership style used by the nurse manager in charge of the nursing service?
- How much control is used?
- Is the main leadership style adapted to changing circumstances when needed?

6. Rewards/acknowledgement

- What type of rewards are given?
- Which people are rewarded?
- What are the effects of rewards or non-acknowledgements on employees in general?

ORGANIZATIONAL EFFECTIVENESS

Organizational effectiveness is measured by a variety of variables, such as patients' satisfaction with their care, staff satisfaction with work, and management's satisfaction with staff. Effectiveness can be enhanced by the following:

- enlarging jobs qualitatively to make them meaningful, interesting, and challenging;
- making the structure more manageable by increasing the clinical nurses' autonomy;
- increasing the manager's span of control;
- flattening the structure;
- employing a participative management style;
- decentralizing authority;
- increasing the employee's responsibility for her own performance;
- increasing creativity and innovation;
- replacing direction and control with advice;
- trying to meet the needs of the employees as far as possible.

CONCLUSION

There are a variety of organizational structures which can be used to achieve success. Each type of structure has its advantages and disadvantages. The nurse manager needs to be astute and pragmatic and should design a structure with a variety of components which will best meet patients' and nurses' needs. The culture and climate of the organization in which she is functioning should be carefully assessed and should then be utilized in order to achieve effective results.

References

Barker, A. M. (1990). *Transformational Nursing Leadership*. Williams and Wilkins: London.

Conway-Rutkowski, B. (1984). Labour relations: how do you rate? *Nursing Management,* volume 15, number 2, pp. 15–16.

Del Bueno, D. and Vincent, P. M. (1986). Organizational culture: how important is it? *JONA,* October 1986, volume 16, number 10, pp. 15–20.

Fuszard, B. (1983). 'Adhocracy' in health care institutions? *JONA,* 10 January 1983, pp. 14–19.

Hein, E. C. and Nicholson, M. J. (1986). *Contemporary Leadership Behaviour: Selected Readings.* Scott, Foresman: Illinois.

Hughes, L. (1990). Assessing organizational culture: strategies for the external consultant. *Nursing Forum,* volume 25, number 1, pp. 15–19.

Jacobsen-Webb, M. (1985). Team building: key to executive success. *JONA,* February 1985, pp. 16–19.

Shehnaz, A. and Funke-Furber, J. (1988). First-line nurse managers: optimizing the span of control. *JONA,* volume 18, number 5, pp. 34–9.

Sullivan, E. J. and Decker, P. J. (1992). *Effective Management in Nursing.* Addison-Wesley: California.

Swansburg, R. C. (1990). *Management and Leadership for Nurse Managers.* Jones and Bartlett: Boston.

Tappen, R. M. (1989). *Nursing Leadership and Management: Concepts and Practice.* F. A. Davies: Philadelphia.

Thomas, C., Ward, M., Charba, C. and Kumiega, A. (1990). Measuring and interpreting organizational culture. *JONA,* volume 20, number 6, pp. 17–24.

CHAPTER 8

JOB EVALUATION

S. W. Booyens

CONTENTS

INTRODUCTION

The nurse manager is, among other things, responsible for ensuring job satisfaction among the nurses employed in her institution, for moving nurses between different positions, for appraising the work performance of the nurses, and for making recommendations regarding salaries and salary increases for her personnel. The evaluation of the different jobs within the nursing manager's jurisdiction is of primary importance for the fulfillment of the above responsibilities. Job evaluation consists of two main pillars — *job analysis* and *job description,* which will be dealt with in the following pages.

JOB ANALYSIS

A job analysis 'identifies, specifies, organizes and displays the duties, tasks and responsibilities actually performed by the incumbent in a given job' (Ignatavicius and Griffith 1982: 37). In the past, job analysis was viewed in a rather narrow sense. Time and motion studies were seen to form its basis. Although time and motion studies have an important role to play to quantify certain physical actions, 'it is only a small facet of the ever-growing range of techniques and methods available to managers for the systematic accumulation of data about jobs, tasks and roles' (Pearn and Kandola 1988: 2).

Uses of job analysis

The usual outcome of job analysis is a job description. Job analysis also gives rise to job specifications. When a job description and specifications have been formulated, it is easier to evaluate the performance of an employee who is working at a particular job.

The analysis of a job facilitates the identification of its initial training requirements. The ongoing developmental training needs for a particular job will also be identified, thus facilitating in-service education programmes.

If one has a proper idea of what a particular job consists of, it is easier to make correct choices when an employee is considering career changes or career movements.

With the specific details of a job spelt out, and with the personal attributes necessary to do the job identified, it becomes easier for those who are recruiting to give the exact facts about jobs. The knowledge of what is really needed for each specific job makes the selection process and the placement of new employees easier (Ivancevich and Glueck 1986: 127).

Accurate job descriptions supply the information needed to decide on the different pay levels and scales for the different jobs in a particular organization. Job descriptions are necessary to be able to conduct wage surveys in order to compare wages of similar jobs between different organizations (Gerber, Nel and van Dyk 1987: 129).

Job analysis provides information about what the job entails and how and where it is performed. It is thus possible to identify restraints such as noise, wrong equipment, incorrect layout, and outdated standards which will hinder the performance of the job. This will facilitate an adaptation of the climate in which the worker has to perform the work, and will eventually increase effectiveness on the job.

Job analysis provides a framework for the evaluation of the performance of workers and for rating merit on an objective level consistent with the requirements of the particular job. Managers who are confronted by trade union representatives about the apparent disparity between the pay levels of certain employees will have a powerful case to put forward when merit rating is done according to scientific job analysis.

Research has shown that employees possessing a realistic image of the job and the circumstances in which they will work before accepting a post tend to stay longer in such a post. These employees also derive more job satisfaction from their work.

Analysis of jobs will show up deficiencies in structures — for instance the overlapping of tasks. When there is too much overlapping of tasks between two posts, one of the posts may be discarded or more meaningful tasks may be found for one of the posts (Vermaak and Dednam 1987: 34).

Steps in the job analysis process

Job analysis is usually carried out in eight steps. These steps are as follows:

Step 1

It is first necessary to identify the place of the job in the organization as a whole. This is done by looking at the existing organogram of the organization to see where the job to be analysed fits in. Process charts may also be used in this step to see clearly which jobs are specifically connected to the one in question. (A process chart shows the job relationships of a specific type of job.)

Step 2

A decision must be made here regarding how the information obtained from the job analysis efforts will be used — eg for recruitment purposes, for merit-rating purposes, for salary-determination purposes, etc. This step is extremely important because the aim of the job analysis effort will, to a large extent, determine how data will be selected for the job analysis.

Step 3

The jobs to be analysed are now selected. It is customary to select a representative sample of similar types of jobs for analysis purposes.

Step 4

This step involves the collection of data by making use of acceptable job analysis techniques. Data concerning the specific characteristics of the job, required behaviours, the necessary employee characteristics, and the conditions in which the job must be performed are collected (Ivancevich and Glueck 1986: 126).

Step 5

The information obtained in step 4 is now used to compile a job description for a particular type of job.

Step 6

The job specification is now compiled from the information obtained in step 4. The job specification spells out the minimum skills, knowledge, and abilities that an employee would need to be able to perform the job (Gerber, Nel, and Van Dyk 1987: 130).

Step 7

The information from steps 1–6 is now used to engage in job design. The job in question is designed or structured in such a way that the employee will get satisfaction from doing the job, and in a way that will promote effectiveness in the performance of the job (Gerber, Nel and van Dyk 1987: 130).

Step 8

In this step, the success or failure of the job design as carried out in step 7 is evaluated and the job design is then modified where necessary (Ivancevich and Glueck 1986: 126).

DEFINITIONS

A number of key terms are defined in order to promote the understanding of the job evaluation process.

- *Job evaluation.* This is the formal process by which the relative worth of the various jobs in an organization is determined for the purpose of determining wage and salary structures. Job evaluation rates the job, not the worker. It is an attempt to determine and compare the demands which the normal performance of particular jobs makes on the normal or average employee (Thomason 1980: 3).

- *Job analysis.* Job analysis is the process of determining, through scientific study, the tasks, responsibilities, and prescribed behaviours of a job, and of specifying the education, abilities, experience and personality traits needed for it.

- *Job description.* This is a written picture of the specific duties, responsibilities, organizational relationships, and working conditions of a particular job (Gillies 1982: 137).

- *Job specification.* This consists of an outline of the minimum skills, knowledge, experience, and the required personality traits which are necessary for the successful execution of a particular job.

- *Job classification.* This is the bracketing or grouping of different jobs which have the same level of difficulty, demand, and responsibility attached to them for the purposes of determining financial compensation (Gillies 1982: 137).

- *Job design.* Job design is the process of structuring tasks and responsibilities on the one hand and the qualifications necessary to do the job on the other hand in such a way that the maximum satisfaction and effectiveness is derived. There are a number of approaches which are commonly used to achieve this.

- *Job simplification.* The job is divided into smaller units for the benefit of poorly-trained employees (Gerber, Nel and van Dyk 1987: 126).

- *Job rotation.* The employee is rotated between different jobs for specific periods of time. This is usually done for professional growth purposes.

- *Job enlargement.* This is the opposite of job simplification. Simple tasks are combined in order to create a more meaningful job which can be done by the better-trained employee (Gerber, Nel and van Dyk 1987: 127).

- *Job enrichment.* The job is enlarged vertically and horizontally. The employee participates to a greater extent in decision-making, and the control over the employee is lessened. This is done to increase an employee's sense of job satisfaction and to add to her motivation (Dienemann 1990: 332).

JOB EVALUATION COMMITTEE

Ideally, an institution should have a job evaluation committee. The task of such a committee would be the analysis of specific jobs, writing job descriptions after analysing the jobs, determining job specifications, and making recommendations to the nursing service manager regarding job design and salary structures. It is also the task of this committee to communicate clearly to every employee in the organization about the purposes, methodology and ultimate utilization of the job analysis efforts. The committee should consist of at least one member from the employee group where the jobs are to be analysed, a nursing supervisor or manager from this group, a representative from the personnel department, and an experienced job analyst (ie a person with a degree in industrial psychology and experience in job analysis) as the leader. It is important to note that conducting a reliable and valid job analysis is a task for a trained professional. Individuals who conduct job analysis must understand people, jobs, and the total organizational system. It is also important to understand how the work flows within the organization (Ivancevich and Glueck 1986: 129).

COLLECTING DATA FOR JOB ANALYSIS PURPOSES

A number of techniques can be used to collect data for job analysis. These include observation, interviewing, job diaries, and questionnaires. A short discussion of each now follows.

Observation

When an analyst observes the work as it is being done, the data collected can be very useful if the whole cycle of activities can be observed and if the employee is not affected in any way by the presence of the observer. Observing the work as it is being done does not, however, reveal the importance of the work being done, nor its level of difficulty. Observation is a most time-consuming way of collecting data, and the reliability of observations cannot always be proven. Observing a job can be very useful, however, if the analyst is going to conduct interviews with the employees observed afterwards. Observation often offers the best way of identifying the different types of behaviours displayed by employees doing a particular job.

Interviewing

Interviewing employees about the jobs that they are performing can prove valuable to the analyst. When an unstructured interview is conducted by an analyst who is an experienced interviewer, the unobservable thinking processes which are part of the job — eg decision-making and problem-solving — may be pointed out by the employee. Sensitive aspects of the work can be probed. The employee can also point out to the interviewer which aspects of behaviour traits are more important in the particular job than others. It is, however, easy for the employee to miss out on some of the less frequently performed activities in a job, the employee and interviewer might not be on the same wavelength, and/or the employee might give wrong information about the job to the interviewer in an attempt to 'blow up' the importance of the job. It can thus be seen that, although interviewing employees about the jobs they perform can yield important information, the interview cannot be used as the sole method of data collection on any given job. It should be combined with another method (Pearn and Kandola 1988: 23–5).

Job diaries

In this method, the employees or jobholders are requested to record their activities over a given period. A number of people doing the same job must keep a diary of their daily activities for perhaps a month or a two-week period and must then present the analyst with a list or a description of the activities that they were engaged in for that period. It is important that the analyst explains to the employees in exact terms what is really needed and what will be done with the collected information.

This method depends entirely on the co-operation of the employees. It is thus possible to get useful information, but the information will be incomplete and biased if the diaries are not completed on a regular basis. The main difficulty with this method is the tendency of jobholders to concentrate only on those areas of the work which they consider important and to omit from their diaries activities which are frequently performed but which are considered less important.

Job diaries work best in jobs where the tasks are more managerial in nature and where the cycle of activities is too great for an analyst to observe it. It is possible for a jobholder to record the different decisions made, and why and when they were made (Pearn and Kandola 1988: 20–1).

Questionnaires

The use of questionnaires to elicit information about a job is the cheapest way to analyse a job. It is an effective way to gather a large amount of information in a short period of time (Gerber, Nel and van Dyk 1987: 131). It is important to remember that the questionnaire must first be tested before it is given to employees to complete. This will allow for refinement of questions which are stated ambiguously, the inclusion of relevant questions that were forgotten, and the exclusion of irrelevant and unnecessary questions.

The Position Analysis Questionnaire (PAQ)

This is a structured type of questionnaire developed by the Perdue University in the USA, consisting of 194 job questions. Of these 194 items, 187 relate to job activities and seven relate to information such as pay rates, etc. The items are organized in six divisions (Pearn and Kandola 1988: 58–9), namely:

- Information input — where and how does the worker get information?

- Mental processes — what reasoning, decision-making, and planning is involved?

- Work output — what physical activities are performed?

- Relationships with people — what relationships with other people are required in the job?

- Job context — in what physical and social contexts is the work performed?

- Other job characteristics — ie what other activities and conditions are involved which affect the worker?

Each item is rated on a specific scale which will vary depending on the item evaluated. The scales are: importance to the job, the amount of time taken up by the activity, the extent of use in the job, the possibility of occurrence in the job, and the applicability of the item.

The job analyst must be familiar with the items of the questionnaire and the job to be analysed, and must construct a similar questionnaire eliminating all the items which will not apply to the particular job (Pearn and Kandola 1988: 58–64).

The PAQ-method can be used to analyse a wide variety of jobs, from basic manual jobs to management posts. This questionnaire is useful for providing a broad picture of a job. It is difficult to construct job descriptions from it, however. The data must be analysed by a computer. The PAQ must be used together with a structured interview.

The Management Position Description Questionnaire (MPDQ)

Although the PAQ does provide items for managerial jobs, this is not the questionnaire's strongest point. Another version, the MPDQ, was therefore developed. This questionnaire is structured to analyse managerial jobs in different industries and consists of 208 items, divided into 10 groups (Gerber, Nel, and van Dyk 1987: 133):

- general information;

- decision-making;

- planning and organizing;

- supervision and control;

- advice and innovation;

- contacts;

- monitoring of business indicators;

- overall judgement;

- expertise;

- organization chart.

Administering and analysing the data collected with these two questionnaires is costly (Gerber, Nel, and van Dyk 1987: 134).

METHODS OF JOB EVALUATION

Job evaluation methods are traditionally divided into non-quantitative and quantitative methods. There are, however, recent job evaluation methods which contain elements of more than one of these approaches.

Non-quantitative methods

Job ranking

This is the simplest and easiest method of job evaluation, but it only provides a rough evaluation of the jobs in a particular organization. The different jobs are assessed by a panel of assessors who then rank the jobs in a hierarchical order from the lowest to the highest in accordance with the value they would ascribe to each. The evaluation is subjective because there are no predetermined scales or criteria against which the jobs are evaluated (Gerber, Nel, and van Dyk 1987: 395).

Ranking is carried out for financial remuneration purposes. Although ranking distinguishes between jobs which are of greater and lesser value to the organization, it does not state the degree of difference which exists between any two jobs in the line organization (Gillies 1982: 144). It is thus difficult to arrive at proper pay differentials (Bartley 1981: 15).

The main disadvantage of this type of evaluation is that it is so easy to rank jobs according to one's inclination that the analysts or assessors might be tempted not to study the job content of the different types of jobs beforehand. Their ranking may thus not reflect the true order of things, and employees may become dissatisfied (Gillies 1982: 144).

Job classification

When job classification is carried out, the different jobs in an organization are measured against a predetermined assessment scale and grouped. Each group is called a *grade* and a predetermined description of what each grade consists of is produced. The appropriate salary scale for each grade is also predetermined. It is necessary to define each grade. The differentiation between the different classes or grades is usually made between the areas of difficulty of the work, job responsibility, qualifications and training required, the amount of supervision received, and the need for the use of judgement (Bartley 1981: 40).

The assessors must study the job description of each type of job and then decide in which of the predetermined groups or grades it must be placed. The number of grades in an organization will vary according to the size of the organization and according to the skills and responsibilities found in the total workforce (Gillies 1982: 144).

According to Gerber, Nel, and van Dyk (1988: 395–6) the job classification method has two major disadvantages. The first is that large scale generalizations about jobs have to be made in order to fit them in a specific grade. Secondly, where jobs in a grade differ because they are in widely different fields, it is necessary to look at all the finer details of the different jobs. For example, it is difficult to compare the work in the production section with that in the general administration office.

Quantitative methods

Factor comparison

In this method a group or set of 'factors' is chosen against which all jobs in an organization are measured. Every job in the organization is compared with every other job in the organization, one factor at a time. The following five factors are generally used to compare jobs with each other: skill requirements, mental requirements, physical requirements, responsibility, and working conditions. Before a job can be evaluated against any of these five factors the committee performing the evaluation must first define precisely what is meant by each factor — eg 'working conditions' may be defined as:

- conditions which make the work pleasant or unpleasant;

- job hazards;

- conditions which make the work safe or unsafe.

The next step in this evaluation process is the selection of key jobs, also called 'benchmark' jobs. Key jobs have the following characteristics (Bartley 1981: 65):

- they are well known throughout the organization;

- the proper salary scale for the job is undisputed;

- preferably more than one employee should fill such a position.

The key jobs must be selected from the different levels in the job hierarchy.

The committee now ranks the key jobs in order of their importance on each of the five factors. The job descriptions and specifications, and the predetermined factor-definitions are compared. A rating scale where each benchmark job is rated against each of the five factors is useful in arriving at an end figure for each job, (see figure 8.1).

Figure 8.1: Committee's average rating factors

Job title	Skill	Mental requirements	Physical requirements	Responsi- bility	Working conditions
Sister-in-charge	5	10	4	10	10
Nurse auxilliary	3	4	8	2	3
– Sister-in-charge = 39 – Nurse auxilliary = 20					

The next step is to tie a monetary value to each factor for each benchmark job. The present salary scales of the jobs are used as the departing point. The ranking of each key job, and the assignment of the monetary value for each factor per job, constitutes a yardstick against which the other jobs in the organization are measured. A job comparison table is constructed where each key job appears five times (ie under each factor). Monetary values, eg R10.80, R10.60, R10.40, R10.20, R10.00, R9.80, R9.60 etc., in a descending order, and each job's five factors are slotted in according to the rand value assigned for the particular factor for the specific job.

The committee reads the job description for each of the other jobs in the organization and, one by one, each different job is slotted in on this job comparison table, with the result that the jobs in an organization are actually compared with one another on this table/ scale (Bartley 1981: 69–71).

The disadvantages of this are that it is rather subjective in nature and that it is hard to find key jobs which are correctly compensated.

The salary scale attached to a job is usually a debatable issue (Gerber, Nel, and Van Dyk 1987: 396).

The point method

This is the most popular approach used for job evaluation. In the point method, each job is evaluated against a predetermined set of factors. After evaluation each job has a total point score according to which its value for the organization and the financial compensation which it merits can be judged.

The evaluation committee has to study the job descriptions and job specifications of the different jobs in the organization and then compile a list of factors. Each factor is subdivided into several subfactors. Each factor is also 'weighted', ie each factor is evaluated separately for its relative importance in the organization. An example would be: responsibility 20%, education 25%, job conditions 15%, levels of decision-making 30%, supervisory responsibilities 10%.

The percentages are now multiplied by any number from three to ten to get the number of points for each factor. Each percentage must be multiplied by the same number, eg

— Responsibility 20% × 4 = 80 points
— Education 25% × 4 = 100 points
— Job conditions 15% × 4 = 60 points
— Levels of decision-making 30% × 4 = 120 points
— Supervisory responsibilities 10% × 4 = 40 points

Total: 100% × 4 = 400 points (Bartley 1981: 149).

Each factor weight (ie number of points) is now further subdivided into various levels or degrees, to which another specific point is assigned. An example would be: education = 100 points (factor weight), divided in four levels, each counting 25 points. These subfactors or levels for each factor are now defined accurately and the points adjusted as follows:

Factor: education:
Sub-factors/levels/degrees:

— Matric certificate 10 points
— Post-matric college certificate 20 points
— Basic university degree 30 points
— Masters degree 40 points

The evaluation committee now evaluates each job against the various factors and sub-factors. The scores/points of all the sub-factors are added, and the job scores a total point value.

The advantage of this method is the common standards which are set against the rates which evaluate the different jobs. This method is seen to be reasonably objective (Gerber, Nel, and Van Dyk 1987: 397).

SOME JOB EVALUATION METHODS USED IN SOUTH AFRICA

Three of the generally-known job evaluation methods used in public and private organizations in South Africa are:

- the Paterson system;
- the Peromnes system;
- the Hay–MSL system.

The Paterson system

In this system only one factor, decision-making, is used to evaluate various jobs in an organization. This system assumes that an employee's decision-making abilities are the most important aspect of his job (Gerber, Nel and Van Dyk 1981: 398). There are six types of decisions listed, and 11 different job grades. The disadvantages are that only one person analyses jobs and the types of decision-making abilities and job grades are predetermined, universal, and not open to variations (Gerber, Nel, and Van Dyk 1987: 399–400).

The Peromnes method

This method uses six job levels, a grading structure, a points system, and eight factors (Gerber, Nel, and Van Dyk 1987: 401–2), eg:

- problem solving (decision-making);
- consequences of errors of judgement;
- work pressure;
- knowledge;
- diligence;
- understanding;
- educational qualifications;
- training/experience.

This method has the following disadvantages (Gerber, Nel and Van Dyk 1987: 401):

- the evaluation process is unstructured;
- the cut-off points on the point scale is arbitrarily determined;

- it is an expensive, time-consuming method;
- the evaluation process is not linked with job descriptions;
- there is too much inbuilt subjectivity.

The Hay–MSL method

This method rates a job against three factors: 'know-how', 'problem-solving', and 'accountability'. Each factor is further subdivided into sub-factors (Thomason 1980: 87), eg:

A. Know-how:

1. Technical, professional, manual know-how.

2. Managerial know-how.

3. Human relations know-how.

B. Problem-solving:

1. Environment in which thinking takes place, ranging from routine to completely unstructured.

2. Type of thinking to be done ranging from repetitive thinking to 'blue-sky' creativity.

C. Accountability:

1. Degree of freedom to act.

2. Value of the areas affected by the job.

3. The directness of the impact of the job.

An evaluation committee, guided by an experienced evaluator, evaluates each job according to three guide charts (one for each factor). Each guide chart is in the form of a grid which must be completed. The depth and breadth of each factor is thus determined for each job (Thomason 1980: 88–9).

When the assessments have been made on the prescribed grids, a total score for each job can be reached by adding the different numbers obtained in the grids for each factor and sub-factor. Another aspect of this method is the 'profiling' element. Jobs are profiled according to the total scores obtained in the three sub-factors. If, for example, a job scored high on know-how, but decidedly lower on accountability and problem-solving, the job might be defined as a routine job (Thomason 1980: 90). A distinct advantage of this method is the 'data-bank' of information on salaries paid at July 1 each year within about 400 organizations. This gives the user-organization the opportunity to do a survey of similar jobs against which it can compare its own salary levels and structure (Thomason 1980: 87).

The steps in this method are (Thomason 1980: 92):

1. Selecting a number of benchmark jobs which represent the different levels and families of jobs in the organization.

2. The preparation of job descriptions by trained job analysts after discussions with the employees. After the descriptions have been compiled they must be validated by the employees as well as their immediate supervisors.

3. Profiling of all benchmark jobs, followed by a comparison of the individual profiles produced.

4. The rating of all jobs on the three dimensions.

5. A comparison of the results of the evaluation with the existing pay rates using a scatter diagram.

6. A comparison of the existing pay rates with the salaries paid in the other companies for the same type of job.

7. Establishment of a pay policy and pay structure.

CHOOSING AN EVALUATION SYSTEM

All evaluation systems have both strong and weak points. The selection of a system depends, among other things, on the following (Bartley 1981: 57):

1. Number and complexity of the jobs.

2. Availability of funds.

3. The level of the jobs to be evaluated.

4. The availability of knowledgeable persons to be in charge of the programme.

5. The acceptance of the job evaluation methods by the employees.

JOB DESCRIPTION

The main aim of job descriptions is the recording of information in a systematic format which can then be used for the comparison of jobs. Job descriptions are, however, useful for a number of other purposes (Berenson and Ruhnke 1976 as quoted by Bartley 1981: 120), eg:

- to clarify relationships between jobs;

- to assist in the evaluation of job performance;

- to aid in the orientation of new employees to their jobs;
- to assist in the appointment and placement of employees;
- to forecast the training needs for a particular job;
- to improve the work-flow;
- to serve as a basis for human resource planning;
- to show the proper channels of communication;
- to help employees to get a better understanding of their jobs.

A general job description for all professional nurses in an organization might be useful as a base document for analysis purposes, but the final job description must be individualized to fit the actual job. The job description of the professional nurse in a medical unit should thus be different from the one of the professional nurse working in a surgical unit.

Some important points to remember when writing job descriptions are the following:

1. The job must be named specifically, eg 'professional nurse: second-in-charge — oncology unit'.

2. The date when the job description was compiled should be indicated.

3. It is recommended that job descriptions are revised yearly.

4. Each specific task must be isolated.

5. The job must be defined precisely.

6. Steer clear of broad, generic statements, such as 'provide clinical supervision to all staff as needed and assist in their development' (Ignatavicius and Griffith 1982: 38).

7. Be specific and divide the tasks contained in the job description into definite items, eg:
   - identify professional development needs of unit members;
   - set individual professional development goals co-operatively with unit members;
   - monitor direct care delivery activities of unit members for conformity to hospital standards;
   - teach unit members clinical skills when skill discrepancies occur (Ignatavicius and Griffith 1982: 38).

8. Each task must be carefully worded. The wording must capture the intent of the task and describe the behaviour or action, eg 'directs the implementation of physician's orders by assigning patient care to specific staff members' (Ignatavicius and Griffith

1982: 38). Action verbs must be selected from lists to assist in wording tasks correctly.

9. Tasks must be listed under proper headings or categories, eg managerial, supervisory, direct care, interpersonal communication, and maintenance. The tasks should be categorized in order to provide a logical structure in the job description.

10. The duties within each category must be prioritized as well as the categories themselves. 'If job descriptions do not organize the tasks coherently, inefficient performance and performance appraisals that focus undue attention on trivial aspects result' (Ignatavicius and Griffith 1982: 39).

11. Each task should be described separately and should not be combined with a related task — eg do not combine tasks by an 'and/or' such as 'plans and/or implements patient care plans'. If both need to be done, state each one separately.

12. Each task must be described in specific terms, eg 'teaches patients about medication regimen' should be specified by 'at the time of discharge' or 'using the standard prescribed patient teaching procedure' (Ignatavicius and Griffith 1982: 39).

13. Eliminate unnecessary items which do not really belong to the main aim of the job and place them in the job description where they really belong — eg 'serve as public relations liaison with the community' does not really fit in the job description of the sister-in-charge, but does fit into the chief nursing officer's description (Ignatavicius and Griffith 1982: 40).

14. 'A job description should record the major and important elements of the job, not all of the tasks assigned' (Bartley 1981: 121).

15. The same style or format should be used for all the job descriptions in an organization.

16. The required knowledge, skills, and abilities should be included under a specific heading.

17. Reporting relationships should be recorded, ie the supervision received and/or given.

18. The conditions under which the job must be performed must be stated in clear terms, eg broken hours of duty, extra compensation for work after hours, etc.

19. Special risks which are inherent in the post should be mentioned, eg noise or social factors such as time pressure and stress.

20. Job descriptions are only useful when they are in written form, when they are realistic regarding technical and human resources, and when they relate to practical requirements of the job.

21. The job summary must describe the care functions and must give an overall view of what the job entails in order to be used in advertisements for posts or when general enquiries regarding the job are made (Vermaak and Dednam 1987: 37).

JOB SPECIFICATIONS

A job specification for a particular job stems from the description of the job. It specifies the minimum required abilities (personal attributes), knowledge, skills, training, experience, and qualifications that a person must possess in order to do the job, thus giving clear directives for recruitment and selection. When writing a job specification, each duty or item in the job description must be analysed and the required behaviour, skill, or training must be determined. Items which usually appear on job specifications include the following (Bartley 1981: 194–5):

1. Mental requirements
   - type and amount of special education;
   - kind of work instruction provided;
   - distractions;
   - experience;
   - intellectual abilities;
   - concentration span;
   - emotional characteristics;
   - communication responsibilities.

2. Physical requirements
   - nature of physical effort;
   - rest periods;
   - minimum height;
   - maximum age;
   - endurance;
   - appearance;
   - percentage of time standing, sitting, walking.

3. Responsibility
   - for equipment;
   - for records;

- for public contacts;
- for the work of others.

4. Working conditions
   - place, eg indoors;
   - type, eg desk;
   - surroundings, eg orderly;
   - atmosphere, eg ventilated;
   - hazards, eg muscular strains;
   - type of co-worker;
   - regular or irregular working hours.

A recent computer program developed in the USA and which is used by some organizations in South Africa to identify the necessary behavioural requirements on the job, is the ICS-program (identifying criteria for success). This program is used in conjunction with the Hay-MSL-job evaluation method.

CONCLUSION

It is the responsibility of nursing management to ensure that high quality patient care is achieved through the optimum performance of each nursing staff member. Optimum performance by the nursing staff presupposes that the abilities of each incumbent of a post will correspond with the requirements for the post she occupies. To achieve such a 'match' between incumbent and post it is necessary to analyse the contents of the different jobs in the organization, to arrive at effective job descriptions afterwards, and to evaluate jobs properly in order to pay the incumbents of the different posts according to the required performance which is expected for each post.

References

Ash, R. A. Job plements for task clusters: arguments for using multi-methodological approaches to job analysis and demonstration of their utility. *Public Personnel Management Journal,* volume 19, number 5, pp. 80–9.

Ash, R. A. and Levine, E. L. (1980). A framework for evaluating job analysis methods. *Personnel,* volume 57, parts 11/12, pp. 53–9.

Atchison, T. J. The concept of job analysis: a review and some suggestions. *Public Personnel Management Journal,* volume 19, number 8, pp. 134–42.

Bartley, D. L. (1981). *Job Evaluation: Wage and Salary Administration.* Addison-Wesley: California.

Brien, E. P., Goldstein, I. L. and Macey, W. H. (1987). Multidomain job analysis: procedures and applications. *Training and Development Journal,* August 1987, volume 21, number 8, pp. 68–72.

Dienemann, J. (1990). *Nursing Administration. Strategic Perspectives and Application.* Appleton and Large: Connecticut.

Gerber, P. D., Nel, P. S. and van Dyk, P. S. (1987). *Human Resources Management.* Southern: Johannesburg.

Gillies, D. A. (1982). *Nursing Management. A Systems Approach.* Saunders: Philadelphia.

Ignatavicius, D. and Griffith, J. (1982). Job analysis: the basics of effective appraisal. *JONA,* volume 12, numbers 7–8, pp. 37–41.

Ivancevich, J. M. and Glueck, W. F. (1986). *Foundations of Personnel/Human Resource Management.* Business Publications: Texas.

Pearn, M. and Kandola, R. (1988). *Job Analysis: A Practical Guide for Managers.* Institute of Personnel Management: London.

Schreider, B. and Kanz, A. M. (1989). Strategic job analysis. *Human Resource Management,* Spring 1989, volume 28, number 1, pp. 51–63.

Thomason, G. (1980). *Job evaluation: Objectives and Methods.* Institute of Personnel Management: London.

Vermaak, M. and Dednam J. (1987). Taakspesifikasie. *Nursing RSA,* volume 2, number 8. pp. 34–5.

Vermaak, M. and Dednam, J. (1987). Die taakbeskrywing. *Nursing RSA,* volume 2, number 7, pp. 36–7.

Vermaak, M. and Dednam, J. (1987). Taakanalise (4): gebruike en voordele. *Nursing RSA,* volume 2, number 9, pp. 34–5.

Wright, P. M. and Wesley, K. N. (1985). How to choose the kind of job analysis you really need. *Personnel,* May 1985, volume 62, number 5, pp. 51–5.

CHAPTER 9

GROUP

DYNAMICS

M. H. Hart and

S. W. Booyens

CONTENTS

INTRODUCTION

The nature of nursing is such that most nurses work in groups and are continually interacting with colleagues, patients, or members of the community. Despite the importance of this interaction, insufficient emphasis has been given to group dynamics in nursing and the subject has only recently been introduced into nursing textbooks. A knowledge of the many aspects of groups and group processes is a very important aspect of management which can enhance the effectiveness of the nurse manager. With this in mind, the present chapter outlines important characteristics of human groups and relates these to the nursing profession.

THE CHARACTERISTICS OF GROUPS

Groups may be of different sizes, they may have different structures, and they may have different activities, but they have a common element in that they reveal an interdependence among their members. Members of groups 'have relationships to one another that make them interdependent to some significant degree' (Cartwright and Zander, in Forsyth 1990: 7). A group can also be seen as a number of people sharing common interests and norms who interact with one another on a regular basis for the purpose of the achievement of a common goal or goals.

Interaction

The observation of groups reveals the ways in which group members influence each other as a consequence of interaction. It has been said that the behaviour of every member of a group can potentially affect all the other members (Bonner, Homans, and Stogdill, in Forsyth 1990: 9). In fact interaction is the key feature of group life, be it physical, verbal, nonverbal, or emotional.

As shown by Bales and Slater (in Gillies 1989: 199), when groups are engaged in problem-solving behaviour, their members tend to give opinions, make suggestions, provide information, evaluate, analyse, express feelings or wishes, clarify uncertainties, and confirm decisions taken.

When they are engaged in negative behaviour there tends to be disagreement, formality, withdrawal, and antagonism between group members with the result that when assistance is required it is withheld, passive rejection is shown, and group members tend to assert themselves and deflate the status of other group members.

When the group is engaged in positive behaviour there tends to be solidarity among the members, with the result that help is given, understanding and agreement are reached, tension is released through jokes and laughs, and group members are supported by one another. They show satisfaction with accomplishments, and there is compliance with assignments (Gillies 1989: 199).

Structure

Ephemeral groups lack structure because of their transient nature. All other groups develop stable patterns of relationships among their members. Forsyth (1990: 9) uses the terms 'role', 'status', and 'attraction relation' to describe group structure.

An example of group structure might be an advisory group in which committee members adopt particular roles. Some might be supporters, some defenders, and some abstainers, while others might be critics. The behaviour expected of group members is defined by these roles, as are the patterns of authority and attraction. Some group members might command more respect than others, while some might be better liked. Another group structure, constituted differently and with members therefore playing different roles, might make different decisions (Forsyth 1990: 9).

Size

Groups occur in different sizes and these were classified by Simmel (in Forsyth 1990: 9) as the dyad (2 members), triad (3 members), small group (4 to 20 members), the society (20 to 30 members), and the large group (more than 40 members). James (in Forsyth 1990: 9) found that, on average, group size in public settings was 2.4, while in deliberately-formed groups, such as found in work settings, the average size was 2.3. Most groups tend to be small, with groups of 5 to 7 members being the most effective. Groups with more members seem not to achieve their objectives. Low job satisfaction, and higher absenteeism and turnover are associated with larger groups (Sullivan and Decker 1992: 258).

As far as group communication and productivity are concerned, the larger group is generally in a position to be more productive than the smaller group because there is a greater variety of experience among the members. The members may also feel more free to give their opinions and voice their objections to recommendations. It is, however, difficult for the group leader to gain effective control or to get the group members to achieve consensus on an issue, because of the great diversity of opinion. It is thus easier for a smaller group to reach a decision, although the decision may be reached without the variety of input of ideas which is found in the larger group. The group leader tends to have more influence on the smaller group, and the morale of group members in the smaller group tends to be better than in a larger group because each group member has the opportunity to present his ideas in detail (Gillies 1989: 191–2).

Goals

Why do groups exist? There is usually a reason and this reason is often that individuals have a common goal. Throughout history, people have used groups to achieve goals. Groups of humans gather for protection, for business and commercial practices, for legal and religious reasons, to achieve military and strategic objectives, and to achieve technological accomplishments. In fact, much of the world's work is done by groups rather than by individuals. So groups make it easier to attain human goals.

Cohesiveness

Cohesiveness in groups describes group strength, group bonds, and the power of the network holding the group members together and sustaining them. Durkheim said that groups with greater solidarity had more influence over their members than loosely-structured groups. Lewin believed that cohesion came from processes operating at the individual level. At this first level, cohesiveness comes from the attraction which each member has for other group members. At the second level it is the feeling of common identity which welds the group. This can be shown in the 'town versus gown' syndrome so often found in university towns. The townsfolk identify themselves as a separate cohesive group which clearly distinguishes itself from the university community despite the fact that the lives of the town and the university are intimately interwoven — geographically, economically, and socially (Forsyth 1990: 10).

As group cohesiveness increases, so too does individual enjoyment and satisfaction. The same can be said of communication and participation. Members of cohesive groups experience heightened self-esteem and lowered anxiety levels. This comes from the security and protection which the group with a cohesive structure affords its members. Also important is the fact that cohesive groups have a greater capacity to retain members than loosely-structured groups. Thus cohesiveness becomes a centripetal force. It creates potency and vitality and it increases the significance of membership for group members. Extreme cohesiveness can be detrimental because it makes the group uncritical of its own capacity and abilities. Cohesiveness is adversely affected by conflict, apathy, non-participation, or inadequate decision-making (Hall 1988: 373).

Temporal change

The final characteristic of groups is temporal change. Groups change over time because they are made up of interdependent human beings. Developmental changes in groups follow one of two kinds of model. The first is the *cyclical model* in which issues may dominate group behaviour, giving way to work-centered behaviour. The second is called the *successive-stage model*. An example of this is Tuckman's approach where it is assumed that groups pass through five stages. Phase one is a formative and orientative phase where group members join together and become familiar with each other. Phase two is a conflict phase, necessitating a resolution of conflict. Phase three is one in which norms and values develop so that human behaviour becomes regularized. Phase four is one in which the group functions as a unit and starts to achieve goals. Phase five is one of adjournment, where goals have been attained and the group's cohesiveness dissipates (Tuckman, in Forsyth 1990: 12).

GROUPS AND NURSING ADMINISTRATION

We now apply the ideas presented above to the nursing profession with special reference to nursing administration. From the viewpoint of the nurse manager the following dimensions of group behaviour are noteworthy: goals, background, participation, communication patterns, cohesion, membership, climate, norms and decision-making procedures.

Goals

Goals can be formal or informal, and they represent the group's tasks. The way the group accomplishes its tasks is its 'group behaviour'.

Background

The group's background is represented by its history and traditions, and the nurse leader takes these into account in handling the group. In fact, the nurse leader who is conversant with group dynamics recognizes the importance of traditions, norms, procedures, and activities, and studies them to see how they impinge upon the present. The leader fosters their positive aspects and develops a strategy to counteract past negative dimensions.

Participation

The leader facilitates group participation to the fullest degree. This encourages all members of the group to contribute their energy and so maximize output. The nurse manager applies motivation theory to accomplish this aspect of group behaviour.

Communication patterns

Finally, there is the question of communication patterns. Here the nurse manager addresses the issues of who is talking with whom, what is said, how it is said, and who is listening (or not listening). She also takes note of non-verbal behaviour which can be an important way of sending signals or messages. Communicating with individuals is quite different to communicating with a group. When communicating with a group, its size, composition, sophistication, organization, and structure must be considered (Gillies 1989: 191).

La Monica (1986: 145) provides three examples of communication networks which affect the nurse manager's ability in areas such as the speed with which tasks are performed, their accuracy, the satisfaction attached to the job, and its flexibility. The three communication networks are reproduced below.

Figure 9.1: Classic communication networks (La Monica 1986)

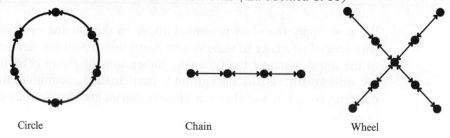

Circle   Chain   Wheel

Bowles, Barrett and Leavitt (in La Monica 1986: 45) found that the circle network yielded slow group speed, poor accuracy, and no informal leader, but good job satisfaction and rapid adaptation to change. The chain, by contrast, gave speedy performance, good accuracy, an increased probability that a leader would emerge, but poor job satisfaction and a slow adaptation to change. In the case of the wheel (so-called because all instructions must go through the central person) the leader is the dominant figure in the group. Performance here is speedy, and accuracy is of a high order. Despite this, job satisfaction tends to be poor and adaptation to change is slow. The nurse manager takes the choice of communication network into account in maximizing efficiency and satisfaction.

Group cohesion and membership

Group cohesion describes the measure of attractiveness of the group to its members. If members feel accepted and liked by others, and have similar qualities, attitudes, and values, attraction is increased

(Stanhope and Lancaster 1988: 278). If group members are willing to accept group decisions, this indicates group cohesion. Similarly, if the group demonstrates a commitment to a common goal, cohesion exists.

The nurse manager's task is to facilitate this cohesive quality in the interests of favourable outcomes to group activity. Sometimes subgroups form within the group and these are called *cliques*. It is in the interests of the nurse manager to identify clique-forming behaviour which usually comes from friendships or from common needs. These common needs may be at variance with the overall goals which the nurse manager wishes to achieve. When cliques form, factions develop. These split the group and the potential for disharmony is considerable, if not inevitable. Lippitt and Seashore (in La Monica 1986: 146) say that, ideally, group members should retain individuality within a general framework of group unity. It is the task of the nurse manager, in the interests of group unity, to steer the group towards this ideal, thus optimizing group functions.

When group members become too welded to group loyalty and unity, no matter what the cost, a situation exists which is called *groupthink* (Rosenblum 1982: 28). Characteristics which are exhibited by a group when they engage in 'groupthink' are the following:

- Most or all of the members think that they are invulnerable and this gives them a sense of overconfidence. The result is that they tend to take reckless or dangerous risks.

- Negative feedback is ignored or, if it is not ignored, the group members rationalize their decisions with the result that they do not consider whether there is really some truth in the negative criticism that is levelled at them.

- Members believe without question in the inherent morality of the group with the result that the ethical consequences of their decisions are ignored (Rosenblum 1982: 28).

- Group members are subjective regarding people who disagree with them. They consider their adversaries to be completely wrong, or weak and badly informed.

- Pressure is placed on any member, even the leader, who expresses any doubt or misgivings about the group's ideas.

- The group members who themselves doubt the value of certain decisions keep these doubts to themselves.

- People who 'groupthink' prefer unanimous decisions. Although they would accept a majority vote, they prefer complete consensus among group members.

How can the nurse manager recognize the symptoms of 'groupthink' and what can she do to counteract them when she has made the diagnosis?

1. When a leader or a group is too task-orientated, it wants to finish each item on an agenda and make decisions without a full discussion of all the alternatives. The discussion then typically centres around two alternatives, without a critical analysis of a wide variety of possibilities. The result is a decision which everybody agrees with, but which is ineffective. The solution would be to be less hurried, to arrange for a second meeting in order for the group members to collect more information, and to think of more alternative courses of action in order to reach a better solution (Rosenblum 1982: 29).

2. Group members do not want to 'reopen an issue' when new information comes to the fore about it. The nurse manager should encourage the group to reopen the issue because the discussion of the new information might lead to completely different decisions on the matter.

3. When group members make little or no attempt to obtain information from experts within an organization who might supply more precise estimates of potential losses and gains, the nurse manager should confront the group members and try to enlist them to go out and collect information from everyone who shares a certain problem. The opinions of a wide variety of nurses are sought regarding a problematic issue — for instance, sending nurses who are unskilled in ICU nursing as relief workers to ICU units. The results of such an opinion poll may then lead to completely different decisions regarding relief for ICU personnel than was taken before when decisions were only made on limited information.

4. Group members show interest in facts and opinions which support their preferred policy, ignoring facts and opinions which do not support them. Here again, the nurse manager will have to challenge the group to collect all available information, to be open to new ideas and data, and not to close the discussion on the matter until all the information has been considered (Rosenblum 1982: 29).

5. Once the group has made a decision, it spends little time thinking about how the decision might be hindered by bureaucratic red tape, sabotaged by political opponents, or temporarily derailed by common problems. The group must thus be taught to be prepared for pitfalls or barriers that can lead to failure or frustration, it must learn to confront rivals intelligently, and to talk to political

opponents. Talking to rivals or opponents is difficult, but it is educational because one becomes more aware of how they think and what their opinions regarding the issues at stake are (Rosenblum 1982: 30).

Group climate

Are group members in harmony with one another? What relationship exists between them? La Monica (1986: 147) deals with this subject in the following way: are members competitive, tense, polite, friendly, flat, energetic, enthusiastic? Once again, the nurse manager has the task of steering individuals in the group in a direction which creates a climate which is positive. Enthusiasm and energetically co-ordinated behaviour are usually conducive to good results, just as the opposite produces poor results.

Group norms

Norms are ground rules or standards. Group norms can be set by the leader — the nurse manager — when the group's activities are in their infancy. This prevents courses of action which may take the group away from its chosen direction. Usually, however, group norms come from the majority of group members. They decide what behaviour is appropriate and acceptable. Norms may be explicit or implicit. They may even be outside the awareness of individual group members. The leader facilitates awareness and frequent examination of group norms (La Monica 1986: 148).

Group decision-making procedures

What procedures does a group follow in making its decisions? The nurse manager, as leader, is responsible for procedural rules, which have been formalized by Schein (in La Monica 1986: 148):

1. Decision by lack of response (the plop). This occurs when members suggest decisions without due discussion of issues and alternatives; the group simply bypasses the ideas. Then one idea is suggested and the group immediately decides that it is the best. There are usually hidden attitudes operating which are often a lack of commitment to the goal and/or feelings of powerlessness on the part of members. The results of this kind of group decision-making procedure are negative feelings about self and other group members. (It is clear that the competent nurse manager, being aware of the potential for this kind of outcome, can steer the group away from 'the plop' as soon as it becomes clear that decisions are premature and emanate from a lack of discussion.)

2. Decision by authority rule. Authority is delegated to someone in a position of power — the leader. (This may or may not be the nurse manager to whom this chapter is directed.) This type of group decision is fine if the leader communicates that she will make the decision but that she needs advice. If, however, the leader communicates that the group can decide on a course of action and then concludes the session by ignoring the group's suggestions, then the group may feel duped — and rightfully so. Such action results in many negative feelings towards the leader, with harmful long-term effects. (Clearly the nurse manager, if she finds herself in this position, should guard against the type of outcome described here.)

3. Decision by majority rule. One person or more uses pressure tactics to railroad a decision in this decision-making style. The balance of the members are left feeling impotent, helpless and 'out of step'. They may wonder what happened. (This type of leadership may alienate group members and the manager practising it may later find increased levels of animosity among her group and, worse still, a tendency for those most alienated to form cliques or factions which can then attack the leader — perhaps with the intention of removing and replacing her.)

4. Decision by majority rule: voting and/or polling. This is the commonest style of group decision-making. The position of each group member on the issue is requested either formally (by voting) or informally (by polling). A member can be for or against an issue or resolution, or can abstain from deciding. The best group procedure is to state the issue and then facilitate group discussion of all sides of the issue; decision by voting and/or polling follows. If the group must implement the decision — that is, if its members must individually do something in order for the goal to be attained — then group decision by majority rule is not best. Decision by consensus would be better because it is more likely that group members will be committed to the decision and less probable that the decision or task will be undermined during implementation.

5. Decisions by consensus. This is a psychological state in which group members see a rationale in the decision and agree to support it. This operates even though some members may be more or less committed than others.

6. Decision by unanimous vote. This, though desirable, is rarely used in organizations. It is used in jury trials, but consensus is usually sufficient in management situations.

The above allows one to proceed to the more specific question of the leader's role since this individual is usually the initiator, the trend-setter, and the person responsible for the choice of decision-making style or type of decision. If the wrong choice is made, the group response could be one that is not desired or anticipated, and possibly even one that is destructive to group functions, the climate of the group, and future relations within it. It could also lead to 'group disintegration', so leadership style and choice are important.

GROUP ROLES

To increase the effectiveness of group endeavours one must comprehend the role each member plays in the group. One might pose the questions: do members understand their roles; how do they perceive their roles: are they aware of the role they play in the group; is their behaviour juxtaposed against that of other group members? We examine, in the first instance, the role of the group leader (the nurse manager in this case, who plays the most important role in the group) and in the second the roles of group members. La Monica (1986: 149) emphasizes the point that group members may be seen in a number of different roles at the same time or during a particular group session.

Role of the formal leader

A formal leader is in a powerful position for she can assume complete control, or delegate her authority, or pass control to the group. One sees from this that the momentum needed to reach a group's goals can come from two quarters — either from the leader or from the group.

The role which the leader adopts depends on the way in which the system is organized. Stogdill and Coons (in La Monica 1986: 149) offer four leadership styles:

1. High structure and low consideration (leadership style 1).

2. High structure and high consideration (leadership style 2).

3. High consideration and low structure (leadership style 3).

4. Low structure and low consideration (leadership style 4).

Implicit in these four styles is the fact that leadership style 1 represents the immature system where group problem solving is inappropriate. Here the group has neither the knowledge nor the experience to discuss an issue. This knowledge and experience must be gained before two-way communication (leader to group members and group members to leader) can proceed. In the case of leadership style 2, the leader should maintain control since both consideration and structure are high and the system is moving towards maturity. In leadership styles 3 and 4, control shifts from leader to group, with almost complete delegation in the latter case since the group can function with minimal leader intervention.

A leader of a group may be appointed to her position, or a leader may emerge from a 'leaderless' group. This emerging leader comes from the more dominant members of a group and undertakes one or more aspects of the leadership role. The inherent desire for structure within a group causes this emergence of a leader. It is interesting to note that such an emergent leader tends to communicate in a more aggressive and authoritarian manner than the leader who was appointed to her position (Gillies 1989: 195).

The effects of the different leadership styles are the following:

- The autocratic leader is quick to criticize harshly and quick to praise superfluously. Such leaders are orientated to the achievement of the task, keeping the group's attention focused on the goal. Their leadership behaviour creates hostility amongst group members, and weaker members tend to shy away from responsibility.

- The democratic leader tends to stimulate group members towards self-direction, providing them with the necessary information and with suggestions to act upon. They are not as quick as autocratic leaders to praise or to criticize. Democratic leaders produce more group cohesiveness among members.

- The laissez-faire leader tends to throw the responsibility for the achievement of goals back to the group members, without preparing them to handle the responsibility (Gillies 1989: 195).

Roles of group members

Two categories of functions must be performed for group goals to be accomplished. These are task functions and maintenance functions.

La Monica's diagram (figure 9.2) is useful in illustrating the relationship between leader behaviour and group roles:

From figure 9.2 one also notes that the group's task and maintenance functions are linked to goal accomplishment. What are these functions? Task functions are the group's tasks — in essence, what the group hopes to accomplish. The maintenance functions are concerned with how the group carries out its tasks. The leader's input is obviously dictated by the amount of intervention necessary, which is in turn a reflection of group maturity as described above. The task roles include those of:

1. Initiator — defines problems and suggests procedures.

2. Information seeker — expresses ideas and requests information.

3. Information giver — gives information, ideas, and facts.

4. Clarifier — defines terms and clarifies concepts.

5. Explorer — investigates all options, looks for deeper meanings and alternatives.

6. Summarizer — draws together loose threads and ideas.

7. Consensus-maker — draws a group towards a conclusion.

8. Record keeper — records and maintains trends of discussions.

Maintenance roles include those of:

1. Standard setter — maintains standards.

2. Encourager — stimulates acceptance of the ideas of others.

3. Supporter — provides support for group performance.

4. Harmonizer — reduces and removes areas of conflict.

5. Compromiser — maintains group cohesiveness through compromise.

6. Gatekeeper — encourages communication and group participation.

Figure 9.2: Roles of group members

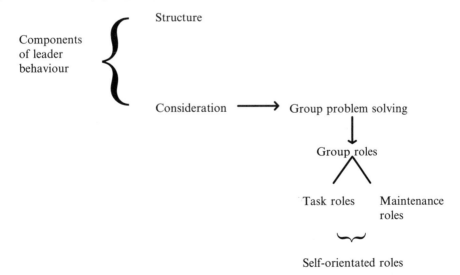

Sometimes group members try to satisfy their own needs using the group as a medium and a platform. In such cases their role becomes dysfunctional. La Monica (1986: 152) lists self-oriented players as follows:

1. The aggressor — displays attacking behaviour.

2. The blocker — negative and stubborn, brings up issues already decided upon.

3. The recognition-seeker — self-centered boastful behaviour.

4. The playboy — cynical and humorous on important occasions.

5. The dominator — authoritative, interruptive and assertive.

6. The help-seeker — requests sympathetic response.

These types are all recognizable by definition, with the possible exception of 'the playboy' who La Monica describes as one who 'displays lack of interest by being cynical and humorous on important occasions' (La Monica 1986: 152).

TYPES OF GROUPS

Three types of groups are recognized in the nursing situation: task groups, teaching groups, and supportive or therapeutic groups (Clark 1986: 4). The various types of groups must not be confused with task and maintenance functions. Regardless of the type of group, task and maintenance functions or roles must be fulfilled for the group to work at its highest level of performance.

Task groups

These are set up to accomplish a specific task, with decision-making and problem-solving as their principle objectives. Health care planning committees, nursing service committees, nursing teams, nursing care conference groups, and hospital staff meetings are all examples of task groups where nurses participate. These groups are problem-orientated and they are usually under pressure to complete a given task within a given period of time. There is frequently underlying conflict because not all members of the group identify the problem in the same way, so there is a tendency to ignore, deny, or try to cover up the conflict.

Teaching groups

As the name implies, teaching groups are set up to pass information on to others: other nurses or clients. One has to take into consideration all the principles of learning — for example, the student's readiness to learn and the student's present knowledge, amongst others.

Supportive or therapeutic groups

The purpose of these groups is to assist members in dealing with emotional stress. The focus here is on the member's thoughts, feelings, and subsequent behaviour. Clark (1986: 7) notes that these groups are not a form of psychotherapy but are educational and should be used to help participants deal with emotional stress.

IMPLICATIONS FOR NURSES

All organizations have objectives and these objectives can be attained through the activities and decisions of the groups that administer the organization. A hospital service is such an organization, and it is the responsibility of the nurse manager to influence group processes to attain the administration's objectives. How can this be done?

In an attempt to increase the interdependence of group members, the nurse manager, as a leader within the system, can plan work and arrange assignments with this goal in mind. This can be achieved by fostering and encouraging the sharing of common interests and by exerting some control over rewards and punishments when work goals are either attained or not attained. In a similar vein it has been shown elsewhere in this chapter that, irrespective of whether a group has a leader or not, the functions of the group members continue to operate. The day-to-day administrative functions of the hospital nurse come to mind in this context. The nurse manager can, however, act as a facilitator by exercising a constructive influence on the group. In this way individual and group performance can be enhanced through leadership behaviour. This role within group dynamics is one of the primary roles of the nurse manager.

The nurse manager must also have a concern for the direction in which groups are moving. She constantly revitalizes and redirects the group's attention towards the goals she has set, particularly when her observations and analyses show that the group has a tendency to lose direction and to lose sight of objectives. Her task is to evaluate progress — a function which cannot be achieved without the assistance and support of other group members — so nurse managers use groups in making decisions (Sullivan and Decker 1992: 257).

In a text by Scandiffio (1990: 77–109), reference is made to the importance of group dynamics in the nurse/manager situation. This author notes that group dynamics play a significant role within any culture, organization, or unit.

Whatever the structure of an organization, it will contain people who have different ideas, different motivations, different backgrounds, and often different agendas, and so a cultural bond must be developed and nurtured. It often happens that one of the group becomes uncomfortable with the culture and begins to change his or her behaviour. This introduces stress for the leader because it is difficult for her to be objective as she sees the cohesiveness of the group falling apart. Under such circumstances she must remember that the employee creating the disturbance is still an integral part of the group and special attention must be given to the employee.

Scandiffio promotes the idea that it is beneficial to perceive the employee who exhibits problematic behaviour as one who needs the benefit of the manager's experience and skills. The employee must not be alienated from the group. At times when there is a divergence of opinion and a potential for conflict, the nurse manager should adopt an introspective perspective and analyse her own views, power, communication, and corporate culture before trying to understand another's point of view.

It is important that the manager should understand her own motivation before offering assistance to another. This recognition of personal insecurities makes it easier to recognize staff dysfunction. It follows that there is a need for the nurse manager to have confidence and feel secure in herself, so that she operates from a secure and stable psychological base before asking her staff to make changes. La Monica (1986: 143) quotes Lippitt and Seashore in saying that the leader's goal is the development of an effective team by facilitating:

1. a clear understanding of purposes and goals;

2. flexibility in how a group accomplishes goals;

3. effective communication and understanding among members — on personal feelings and attitudes as well as task-related ideas and issues;

4. effective decision-making strategies that secure the commitment of members to important decisions;

5. an appropriate balance between group productivity and individual satisfaction;

6. group maturity, so that leadership responsibilities can be shared according to the group's ability and willingness;

7. group cohesiveness, while maintaining the needed measure of individual freedom;

8. the use of the employees' different abilities;

9. the group's ability to solve its own problems;

10. a balance between emotional and rational behaviour — steering emotions into productive teamwork.

The nursing profession, being anthropocentric, creates numerous situations in which nurse leaders and especially nurse managers are called upon to solve group problems. A knowledge of group dynamics can be utilized in the context of nursing leadership, but also as an influence on the health behaviour of patients in a hospital or on clients in the community. La Monica (1986: 152) lists the common nursing groups as staff support groups, teaching situations, procedural issues, patient discussions, conferences on directives which have come from another authority and self-help groups.

COMMITTEES

Much of the work in the nursing service is done through committees. The nurse manager who knows how to use committees effectively can greatly increase the productivity in her service. The manager using a relational style of management, as opposed to a direct management style, sees committee work as valuable, because individuals learn to work with each other, come to understand the challenges and problems of the organization, and tap each other's creativity (Veninga 1984: 43).

Committees are useful when problems need to be solved which require a number of specialists' knowledge or multiple input from various sources for its solution. The manager must bear in mind that committees should not be used to override the authority of line managers. Committees are better at handling larger issues such as major policy changes or long-term planning rather than day-to-day decisions.

The nurse manager, when deciding on committees and their structures, will therefore first have to determine which functions in her service could be carried out more effectively by committees than by individuals. She will also have to decide whether a committee fulfills a vital need/function which is not within the scope of another committee and whether the total number of committees is appropriate for the size of the nursing division and its objectives (Stevens 1975: 15).

Committee powers and membership

Before using a committee, the degree of power to be delegated to the group must first be considered. It is important for committee members to understand clearly the degree and type of power that is vested in them.

A committee should do work, and not merely satisfy the status needs of personnel, nor be merelyt an exercise in democratic management (Stevens 1975: 15). The individuals best suited to the goals of the committee should be selected to serve on it. Care should be taken to prevent the overuse of the same reliable staff members on a number of committees.

A committee should contain the smallest number of people who will be able to meet its objectives. With large projects, the number of committee members can be controlled by creating a small stable executive body responsible for carrying out the work, and giving them the power to co-opt other members as needed during the various stages of the project.

Committee productivity and functioning

It is very easy for committee members to use their time unproductively. The nurse manager must carefully compare the number of hours used on committee meetings with the results achieved by the committee. A committee may be unproductive because there is no real reason for its existence, because the leader lacks appropriate leadership skills, or because the mix of members on the committee is incompatible with its objectives. If the committee members each have a heavy workload, and if they find it difficult to fit participation in the committee meetings into their work programmes, it is also unrealistic to expect good results (Stevens 1975: 16).

The functions which generally form part of a committee's activities are problem-solving, research, setting standards, designing, monitoring, and evaluating. To perform these functions, the committee members must communicate with each other, express their ideas, compromise to reach workable solutions, reason among themselves, and reach consensus regarding decisions. The committee members inform others in the service about their activities by educating them, making recommendations, by clarifying issues, summarizing their activities, and encouraging participation in new projects.

Types of committees

Different types of committees can be found in a nursing service, for example standing committees, ad hoc or design committees, peer group committees, steering committees, and interdivisional or interdepartmental committees.

- Standing committees — eg standards committees, education committees. This type of committee meets on a regular basis and has a continuing function.

- Peer group committees — eg the senior professional nurse's committee. This type of committee meets on a regular basis, is composed of members of the same staff level or group, and deals with day-to-day operational problems.

- Ad hoc committees — eg the nursing audit committee and the annual end-of-the-year function committee. This type of committee is established to handle a specific function or solve a specific problem, and is convened on a temporary basis.

- Interdepartmental committees — eg quality circle committees, hospital management committees. This type of committee consists of members representing different departments in the hospital — eg nursing, the laboratory, medical records, etc. The purpose of such a committee is to identify interdepartmental problems and improve interdepartmental co-operation (Lochhaas 1987: 3).

Advantages of committees

Group problem-solving has some major advantages over individual problem-solving.

1. More knowledge and information is available. When a problem is of such magnitude that no single individual possesses adequate information to solve the problem, a group should be formed — for example quality circles can be formed to improve productivity.

2. More solutions to a problem may be generated. In a group it may be found that some individuals arrive at solutions through concrete experience, some by reflective observation, some through active experimentation, and others through abstract conceptualization.

3. There is an increased acceptance of solutions. When staff members have been involved in the decision-making process they are generally more committed to the implementation of the decisions than when they are not involved.

4. Committees are cost-effective. Group meetings cost less than meetings between the leader and each member of the group because less working time is consumed. Group meetings cost, on average, 54% of the cost of one-on-one meetings between individuals.

5. Groups take risks more readily. Groups tend to be more innovative and daring in their solutions to problems than individuals.

Disadvantages of committees

1. Decisions may be reached prematurely. When group members do not do their homework, when they do not want to spend time discussing a problem sufficiently, and when they reach decisions which are popular but not necessarily effective, the group decision might be inferior to one made by an individual.

2. Individuals with strong personalities might dominate the group. Domination by one or two individuals may dampen the enthusiasm of others, with the result that the other members may become withdrawn, may fail to contribute, may not share in the decision-making, and may not support decisions taken.

3. Disruptive conflicts erode decision-making energy. When some members in a group feel threatened by others, the energy of the group is no longer focused on the accomplishment of tasks, but rather on arguments about position. The reason for the existence of the group is then lost (Veninga 1984: 43–5).

Rules for effective participation

In general, a group will usually tend to be effective when the following conditions are present (Sullivan and Decker 1992: 272):

- the individual members are attracted to it;
- there is mutual trust among the members;
- the norms and goals of the group are in agreement with those of the organization;
- the task to be accomplished or goal to be achieved is matched by the size of the group, its structure, and the diversity of its members;
- group members are motivated to communicate openly with each other and to co-operate with one another;
- the group is rewarded for the attainment of the goal;
- social loafing is reduced.

Committee leadership skills

There are a number of basic rules which the group leader who wants to run effective meetings must adhere to.

Preparing for a meeting

1. Preparation of the physical environment:
   - Reserve a room well in advance.
   - Ensure adequate ventilation and light, comfortable seating, as well as space for writing.

2. Preparation of the agenda:
   - The agenda should clearly indicate the purpose of the meeting.
   - The number of topics to be covered should fit in with the time allowed for the meeting.
   - Each topic on the agenda should have a specific objective.
   - Sometimes discussions during meetings can be expedited by indicating roughly how much time should be devoted to each topic (Stevens 1975: 20).
   - The committee members should receive the agenda well in advance of the meeting in order to have time for adequate preparation for the discussion. (It is, however, unwise to dispatch the agenda fourteen days before a meeting because it will inevitably be put aside and be either completely forgotten or just be grabbed before the meeting is to take place).
   - The agenda should not be too brief. Agendas are also commonly too vague. For example, the phrase 'develop budget' tells nobody very much, but the phrase 'to discuss the proposal for the reduction of the recommended budget items for each unit' helps everyone to get their facts and figures together for the meeting.
   - A long agenda is thus in order if its length is the result of describing each item in more detail.
   - Try to briefly state why each topic is to be discussed.
   - Organize agenda items under such headings as: 'for information', 'for discussion' or 'for decision'.
   - The order of the items on the agenda is important. The items for urgent decision should come before those that can wait for another meeting (Jay 1982: 25).

Other agenda considerations
   - The early part of a meeting tends to be more lively and creative than the end. If an item needs mental energy, bright ideas, and clear thinking it should be put high on the list.

- If one item is of great interest and concern to everyone, it should be held back for a while, and some other work done first.

- Some items unite a meeting and some divide the members. It may sometimes be useful to start with a unified front before entering into division, or at other times it may be useful to do it the other way round. It is necessary to make a conscious choice on this. It is usually a good idea to end the meeting with an item which would enhance unity (Jay 1982: 25).

- It is often found that too much time is spent on trivial but urgent items, leaving little or no time for subjects of fundamental importance which usually have more long-term significance. This can be remedied by putting on the agenda the time when the long-term issue should be started, and sticking to it.

- A meeting usually does not achieve much after an hour-and-a-half. It is good practice to put the starting time as well as the finishing time on the agenda.

- If meetings tend to go on too long, the meeting could be scheduled to start an hour before lunch or an hour before the end of the workday.

- The papers or reports which are circulated to group members in advance must not be too long otherwise they will not be read or studied.

- If papers are produced at a meeting for discussion, they should be to-the-point, brief, and simple for a quick perusal.

- Listing the words 'any other business' on the agenda invites time-wasting. An extra agenda item may well be added at the meeting, but it should be fairly simple and straightforward.

- Decide whether it is necessary to invite anyone who might have specialist or specific knowledge regarding the topics on the agenda. If necessary, invite such people well in advance and discuss their roles with them.

- Develop questions to stimulate discussion. Such discussion should achieve the meeting's objectives, but questions could also be used to move from one topic to the next.

- Additional material or handouts (as well as extra copies of the agenda) which the participants must use in the meeting should be prepared beforehand.

- The strategies (eg brainstorming, or the nominal group technique) to be used during the meeting should be determined and be studied beforehand.

3. Preparation of participants.

- Any statistical data, survey or audit results, or any other documents which will be needed during the discussion, should be gathered in advance. Copies of these materials should be distributed to the members, together with the agenda, for an in-depth study before the meeting is to take place.

- If there are any materials that the participants should bring to the meeting, these must be indicated in advance to them.

- If a specific presentation or contribution is expected from a group member, the request for this should be made to the individual well in advance in order for her to have special time to prepare.

4. Preparation by the leader.

- The agenda topics should be reviewed and the necessary background information and supportive data on the agenda topics should be assembled.

Conducting the meeting

1. If necessary, participants can be supplied with paper, pencils, and name cards.

2. The door should be have a notice on it, specifying that a meeting is in progress.

3. The secretary should take all telephone calls and messages for distribution to participants after the meeting.

4. The leader should welcome everybody.

5. An individual should be appointed to keep the minutes of the meeting.

6. Each topic should be introduced with a summary of past actions, decisions, and what is to be accomplished during the present meeting, or a new topic should be introduced by supplying the necessary background information.

7. The duty of the leader is to see that the participants produce meaningful discussions and reach appropriate decisions regarding the different topics. This could be done by:

- Asking questions. When the pace of a meeting is slowing down, the leader can stimulate the group in this way.

- Encouraging participation. When there are quieter members who are not sharing their opinions with the others, it is a good idea to direct a question to such a person, eg 'Sally, what is your viewpoint on this matter? Perhaps you have an interesting idea to share with us.'

- Clarifying group questions or discussions. The leader should possess sufficient background knowledge to clarify issues which the group is not clear about, or to supply additional information where asked.

- Rephrase group comments. By rephrasing comments made by the group or summarizing what has been discussed and decided at regular intervals during the proceedings, the discussion can be stimulated (Stevens 1975: 20; Lochhaas 1987: 12–13).

8. It is the leader's responsibility to prevent misunderstandings and confusion. Clarification from the speaker should be sought if an argument cannot be followed. If two people are using the same word with different meanings the speaker should clarify the matter.

9. One of the most common faults of the chairman is the failure to close the meeting when nothing more can be accomplished. A meeting should be closed when more facts are required, when the meeting needs the viewpoints of people who are not present, when members need more time to think or discuss a subject in depth, when the time available is insufficient to go over the subject properly, and when two or three members can settle the issue outside the meeting.

10. The leader or chairman should give a brief and clear summary of what has been agreed upon at the end of the discussion of each agenda item (Jay 1982: 26)

Managing the people in a meeting

1. Punctuality. The only way to ensure that meetings start on time is to actually go ahead and start them at the time specified, even if it is known that someone is still to arrive. Punctuality at future meetings can be encouraged by listing all the names of theose people who arrived late in the minutes!

2. Seating arrangements. If members sit face-to-face across a table, this facilitates opposition and disagreement. Sitting side-by-side makes it more difficult to confront a person and disagree with her. Generally speaking, the closer one is seated to the chairman, the more honoured one should feel.

3. Control the long-winded speaker. As chairman you should indicate that time is precious and that if the speaker does not cut her story short the others will not have an opportunity to give their opinions. If the person must be stopped while talking, pick a phrase that she is using, eg 'reaching consensus' and say 'Sister Smith, do you agree that reaching consensus is absolutely necessary?' in order to stop the person by way of interruption.

4. Get the silent person to contribute. By asking the quiet person for her view directly, the chairman may find that a valuable contribution is made or that she has a hostile reaction to the meeting in general, or the process by which decisions are reached. It is better to get the hostility out in the open and to deal with it rather than ignoring it (Jay 1982: 27).

5. Encourage a clash of ideas. A clash of personalities must be discouraged, but a crossflow of debate must be stimulated by the chairman probing, stimulating, guiding, mediating, and summarizing points. If two people seem to get cross with one another, widen the discussion by directing a question to a neutral member.

6. Protect the weaker members. It is the chairman's responsibility to see that junior members get a chance to contribute. When senior members seem to override the junior ones, it is the chairman's duty to make a special comment regarding a junior member's idea and to reinforce that person's contribution by writing the point down to refer to it later in the meeting.

7. Get suggestions from members. It is easy to ridicule suggestions because they are not facts or opinions. It is, however, useful to have as many suggestions offered as possible, because although only a few of them lead to anything, some might, in an adapted version, just lead to creative directions for the organization in future. A suggestion should thus not be squelched — the best part should be picked out and the other committee members should try to build onto it to make it a workable one.

8. Let the senior people contribute at the end. When a senior member makes a contribution at the beginning of a meeting, the junior members become inhibited. It is thus wise to get the viewpoints of the junior members before giving seniors a chance.

9. Stop side conversations. If side conversations are disruptive, stop talking until the culprits stop.

10. Keep the meeting focused. If a member strays and does not keep to the point under discussion, restate the main points under discussion and thank the person concerned for her comments.

11. Manage domineering members. When one member does not allow others to express their views, the chairman should direct specific questions at the other members, ask the person concerned to wait until the others have expressed their views, and address specific detailed questions regarding the topic to her (Lochhaas 1987: 84).

12. End the meeting with a note of achievement. Even if the final item remained unresolved, the chairman can refer to an earlier item which was well resolved as she closes the meeting and thanks everybody for their contributions. If a date for a next meeting must be set, it is wise to decide on it with the diaries of every member at hand (Jay 1982: 27).

Recording of minutes

1. The minutes of the meeting should include the official name of the meeting or committee, the time it commenced and the time it ended, the date, the chairperson, the recorder of the minutes, the names of all present, apologies for absence, and the date, time, and place of the next meeting.

2. The first topic of the meeting is usually the approval of the minutes from the previous meeting. Corrections should be made in red ink on the original copy.

3. The recording of items discussed should be simple, clear, and as brief as possible. Only relevant information that relates to the topics should be recorded. The actions/recommendations agreed upon should be indicated and the name of the person responsible for the action should be underlined.

4. A copy of the minutes should be sent to each member of the committee whether present or absent.

5. The typing should be double-spaced to make it easier to write in corrections.

6. The minute topics should be numbered consecutively with the agenda items for easy reference.

7. Abbreviations should be avoided. When referring to individuals, their full names should be used.

8. If a meeting or part of a meeting is strictly informational (no decisions required) the information should be recorded under the heading 'discussions'. The information should be brief and clear. If a problem remained unresolved and must be followed-up at a further meeting, it should be entered under the heading 'follow-up' and the name of the person responsible for the

follow-up, if appropriate, should be indicated (Jay 1982: 28; Lochhaas 1987: 23–5).

CONCLUSION

This chapter examined group dynamics in general terms and as they pertain to the nurse manager and the nursing profession. The general concepts underpin the professional realities. The goal is to make groups more effective and to increase the cost-effectiveness of the services (La Monica 1986: 157). Leaders who have studied and understood the complexities of groups have administrative advantages which remove many of the day-to-day problems encountered in the hospital situation where both patients and staff are members of groups. 'Studying group dynamics is ... an essential aspect of the leader's responsibilities — fostering team maturity' (La Monica 1986: 157). So one can say that areas of group behaviour that require observation and study include the following: goals, background, participation, communication, cohesion, membership, climate, norms, and decision-making procedures.

References

Clark, C. C. (1987). *The Nurse as Group Leader*. Second edition. Springer: New York.

Forsyth, D. R. (1990). *Group Dynamics*. Second edition. Brooks/Cole: Pacific Grove.

Ganong, W. L. and Ganong, J. M. (1972). Reducing organizational conflict through working committees. *Journal of Nursing Administration,* volume 2, number 1, pp. 12–19.

Gillies, D.A. (1989). *Nursing Management: A Systems Approach*. Second edition. Saunders: Philadelphia.

Hall, J. (ed) (1988). *Models for Management: the Structure of Competence*. Second edition. Woodstead Press: The Woodlands.

Jay, A. (1982). How to run a meeting. *Journal of Nursing Administration,* volume 12, number. 1, pp. 22–8.

La Monica, E. L. (1986). *Nursing Leadership and Management. An Experiential Approach*. Jones and Bartlett: Boston.

Lochhaas, T. (ed) (1987). *Group Leadership Skills for Nurse Managers*. Mosby: St Louis.

Rosenblum, E. H. (1982). Groupthink: one peril of group cohesiveness. *Journal of Nursing Administration,* volume 12, number 4, pp. 27–31.

Scandiffio, A. L. (1990). Group dynamics. *Nurse-Manager's Bookshelf,* volume 2, number 4, pp. 77-109.

Stanhope, M. and Lancaster, J. (1988). *Community Health Nursing. Process and Practice for Promoting Health.* Second edition. Mosby: St Louis.

Stevens, B. J. (1975). Use of groups for management. *Journal of Nursing Administration,* volume 5, number. 7, pp. 14–22.

Sullivan, E. J. and Decker, P. J. (1992). *Effective Management in Nursing.* Third edition. Addison-Wesley: Redwood City.

Sundeen, S. J., Stuart, G. W., Rankin, E. A. D. and Cohen, S. A. (1989). *Nurse Client Interaction Implementing the Nursing Process.* St Louis: Mosby.

Veninga, R. L. (1984). Benefits and costs of group meetings. *Journal of Nursing Administration,* volume 14, number 6, 42–6.

CHAPTER 10

COMMUNICATION

S. W. Booyens

CONTENTS

INTRODUCTION

More than 80% of the top level executive's time is spent on communication — 16% reading, 9% writing, 30% speaking, and 45% listening (Swansburg 1990: 385). It is thus clear why the top level nurse manager needs to develop her communication skills.

Communication involves a sender of a message, the message itself, and a receiver of the message. Effective communication only occurs when the recipient of the message interprets the meaning of the message in the way intended by the sender. It is, however, a fact of life that communication often fails to achieve its intended objective. This is because people perceive things in different ways and therefore vary in their interpretation of a message.

In order to communicate, the sender must know what the recipient expects to perceive and hear because the human mind tends to perceive what it expects to perceive. Even where a person has perceived the intended meaning of a message, messages are usually retained selectively because of the individual's emotional association with them. Messages may also be retained or rejected according to whether they give rise to good or bad emotional associations within a particular individual (Swansburg 1990: 388).

CLIMATE FOR COMMUNICATION

The traditional nurse manager, who is unable to break through the barriers of the bureaucratic organization in which she is operating, creates a *defensive climate* for communication. In this type of climate, the assumed superiority of the leaders is supported by a hierarchical structure and chain of command. The nurse's work performance is usually evaluated annually and the evaluation consists mainly of one-way communication. Strategic planning is carried out at top level, with no input from subordinates, and there is a tendency for standardization of most of the procedures — even orientation procedures. The view of the supervisor is usually emphasized through control measures (Beck and Beck, referred to by Swansburg 1990: 387).

By contrast, the *supportive communication* climate fosters an acknowledgement of the ideas of many individuals and thus encourages employees to ask questions and to give solutions to problems. Every employee is free to talk to managers at any level of the organization without fear of any kind of retribution. Opportunities for this are planned and communicated to all staff members. There is a spontaneous atmosphere in the organization, and experimentation is encouraged. Management by objectives is usually practised — the employee sets objectives to be attained with the help of the supervisor (Beck and Beck, as referred to by Swansburg 1990: 387).

Research concerning the characteristics of organizations and the communication between superiors and subordinates revealed the following:

- subordinates in the lower levels of the organizational hierarchy perceive less openness in superior–subordinate communications than subordinates at higher levels of the hierarchy;

- openness in communications decreases as organizations increase in size, particularly if they have more than 1000 employees;

- although the employees in large organizations perceive communication to be less open in nature, more communication takes place in big organizations than in smaller ones;

- from the observations made about openness in relation to span of control, it was concluded that the quality of interactions may be more important than their quantity (Joblin 1982, as referred to by Swansburg 1990: 386).

The climate of the organization also determines whether an open- or closed-door policy will reign. When a nurse manager operates an open-door policy this implies that a nurse or sister can walk into her office at any time to discuss matters that they have on their minds. In practice, however, the person who walks into the nurse manager's office will find her attending to her own schedule of work which cannot be interrupted easily. Therefore it is always more convenient for both the employee and the manager if appointments are made (Swansburg 1990: 387).

When a nurse manager wants to apply an open-door policy, she will clearly state the rules for such a policy, including whether the employee needs the permission of anyone to make an appointment with her. Such a manager will also know how to deal with confidential facts entrusted to her, and will protect both the employee and her supervisor (Swansburg 1990: 387).

FORMAL AND INFORMAL COMMUNICATION IN ORGANIZATIONS

Formal communication in health organizations occurs through various reports — eg audit reports, monthly statistical reports, reports to higher authorities, committee's monthly or annual reports, incident reports, memorandums, newsletters, and official notices regarding policy decisions or policy amendments in the organization. Formal communication would also include formal meetings between physicians and nursing staff, or between the chief professional nurse and the senior professional nurses in charge of units, or the wide variety of meetings which take place between the different professional groups in a health care setting and between the nursing staff and the supporting services.

The informal communication network — ie the grapevine — is an inherent part of the organization. This network helps employees to make sense about the world around them and in this way it provides a relief from emotional stress. If left unguarded, the grapevine can become an organization's worst enemy, but when it is managed properly it can significantly increase the productivity and job satisfaction of employees (Simmons 1985: 39).

The grapevine's communication does not really concentrate on gossip regarding individuals; about 80% of it pertains to business-related politics. It is also interesting to note that 70–90% of a message's details are usually correct. The rumours that are spread along the grapevine are in direct proportion to their importance to the employees and to the lack of information on the subject from official sources. Sending or receiving information on matters such as who is going to be transferred, who is in line for the big promotion, and which new jobs are available, fulfills a basic human need in the workplace (Simmons 1985: 41).

The grapevine can be managed — ie controlled — by the following measures:

- accept its existence and pay attention to the rumours spread;

- act promptly to determine how far a rumour has spread;

- keep employees well-informed by using the formal communication system, thereby limiting rumours;

- develop faith of the employees in the communication which comes from the managers;

- managers should make themselves available to answer questions;

- determine the cause of a rumour in order to understand employees better;

- inform key personnel of important organizational changes and decisions as soon as possible, so that they can inform everyone and get opinions from everyone;

- present negative information honestly, without sugar-coating the facts;

- a rumour cannot be stopped by silencing key communicators since the grapevine is more a product of a situation than of people (Simmons 1985: 42).

ORAL COMMUNICATION

What are the criteria for sending effective messages? In his series of articles on communication, Felix Bosch recommends the following:

- If the words used are chosen carefully the meaning of the message will be clear and accurate.

- Use language that is appropriate to the audience or listeners.

- Use the simplest words that will convey the meaning accurately in speeches and presentations. A strange word used during a speech may hamper concentration and comprehension.

- One must try to be original and develop one's own speaking style. Avoid clichés.

- Try to use well constructed, grammatically correct sentences. The length of sentences should be limited to about twenty words.

- Avoid excessive use of foreign words and phrases. Use only those that are appropriate and well known, and only for a special purpose.

- The judicious use of idioms, quotations, and similes will enhance a speech or presentation considerably. They must, however, be used correctly.

- When speaking, varying one's voice and using pauses is necessary to enhance understanding and interpretation.

- When using unfamiliar or strange words, make sure that they are pronounced correctly.

- The words used should be appropriate for the purpose of the speech or presentation (Bosch, 1992: 13).

PUBLIC SPEAKING

The successful nurse manager should master the skill of public speaking and should be able to present her views on a number of issues before the public. This essential skill is one which can be mastered by following a number of guidelines.

The major factor in effective presentations is adequate preparation. The speaker must know what the purpose of the presentation is — eg is it to inform, to persuade, to entertain, or a combination of these?

During the preparation phase the speaker must gather enough information about the topic in order to deliver an interesting speech as well as to be able to answer related questions. It is boring for the participants if they know more about a subject than the speaker, and the audience can thus become apathetic. If you give all the information in the presentation, however, then you might not have sufficient information to answer questions.

The preparation must be started well in advance so that the material can be read and adjusted to provide a smooth flow of ideas. Outlining a presentation helps to organize it. Most presentations include an introduction, a preview, a main part, and a conclusion.

The introduction must spark the interest of the audience. Humour often helps but should preferably be related to the topic. Care should be taken to avoid derogatory or cynical remarks and references to sex, religion, and other controversial issues should be carefully selected, if used at all. It pays to work hard on the introduction because it builds the confidence of the speaker when it is apparent that the audience's attention has been captured.

A preview is often used between the introduction and the main part to give the audience an idea of what is going to be discussed — this could consist of the headings under which the body of the speech is organized.

The main part or body of the presentation contains the main message and is usually broken into several main points or subsections. For each major point, adequate supportive evidence such as statistics, testimonies, practical examples or explanations should be used. 'Specifics hold an audience's attention much better than generalities' (Lancaster 1985: 32).

The conclusion ties the message together, either by way of a summary, a request, a warning, a prediction, a plea, or a motivation for future action. It should leave the audience where you want them to be left (Lancaster 1985: 32; Bosch 1992: 7).

Audiovisual aids

Organization and preparation involve deciding upon and developing the audiovisual aids that are to be included. The speaker should find out who the audience will be, what resources are available, and how long the presentation should last by discussing these matters with the host or organizer.

Visual aids help the audience to concentrate on key points, understand complex information, and recall what was presented (Lancaster 1985: 32). High-quality visual aids can help speakers feel more confident, can create interest, and can draw attention away from the speaker momentarily. Poor visual aids harm a good speech. They should thus be clear, simple, and visible to the entire audience, and they should be tailored for each situation (Lancaster 1985: 32).

Tailoring the message to the audience

Good speakers know who their audience is and try to provide useful and welcome information. Effective speakers usually keep the following questions in mind:

1. To whom am I speaking?

2. What do I want them to know, believe, or do as a result of my speech?

3. What is the most effective way of organizing and delivering my presentation to accomplish the goal (Lancaster 1985: 32)?

Ideally the speaker should know the expected size of the audience, their sex, age, language distribution, occupation, employment, cultural background, likely level of knowledge regarding the topic, and level of interest in it. This is not, however, always possible.

The larger the audience, the more formal a presentation should be. Question-and-answer-sessions and dialogue between speaker and audience are more easily accomplished if the groups consist of less than 40–50 participants (Lancaster 1985: 32).

The attitude of an audience towards the topic and speaker will also affect the presentation. If the audience is eager to hear the information and considers the speaker an expert on the topic, the presentation is easier than when the audience is hostile or when it considers the speaker arrogant or uninformed (Lancaster 1985: 33).

Preparation of the environment

Surroundings are important and, if you are in a position to have some input in their selection, you should check the following:

- the lighting and sound equipment;
- that the table or podium are in place;
- the audiovisual equipment;
- the removal of unnecessary barriers between you and the audience such as furniture and flower arrangements.

Present yourself in conventional clothes, but appear well groomed. A good night's sleep beforehand and a planned schedule leaving time to relax before addressing the audience are recommended.

The presentation

1. Speak to be heard.

2. Use voice inflection and different levels of volume to highlight key ideas and counteract the hypnotic effect of monotones.

Varying the rate of speaking also serves to hold the interest of the audience (Veehof 1985: 37).

3. Eye contact with the audience makes them feel that you are talking to them, and not at them. Eye contact adds a personal touch to a speech.

4. Smiling with the audience extends warmth and adds friendliness to a presentation.

5. Keep the space between you and the audience open by presenting the talk enthusiastically and showing interest in the audience's responses.

6. A pause of typically two seconds here and there helps emphasize important points.

7. It is necessary to make use of 'bridges' — ie statements which can serve as a bridge between one section and the next — in order to get the message across in a smooth and flowing manner.

8. The presentation must be made to sound natural even if it is read.

9. Know where your hands and feet are at all times.

10. Facial expressions, hand movements, or body movement should all convey warmth, openness, energy, approval and interest (Swansburg 1990: 394).

11. Adapt to audience feedback and be sensitive to its mood and level of interest as portrayed by the body language of the members of the audience — shifting in seats, whispering, facial expressions, gestures, and body movements are all important cues.

12. Be prepared to answer questions. Questions from a large audience should be repeated for everybody to hear before they are answered.

13. If the audience is treated with respect, they will perceive the speaker as genuine (Swansburg 1990: 395).

EFFECTIVE COMMUNICATION THROUGH FEEDBACK

It is usually the perceptions of the receivers of a message which determine the effectiveness of communication. If they do not understand the message they will not receive it. It is thus necessary for the nurse manager to find out what the nursing personnel — ie the listeners or receivers of the communication coming from her — can perceive, expect to perceive, and want to perceive. It is far more effective if the nurse manager, in her communication, focuses on the aspirations, values, motivations, and needs of her nursing personnel than if she focuses on what *she* wants to get across to them.

By giving feedback to employees, the communication cycle is completed, making it two-way communication. Effective communication — ie two-way communication — can only be accomplished in an atmosphere of mutual respect and confidence. In such an atmosphere, where suggestions are given and received, an effective exchange of opinions and information is accomplished (Swansburg 1990: 389).

When one-way communication prevails in an institution — ie the nurse manager *telling* her nursing personnel what she expects from them, *giving* them information about the new policy decisions, *asking* them to co-operate and be loyal to the profession and the organization, and *thanking* them for their contributions in the past — little or no interaction takes place between the manager and her personnel because she is talking *to* them, but is not getting real involvement *from* her personnel in the form of shared opinions or interests. This type of communication worked well in the past, but with today's workers, who are better educated, more affluent, who retire earlier and who prefer to work in a more democratic environment, it does not promote understanding and internalizing of the messages that are sent.

This type of one-way communication prevents input, feedback, and interaction. The effects are numerous and are seen in a depersonalization of patients, conflicts and barriers between nurses and doctors, distorted communications, and the resultant distortion of feedback, frustration, stress, scepticism, emotional blow-ups, and scapegoating (Swansburg 1990: 389).

Sufficient feedback to employees from the manager is one of the most important measures to improve productivity and performance. Such feedback should help the individual to set specific goals for improvement, set measurable targets which must be met at specified deadlines, and describe the methods of attaining them. Involving the individual in the goal-setting process produces the best results (Levenstein 1984: 64).

The feedback provided to employees regarding their general work performance should ideally take place not at yearly intervals but rather at four-to-six monthly intervals. These reviews of work performance should also be kept as distant as possible from the dates when salary increments and promotions are considered. Coaching and other forms of on-the-job training should be carried out continuously and will yield the best results when linked to specific acts, omissions, or performances which are below expected standards (Levenstein 1984: 64).

Research regarding the effects of feedback on employees in health care settings has shown that an increase in productivity is marked where sufficient feedback is given, eg ranging from 83% over 23 weeks to 163% over a period of 38 weeks (Levenstein 1984: 64).

Although managers are often reluctant to give the necessary feedback, because they fear that positive feedback might lead a person to ask for a pay increase or promotion and that negative feedback may lead to unpleasant arguments, research has shown that these fears are unwarranted. Most people want to know about themselves and are sincerely grateful when supplied with the information (Levenstein 1984: 66).

THE ART OF LISTENING

As managers, we spend about 80% of our time communicating. More than half of this time is spent in listening to employees. Poor listening habits — a frequent occurrence among managers — lead to distorted communication. Listening is often seen as a passive activity whereas, when done properly, it is just as active as speaking (Morgan and Baker 1985: 34).

Listening does not mean that you just keep quiet in order to allow the other person to speak, or that you wait for a conversational opening. Listening involves the processes of sensing, interpretation, evaluation, reaction, and retention. Sensing is represented by *hearing* the message; interpretation is represented by *understanding* the message; evaluating means *appraising* the message according to the value we assign to it; reacting is *responding* to the message, and retention means the *storing* of the message in our memory (Morgan and Baker 1985: 35).

Bad listening habits

The following bad listening habits are frequently encountered among managers:

1. A tendency to make inferences from what we hear. It is wrong to evaluate the message in the beginning and to make hasty interpretations about *why* the speaker wants to deliver his message. Good listeners respondsto the face value of the message.

2. Avoiding eye contact with the speaker. Making eye contact with — but not staring at — the speaker, removes mistrust and contributes to the transmission of the total message.

3. Poor retention. We only normally listen at a 25% level of efficiency. Good listeners recognize this and exercise their memories to try to retain a bit more.

4. Premature dismissal. By hearing certain uninteresting 'buzz words', many people 'tune out' what is being said because they think that the message cannot be interesting or that they do not want to hear something again. They focus their attention on something else and do not hear anything, or hear very little, of what is being said. Good listeners may have the same initial reaction, but instead of tuning the message out, they try to see what they can gain from it and often find that they can learn something by what is being said (Morgan and Baker 1985: 36).

Listening mistakes

When listening, one must try to avoid the following:

1. Interruptions. Don't interrupt or change the subject; wait until the speaker finishes and then ask clarifying questions.

2. Preconceptions. Do not let your own biases and preconceptions cloud the issue and make you listen selectively, thereby leading to a misinterpretation of the intent of the message.

3. Argumentativeness (Morgan and Baker 1985: 36). When one listens with the intent of looking for an argument in what the person is saying, a lot of the message is missed as one is planning a response. Good listeners do not jump to conclusions too soon.

4. Listening for facts alone. Poor listeners tend to listen for facts alone, while good listeners focus on central themes and use them to provide sense and meaning to the topic under discussion.

5. Too much note-taking. Too much note-taking sidetracks the listener from what is being said.

6. Distractions. Poor listeners are easily distracted whereas good listeners concentrate on what is being said (Morgan and Baker 1985: 37).

Ways to improve listening

Active methods which one can employ to improve listening are:

1. Be responsive to the speaker.

2. Listen for *what* is said, rather than how it is said.

3. Work at listening.

4. Energy needs to be expended in order to understand the speaker.

5. Open your mind. Do not overreact to emotionally charged words — eg 'strike'; look beyond the words to the overall message (Morgan and Baker 1985: 37).

6. Use thought speed. We can think three to four times faster than we speak. Do not fill in the intervening time by daydreaming, but use it for summarizing, weighing, anticipating what the speaker will say, and looking for further clues to what he wants to convey (Morgan and Baker 1985: 37).

7. Expand your mind. Do not tune out information when the subject is a bit too difficult for you. Work at listening to it to expand your horizon.

8. Use active listening. Active listening uses paraphrasing. This does not mean simply repeating a message; it means putting into one's own words what someone has said. By doing this the speaker knows whether the point was missed and whether further clarification is needed (Morgan and Baker 1985: 38).

According to Morgan and Baker, to listen well is to enter into the private world of another and to see things from that point of view without bias or distortion.

In conclusion, Wlody (1984: 25) puts forth the following nine commandments for good listening:

- Stop talking. (You cannot listen if you are talking.)
- Put the talker at ease.
- Show him that you want to listen (listen to understand rather than to reply).
- Remove distractions.
- Empathize with the speaker.
- Be patient.
- Hold your temper.
- Go easy on argument or criticism (even if you win, you lose).
- Ask questions.

Results of listening

The results of effective listening are:

1. People hear each other.

2. Beneficial information is gathered on which to base the correct decision.

3. A better relationship is established between people.

4. It is easier to find solutions to problems.

5. It helps to relieve stress and burnout.

6. It encourages the co-operation of employees and their acceptance of change.

7. It elicits suggestions that may lead to profitability.

8. It saves disciplinary action when it reveals the real cause of an error (Swansburg 1990: 392).

STRAIGHT TALK

Managers have the responsibility to be honest and direct with employees about their performance, function, goals, good and bad points, where they are going, what they can expect, and what they should do to improve their capabilities. It means making sure that employees are in tune with their abilities, strengths, and weaknesses. It also means making all information known to employees. Managers thus need to praise when praise is due, but also to criticize when criticism is necessary. Although honesty and openness are the key elements of straight talk, this does not mean that managers should not apply tact in their dealings with employees. The manager cannot just say anything that she wants to an employee. Such an approach will breed resentment and hostility (St John 1984: 53).

Many managers are afraid to speak up for fear of alienating the employee. It is, however, impossible for employees to improve on inappropriate conduct and unsatisfactory performances unless it is pointed out to them. When the manager avoids the issue she is making her burden heavier because the gap between the employee's actual and expected performance must somehow be overcome (St John 1984: 53).

Proven methods for effectiveness

According to St John there are four proven methods for making 'straight talk' effective:

1. Control the content of the session. Focus on the sharing of feelings and information, rather on giving advice. Address only one major issue at a time. Say what needs to be said and mean what you say. Once a particular point is raised and understood, drop it and move ahead. Focus on the explanation of alternatives to arrive at the best solution (St John 1984: 54).

2. Focus the session. The needs of the employee, not those of the manager, should be emphasized. Introduce an amount of information that the employee can use rather than everything you want to unload.

3. Make both participants accept responsibility. Make direct eye contact with the employee. Make the employee responsible for her own behaviour. Describe the problem, do not judge. Let the employee identify possible alternative solutions.

4. Avoid damaging the employee's self-esteem. Discuss matters privately. Be positive, helpful, and constructive. Praise the employee, if warranted, before raising an unpleasant issue. Describe behaviour in 'more-or-less' terms which stress quantity, rather than on 'either/or' terms. When you are talking to especially sensitive people, consider giving an example of some of your own mistakes before embarking on a discussion of their mistakes. Give the other person a fine reputation to live up to. Demonstrate faith in the employee. Be encouraging when ending the interview ('I know you can do it', etc.) (St John 1984: 54).

NON-VERBAL COMMUNICATION

Non-verbal messages tend to have a greater impact than words because people are more inclined to believe what they see than what they hear (Bosch 1992: 6).

Elements of non-verbal communication

Kinesics, or body language

This includes gestures, eye contact, eye movement, posture, and body movement.

When making a presentation the speaker should use her hands to emphasize the words, to stimulate participation by the audience, to indicate size, form, movement, and numbers, to dramatize ideas, and to prompt a response from an audience. The hands should at all times be visible to the audience (Bosch 1992: 6).

When presenting a speech, eye contact should be maintained with the group. The focus of the contact should be shifted deliberately but slowly, to include the whole group if possible. When speaking or listening to another individual, eye contact indicates interest and respect.

Eye contact should be broken downwards, unless one deliberately wants to convey a lack of interest in the other person or unless one wants to throw the other person temporarily off-balance by a disconcerting upward glance. On an initial encounter with a person a gaze should not last for longer than three seconds. A violation of this rule can generate a negative impression in the person who is gazed at (Lewis 1989: 82).

Body movement during a presentation could enhance the message or distract from it. Moving in front of an audience is one of the most visible physical actions a speaker can utilize to attract attention. It must, however, not be done without good reason (Bosch 1992: 6).

The posture you exhibit during a presentation will indicate nervousness or confidence. If you want to appear in control of the situation, the posture should be upright, leaning forward slightly, with the feet about 300 mm apart, one slightly behind the other and with shoulders relaxed but not drooped (Bosch 1992: 6).

Physical appearance

The appearance of a speaker should be in harmony with the occasion. Neatness, appropriateness of dress, and a well-groomed appearance are more important than showiness. Large, shining items of jewellery could cause irritating flashes if a speaker is directly below a light (Bosch 1992: 6).

Haptics

Haptics is the use of touch to communicate. Some people like being touched, but others are turned off by it. The manager should remember to use touch only when giving reassurance, support or encouragement (Bosch, quoting Blanchard and Johnson 1992: 6).

Proxemics

Proxemics refers to the space you use around you during communication — eg how close you would put a visitor's chair in your office to your own chair. The public distance which is usually maintained varies between two to three metres. When the nurse manager wants to discuss a confidential matter with a member of staff, she often arranges the seating so that she and the staff member are seated next to each other, but with some space in between.

Chronemics

This refers to the speaker's use of *time* when speaking — ie whether she speaks quickly or slowly; whether she pauses at intervals. It also refers to punctuality when returning phone calls or when arriving for a presentation (Bosch 1992: 6).

Artifacts

The objects that you display in your office or workplace convey a considerable number of non-verbal messages (Bosch 1992: 6). For example, an office decorated with bright flowers in a vase, displayed on a neat little table with a basket of toffees, would convey the message of a neat, empathetic, friendly, open inhabitant.

Paralanguage

This is non-verbal communication conveyed through your use of voice — eg volume, pitch, time, fluency. A deep cultured voice portrays education and sophistication, while hesitancy and tremors indicate lies and half-truths (Bosch 1992: 6).

WRITTEN COMMUNICATION

Writing to be understood or to state one's viewpoint or request in a letter, memorandum, or report poses a challenge to the nurse manager.

There are a number of general rules to follow in order to produce effective written communication which will yield results.

1. Be sensitive to the needs and desires of the person you are writing to. If you are writing to a specific person, the person's name should appear in the salutation as well as in the body of the letter or memorandum. Being sensitive and emphatic also means that the writer must have the ability to see the message as the listener will. It also means being tactful, courteous, and communicating in a tone of general goodwill.

2. Letters should also be written using 'you-centred' instead of 'I-centred' communication. For instance, instead of saying 'I/we would like to inform you', rather say 'you would probably be interested to know ...'

3. Aim for clarity. Simple words, short sentences, and logical reasoning are essential. Your aim should be to create mental pictures using language that is suitable to the experience and knowledge level of the receiver. Ambiguity must be avoided, as well as words which look impressive but which can be replaced by simpler words. It is, however, necessary to remember that a report on a specialist subject, such as nursing matters, should be written in the appropriate 'technical' language.

4. Use the format of the newspaper story: accuracy, brevity, clarity, digestibility, and empathy. The reader's interest can be aroused by an unusual headline as an opener. In the first paragraph a summary that highlights all the significant facts/aspects can be given. The details are given in the rest of the paragraphs.

5. Accuracy is very important. Facts, figures, statements, and statistics used must be accurate. They must be appropriate and must not be outdated. Avoid excessive use of adjectives and adverbs, and be specific when using adjectives. When dealing with quantities it is far better to state an exact amount — eg '100' instead of 'much' or 'a lot'.

6. It is easier and more interesting to read a solid printed page which has been made digestible and attractive by underlining, indenting, boxing in, summarizing, spacing, and capitalizing (Swansburg 1990: 396)

7. It is necessary to be comprehensive in order for the reader to understand the issue clearly. Unnecessary and irrelevant detail should be omitted, but the reader should also not have to guess about certain statements made in the report. A statement must be backed up by sufficient and appropriate facts and figures.

8. Try to use words sparingly. Sentences should ideally not be longer than 20 words on average. The use of too many qualifying words should be avoided. Sentences should each contain one idea. The length of the sentences should be varied.

9. A letter or report should project 'strength'. It is thus necessary to go right to the point. State the purpose of the letter or report directly and ask for a response within a certain time limit, if appropriate.

10. Written communication must often be reread, revised, edited, a draft must be checked and rechecked, typed copies must be proofread, and the logical sequence of the contents evaluated before it can be dispatched.

Guidelines for writing reports and memoranda

The following guidelines may assist in the compilation of reports and memoranda:

1. During the preparatory phase, the nurse manager must make absolutely certain who is to receive the report/memorandum. The individual(s) receiving the report will, to a large extent, determine the type of language which would be appropriate, as well as the general tone of the report.

2. The objective of the report will have to be determined and all the facts bearing on the particular issue will have to be collected from the various sources — eg senior professional charge nurses, doctors, technicians, etc. When all the facts have been collected, they must be weighed up against the policy of the institution or against current practice. Try to identify any shortcomings in the facts collected and check for contradictions (Unisa Study Guide I for NUA 202-R: 1979: 90).

3. The outline of the report/memorandum must now be prepared. Decide on the facts which must be included and consider the different headings under which the information will be organized.

4. Write the first draft. The main objective of the report must be kept in mind constantly. The facts must be arranged under the different headings so that the report/memorandum forms a logical order. The order should be sequential in nature, either in chronological order or showing a cause-effect relationship, or in a format which is increasing in complexity. The sentences or groups of sentences should be linked together using devices such as time-order words — eg 'first', 'later', 'finally' — or guide words — eg 'as a result', 'therefore', 'on the other hand'. In the introduction one may outline the problem/need for the memorandum, give a historical background to the subject, or refer to previous correspondence on the issue.

- If the report is going to a group of people with limited time, such as a board of directors, it may be wise to add an executive summary to the beginning of the report. In this way you highlight what it is you want the readers to act upon. It may speed up their response.

- When writing a memorandum it is necessary to include proposals for implementation. These proposals should include dates and resources — eg time, money, and personnel required (Unisa Study Guide I for NUA 202 R-1979: 92).

- The report or memorandum should end with a suitable conclusion or summary. It is customary to repeat the key issues and main points/aspects in the summary. Recommendations made must be capable of being implemented in practice and must be as specific as possible, otherwise they do not serve their purpose.

- When tables or figures containing detailed statistics are necessary to support the facts, these should be in an annexure at the end of the report or memorandum. If these are given in the text they tend to break the continuity of the report and make it harder to read.

5. When the report/memorandum has been developed it must be edited. It is necessary to read and reread the whole, to consider if all the facts are correct and whether they tie in with the objective of the report, whether the report makes sense, whether it follows a logical order, and whether it is written in a language which is clear and unambiguous, with no unnecessary or irrelevant detail obscuring the essence.

6. Finally, it must be remembered that a memorandum and a report usually has a title page and that the individual to whom it is sent is identified clearly on the first page, as well as the issue or

matter of the report/memorandum and the person who has compiled it. A referral letter usually accompanies a memorandum (Study Guide for NUA 202 R-1979: 93).

CONCLUSION

The ability to communicate effectively is often considered the most valuable skill that a manager can possess. Both formal and informal communication must be heeded in an organization. The effective nurse manager should be proficient in both oral and written communication. Apart from speaking to colleagues and subordinates, the nurse manager should also possess good listening skills in order to understand her nursing staff and to be able to communicate with them in a meaningful way. Her non-verbal communication should serve to strengthen the meaning of her words and not to detract from it.

References

Bosch, F. (1992). Can you make your point? (Part 2). *Nursing News,* volume 16, number 7, p. 6.

Bosch, F. (1992). Can you make your point? *Nursing News,* volume 16, number 9, September 1992.

Lancaster, J. (1985). Public Speaking can be improved. *JONA,* volume 15, number 3, pp. 31–5.

Levenstein, A. (1984). Feedback improves performance. *Nursing Management,* volume 15, number 2, pp. 64–6.

Lewis, D. (1989). *The Secret Language of Success.* Bantam Press: London.

Morgan, P. and Baker, H. K. (1985). Building a professional image: improving listening behaviour. *Supervisory Management,* November 1985, pp. 34–8.

Simmons, D. B. (1985). The nature of the organizational grapevine. *Supervisory Management,* November 1985, pp. 39–42.

St John, W. D. (1984). Leveling with employees. *Personnel Journal,* August 1984, pp. 52–7.

Swansburg, R. C. (1990). *Management and Leadership for nurse Managers.* Jones and Bartlett Publishers: Boston.

Unisa Study Guide for Nursing Administration: Study Guide I for NUA 202-R (1979). UNISA: Pretoria.

Veehof, D. C. (1985). Standing ovation. *JONA,* volume 15, number 10, pp. 34–8.

Wilkinson, R. Communication: learning from the market. *Nursing Management,* volume 17, number 4, pp. 42J–42L.

Wlody, G. S. Communicating in the ICU: do you read me loud and clear? *Nursing Management,* volume 15, number 9, pp. 24–7.

CHAPTER 11

MANAGEMENT OF TIME

J. H. Roos

and

S. W. Booyens

CONTENTS

INTRODUCTION

Time is money. People delivering health care become increasingly conscious about the advantages of good time management for an organization. The way a nurse manager uses her time affects the quality of patient care in her organization.

WHAT IS TIME MANAGEMENT?

Time management means the effective and efficient use of time (McFarland, Leonard and Morris 1984: 264). It is regarded as the effective planning and scheduling of work time to ensure that the most important work is completed and that sufficient time is left for unexpected emergencies and crises that may occur (Sullivan and Decker 1988: 239). It is important to remember that, for all of us, there are 24 hours available for each day of the year

The activities on which one spends one's time are what makes the difference. These activities can be described either as *time-consumers* (those activities that contribute to a large extent to the goals of the organization) or *time-wasters* (those activities that use a person's time without contributing to the goals of the organization or the individual) (La Monica 1990: 292).

The effective manager can distinguish between *urgent* and *important* tasks. Urgent tasks demand immediate action and the important tasks are sidelined to take second place. By concentrating excessively on the urgent tasks, and neglecting the important ones, the manager can expect to be confronted by a looming crisis.

Trying to hurry up or to work longer hours to get everything done is not the solution. When one is in a hurry one is unable to reflect, to evaluate alternatives, to plan, and thus work effectively. When fatigue sets in because of long hours, poor judgement is the result.

The solution to effective use of time lies in:

- Planning and organizing more effectively. Every hour spent in effective planning can eliminate three to four hours in the execution of tasks — and can get better results.

- Concentrating on the few critical tasks/problems which will really produce results.

- Eliminating many trivial activities.

- Delegating responsibility and authority as far as possible.

- Thinking before acting.

To use time effectively, managers should not manage by crisis. It is unnecessary to overreact and to treat every problem as if it has global consequences. Over-responding to every problem causes anxiety, impaired judgement, hasty decisions, and wasted time and effort.

'Working smarter' always beats 'working harder'. Doing the wrong or trivial things 'harder' never helps. It only adds stress and tension and ultimately causes illness (McCarthy, 1981).

STRATEGIES FOR TIME MANAGEMENT

There are a number of strategies which can be followed to ensure that time is utilized constructively.

Using time wisely

The nurse manager who wants to use her time constructively must know what her goals in life are. It is necessary to draw up a list of personal and career goals. These goals should be divided into lifetime goals, five-year goals, and goals to be accomplished in the next six months. If the list of goals is extensive, the manager should try to select only the three most important goals for each period, identify the actions needed to accomplish each one, and set realistic target dates for each. These goals will then serve as guidelines as to when time must be found to pursue them (Tappen 1989: 236).

It is important to identify how one's time is spent and to see how much time is spent on unproductive or minimally productive activities. To achieve this it is recommended that one keeps a time log. The time log is a format where the nurse manager enters her activities at half-hourly intervals from approximately 06:30 until 17:00. The activities must be recorded as accurately as possible for a period of at least three days. The activities could be anything — eg networking, socializing, planning, worrying, daydreaming, talking, conducting a meeting, interviewing, counselling, or compiling statistics for a report.

When this time log is analysed, a pattern should emerge revealing how one normally spends one's time. It is then possible to plan for the elimination of the unproductive hours in order to have more time available for pressing and important issues. The activities which do not contribute to the attainment of personal or career goals should be listed. It is recommended that the exercise be repeated in six months' time because situations are changing constantly.

In addition to the time log, it would also be helpful to keep an interruption log for a week. This detailed log should contain the names of the people causing the interruptions, and the length, reason and importance of every interruption. Once the nature and types of interruptions, and reasons for interruptions are identified, a definite plan of action can be instituted in order to avoid some of them and manage the others. Recommendations regarding interruptions are the following:

- Control time spent receiving telephone calls by focusing the caller to the point under discussion and leaving discussion of personal and family matters for telephone conversations from home.

- Train your secretary to divert non-emergency calls to other managerial staff when the problem is one that could just as easily be handled by someone else.

- Maintain an open-door policy by appointment only.

- Keep unavoidable interruptions short by thanking the person for the information and saying that you must get back to what you were doing.

The nurse manager needs to plan and schedule activities in order to accomplish the set goals. A year-planner which depicts the major responsibilities for the coming year is recommended. It shows at a glance when the budget must be completed, when the monthly staff meetings are to take place, when meriting sessions must be attended, when graduation ceremonies take place, etc. A monthly calendar should be kept where each month's main events and responsibilities are noted. Weekly and daily calendars are of equal importance in streamlining activities to achieve major goals and responsibilities.

It is necessary to allow a few minutes at the beginning of each day to plan the necessary activities for the day in order of importance. It is wise to jot them down in your daily calendar. Another helpful tip is to keep files labelled 'urgent', 'return calls', 'dictate', 'read', 'file', and 'low priority' in order to handle the flow of incoming messages and problems. One should arrange to have certain blocks of free time per day to attend to these files.

The nurse manager should also assess her own bodily 'peak' and 'low' times in order to plan the effective use of her time. For instance, when her most creative time for working alone is in the middle of the morning, she should try to make appointments and schedule meetings for a time either early in the morning or after 11:30. Likewise, if her best time for working with others is in the afternoons, she should arrange staff office visits for that time (Marriner-Tomey 1992: 61).

Communicate effectively to save time

Telephone calls

If a telephone call can be made instead of an office visit or writing a letter, this saves time. Messages can be left if people are not available, and a call-back system can be used to complete the business. Forms which are specially designed for writing down telephone messages do not get lost as easily as other scraps of paper. It is helpful to collect all phone messages in one place. It is necessary to have a list of commonly used telephone numbers handy. Telephone conversations should focus on the business at hand and not on social matters. It also saves time to have a list of all the people one wants to phone and then to phone them in succession, as well as jotting down the major topics for the conversations in order not to forget what it is you wanted to phone about.

Streamline paperwork

It is wise to set aside a block of time without interruptions to answer letters. Standardized replies or letters should be used when the same type of reply or query has to be written repeatedly. One may also return a memo containing a query with the answer on it when it does not need filing. Selective reading, scanning tables of contents, and reading summaries at the end of long reports also saves time. Managers should not concentrate on details unless this is necessary, because they are quickly forgotten and it is usually the major points which must be remembered (Marriner-Tomey 1992: 62).

Recording and reporting

When the records and reports that are written have a functional value, time can be saved. If they do not, they should not be written (McFarland et al. 1984: 282). Excessive record-keeping, unorganized files, a complicated reporting and recording system, an inadequate filing system, failure to purge files of outdated material, failure to use standardized letters or memos where appropriate, and the lack of periodic status reports, are all examples of time-wasters (McFarland et al. 1984: 272). Eliminate the use of unnecessary reports. Standardize letters and memos as far as possible, and keep the filing system as simple as possible.

Meetings

A considerable amount of time spent by managers in meetings is wasted. The manager must first consider the purpose of a meeting — eg morale-building, the sharing of information, decision-making, problem-solving, etc. If the meeting is not necessary it should not take place. Alternatives to holding a meeting — such as sending a memo, making a telephone call, or holding a telephone conference — must be considered. When the nurse manager does not think that her presence at a meeting is absolutely necessary, she may send someone to represent her. In this way, time can be used for more important or pressing issues. The staff member who is representing the nurse manager will probably pick up some management knowledge simply from attending the meeting as the manager's substitute. The manager may also limit the time she spends in attending meetings by only attending the section where she must make a contribution. The purpose of a meeting must be defined and an agenda must be circulated before a meeting is to take place. When conducting a meeting, the manager should ensure that it starts on time, that the agenda is followed, that high-priority items are dealt with first, that interruptions are controlled, that conclusions are restated, deadlines for assignments are set, and that minutes are circulated within a day after the meeting.

Control visiting time

It is easier for the manager to control the time spent by visitors if the visit does not take place in her own office. If she meets visitors in a central reception area she is free to leave whenever she desires. She may also control visiting time by standing up when a visitor enters her office, thereby preventing the visitor from sitting down. She can then decide whether she would like the visitor to sit down for a long discussion, whether she wants to make an appointment with the person for another more suitable time, or whether she just wants to cut short the visit. The manager is also advised to have lunches with her staff members on a regular basis because she may then discuss matters of common interest with them, thus limiting the number of staff visiting her office (Marriner-Tomey 1992: 64).

Other communication time-wasters

- Poor listening habits may give rise to situations where you 'think you know' but do not know at all.

- Excessive/inappropriate socialization may give rise to situations where the work of the organization is neglected while the employees are discussing private matters during working hours.

- Communication overload which makes it impossible for the worker to handle the situation.

- Delayed information may give rise to frustration on the part of the worker.

- Non-assertive behaviour — for instance not standing up for your rights and letting other people talk you into things you do not really want to do.

Solve problems scientifically

When the nurse manager does not apply problem-solving processes, she may waste a lot of time because this may give rise to indecision, delayed decisions, snap decisions, the collection of inappropriate data, failure to clarify/identify a problem, failure to identify and examine alternative solutions, failure to select the most appropriate solution, failure to examine the consequences of selected solutions, failure to utilize the evaluation of the selected action to reformulate the problem, inappropriate use of group decision-making, and acting without thinking (McFarland et al. 1984: 278).

She should thus use the approved techniques of problem solving, but she should also remember that although participative management is regarded highly, it is a time-consuming activity.

Delegate duties and tasks to others

The nurse manager sometimes fails to delegate tasks to other personnel members for the simple reason that in order for the staff member to take over the task from the manager she needs to be supplied with a considerable amount of information which must be communicated to her by the manager herself. This information is stored in the nurse manager's memory and has been obtained over a period of time from many sources — eg higher authorities, networking with other nurse managers, and private conversations with a number of officials. The result is that it is too time-consuming and difficult to give the staff member sufficient information to enable her to execute the task. The nurse manager might also consider some of the information as too confidential to impart to another person.

There are less acceptable reasons why the nurse manager fails to delegate tasks. These might include the following (Gillies 1989: 220):

- Lack of confidence in the abilities of subordinates.

- Fear of losing control over highly valued activities.

- Fear of offending subordinates by increasing their workload.

- Fear that delegating certain tasks would be seen by others as evidence of the manager's inability to fulfil her job expectations.

- Fear that a talented subordinate may execute the job better than herself.

- Reluctance to request help from subordinates.

The result of these attitudes is that the manager becomes overburdened. Failure to delegate is usually seen as a weak point in management. The following principles should be adhered to for delegation to be effective:

- Careful planning is needed in order to decide which duties to delegate, to whom each duty should be delegated, and how to empower and motivate staff members to execute duties satisfactorily.

- Responsibilities for strategic planning, evaluation, and the disciplining of immediate subordinates should not be delegated.

- It is advisable to delegate a complete task or project to a subordinate, not just certain aspects of it. The subordinate becomes far more committed to executing the job to the best of her abilities when the manager does not retain certain aspects of it. By delegating a complete project the manager shows confidence in the abilities of the individual. The result is that the person becomes motivated to use her initiative to execute the job to the best of her abilities.

- The manager and subordinate should discuss the project. They should agree, and put in writing, the scope of duty, the amount of authority granted for the execution of the project, the specific results which should be achieved, and the criteria against which the results will be evaluated.

- The manager should notify all the significant members in the organization in writing about the delegation and the subordinate who has been entrusted to execute the project in order for the individual to be able to request the necessary resources and issue orders without unnecessary hindrances.

- To motivate subordinates to accept delegated duties and perform them effectively the manager should carefully select the most appropriate person for the job, provide direction and support when needed, and reward the delegated person for excellent work (Gillies 1989: 221).

The development of personnel should always be one of the manager's top priorities. This, however, can only be achieved if the manager delegates properly — that is if she discourages subordinates from depending on her answers — otherwise she will end up by doing much of the delegated work herself (McCarthy 1981: 63).

Directing, controlling, and evaluating

The nurse manager must aim to motivate her staff. Incomplete or unclear directions, lack of performance standards, unclear or inappropriate performance standards, not requesting progress reports and feedback on the performance of a job frequently enough, not providing needed feedback on job performance, discussing tangential issues while providing job guidance to a subordinate, issuing inaccurate or inadequate information, reviewing subordinates' performance excessively, conveying an overly critical attitude and rigid expectations, and an adherence to 'the way things have been done' may all demotivate a subordinate and may lead to time being wasted. The nurse manager must control her service in such a way that it motivates her personnel. It is also necessary to set standards for performance.

Foster constructive human interaction

Poor conflict management, non-assertive communication, creating a 'bottleneck' for co-workers, not intervening, inappropriate interpersonal behaviour, failure to assess personal traits, creating interpersonal friction or conflict, and failure to discuss interpersonal difficulties openly, will all give rise to excessive amounts of time spent on conflict. It is the nurse manager's obligation to intervene and arrest non-productive behaviour from her personnel. Interpersonal difficulties should be discussed openly. She should create an open, supportive system where staff feel free to express their feelings and where assertive communication is encouraged.

Motivating

Lack of motivation, or job dissatisfaction, may give rise to a situation where staff often waste time on unimportant issues. Attention should be given to factors that may cause a lack of experience, use of inappropriate change strategies, lack of motivation towards achieving organizational goals, use of inappropriate rewards, excessive criticism, inappropriate use of negative feedback, assigning job tasks and activities inappropriately, and not giving enough recognition good work (McFarland et al. 1984: 270).

The nurse manager should thus give attention to the type of supervision which is used, personnel policy and procedures, job circumstances, and salaries. The nurse manager may even find it necessary to attend seminars to improve her leadership style.

Managing the work environment

It is important that the work environment should enhance productivity. Factors that may prove to be stumbling blocks are an indiscriminate open-door policy, inadequate storage space for essential materials, inadequate workspace, excessive or distracting noises, disorganized workspace, permitting unessential materials to accumulate, and the non-functional arrangement of furniture and materials needed for work (McFarland et al 1984: 270). The nurse manager should thus give attention to the arrangement of furniture, she should secure enough supplies for use, and should avoid unnecessary documentation.

Organizing

An organizational structure that facilitates goal-achievement saves time. Aspects that may be disruptive to organizing are nebulous job descriptions, resources for job performance which are not readily accessible, confused authority, frequent crisis situations, unclear lines of formal authority, under-defined or over-defined roles and responsibilities, the duplication of tasks, focusing on unimportant or unessential tasks, a failure to break complex tasks into their component parts, personal disorganization and clutter, failure to use prime time for priority tasks, red tape, not doing the right job, and an exclusive focus on the component parts of complex tasks (McFarland et al. 1984: 270). The nurse manager should develop an organizational structure that encourages attainment of objectives — for instance clear job descriptions, avoiding red tape and duplication of tasks, and keeping enough supplies at hand.

Evaluation of personal habits and traits

It is good to evaluate yourself to assess whether you have habits like the following: procrastination, perfectionism, lack of self-discipline, poor reading skills, excessive need for recognition, complaining, inattention, an 'I don't care' attitude, a negative attitude, resentment, carelessness, a high state of tension, lack of self-confidence in achieving goals, loafing or daydreaming, not assessing personal or group time-wasters, excessive attention to routine and detail, inability to communicate assertively, gathering or distributing gossip about co-workers, failure to consider personal vulnerabilities and weaknesses, setting unrealistic goals, expecting everything to be done immediately, feeling 'pulled in all directions', frequent absenteeism or tardiness, making mistakes and producing poor quality work, inability to say 'no', and mental blocks (McFarland et al. 1984: 271).

The manager should identify which tasks are usually put off and why, and determine whether it is not better to delegate. A plan of action should be developed to complete a task.

The nurse manager should unlearn certain attitudes and behaviours which have been acquired during earlier nursing experiences. For example, a nurse manager who has worked as a professional nurse in an intensive care unit and has become a valued nurse because of her ability to handle crises effectively may become a manager who puts greater value on an immediate and effective response to a crisis than on thoughtful planning. When planning is neglected, crises tend to increase in number and severity, so that most of the manager's time is spent in fighting the erupting fires. Nurse managers who are used to this type of management see themselves as 'rescuers' and they find it more difficult than other managers to say 'no' to another person's request for assistance (Gillies 1989: 223).

Most people find it difficult to say 'no' to a reasonable request from a co-worker. It is however necessary for the nurse manager to refuse to undertake additional responsibilities which do not form part of her duties under the following circumstances:

1. When the activity will not contribute to the manager's own professional or occupational goals.

2. When the activity requires time and skills which the manager does not possess.

3. When the activity does not interest the manager.

4. When undertaking the activity will prevent the manager from having time and energy for involvement in more attractive or rewarding activities.

To avoid guilt feelings and to prevent unfavourable responses, the manager should learn to say 'no' firmly and tactfully. The most effective way of doing this is to look the person voicing the request straight in the eye, and to say 'no' with a pleasant expression on the face. It is advisable not to give reasons for the refusal because when reasons are offered the person making the request might be prompted to suggest ways of overcoming the mentioned obstacles with the result that guilt feelings are engendered (Gillies 1989: 223).

Bad personality traits which have been identified may be discussed with a trusted colleague who may give constructive criticism and advice in order to modify certain behaviours. Some negative personality traits may require skilled counselling (McFarland et al 1984: 281).

Goal-setting and planning

When a person working in an organization spends the day working on a project that does not serve organizational or personal goals, she is wasting time (McFarland et al 1984: 281). Situations that may give rise to this include the following (McFarland et al. 1984: 271-2):

- absence of, or unclear, organizational and subsystem goals and objectives;

- failure to set, plan, or schedule daily activities;

- absence of, or unclear, priorities;

- treating all tasks as priorities;

- unrealistic time frames (attempting too much or too little);

- failure to identify viable alternatives;

- failure to work on priority tasks

- immersion in detail and process without attention to objectives;

- neglecting to plan because of pressure;
- concentrating on staying busy while losing sight of objectives;
- lack of contingency plans;
- leaving tasks unfinished;
- trying to accomplish too many things at once;
- no self-imposed deadlines.

To overcome these habits which waste time, a list should be drawn up of all those activities that do not contribute to the attainment of personal or career objectives. Daily activities should be arranged in order of priority, and the most important activities should be worked on during one's peak performance hour.

Staffing and staff development

It is necessary that the nurse manager should have an input to ensure that the staff in her department are selected, placed, and developed (McFarland et al. 1984: 272). Much of her time (and that of other personnel) may be wasted if:

- inadequately prepared staff are selected;
- there is a problem in staff development, continuing education, and direction and guidance;
- there is an inappropriate assignment of responsibilities;
- poor assignment of personnel takes place;
- high staff turnover or absenteeism occurs;
- there is an inadequate number of personnel;
- there are inadequate support staff;
- tardiness occurs;
- there are inappropriate types of assignments;
- she cannot involve staff in ways to expand their abilities.

The nurse manager should have as much say as possible when selecting and placing staff. A lot of time may be saved through in-service education and appropriate delegation.

Utilizing facilities and non-human resources; budgeting

The nurse manager needs to do a comprehensive assessment of the work environment, otherwise she may waste valuable time by the frequent ordering and obtaining of supplies, ordering inadequate or improper supplies, through mechanical failures or ordering non-usable supplies, failure to acquire adequate facilities, resources, or finance, through input exceeding requirements of throughput and output, and through not having appropriate resources available for doing a job (McFarland et al. 1984: 272–3). By ensuring enough supplies and storage space and an adequate budget, time may be saved.

General considerations regarding utilization of time

The next step entails studying the list of the time-wasters most commonly encountered. For every identified time-waster there is a managerial solution. If unnecessary or unproductive meetings are a problem, attention should be given to procedures followed at meetings, the effective use of agendas, and sticking to the time schedule for the meetings. The nurse manager will be surprised to discover what effect her own poor management and leadership style may have on the use of time in her department. McFarland et al. (1984: 274) point out that one person's poor time management habits may have a ripple effect on the rest of the organization, and they suggest that group analysis be used to identify and diagnose major problems in time management. The group must then decide which intervention strategies to use.

After a period of time it is necessary to evaluate the results of the time-saving strategies. If the result is not satisfactory, another approach may be needed.

CONCLUSION

Time management is an important tool that can be successfully applied in nursing management. For best results, teach subordinates to apply time management techniques in their personal lives too. When subordinates waste personal time, they will try to catch up during working hours, a situation that may prove to be very unproductive.

References

Gillies, D. A. (1989). *Nursing Management: A Systems Approach*. Saunders: Philadelphia.

La Monica, E. L. (1990). *Management in Nursing. An Experimental Approach that makes Theory Work for You*. Springer: New York.

Marriner-Tomey A. (1992). *Guide to Nursing Management*. Fourth edition. Mosby: St Louis.

McCarthy, M. J. Managing your own time: the most important management task. *JONA*, volume 11, number 11, November/December 1981, pp. 61–5.

McFarland, G. K., Leonard, H. S. and Morris, M. M. (1984). *Nursing Leadership and Management — Contemporary Strategies*. John Wiley: New York.

Sullivan, E. J. and Decker, P. J. (1988). *Effective Management in Nursing*. Second edition. Addison-Wesley Publishing Company: Menlo Park.

Tappen, R. M. (1989). *Nursing Leadership and Management: Concepts and Practice*. Davis Co: Philadelphia.

PART THREE:

STAFFING

CHAPTER 12

METHODS OF PERSONNEL ASSIGNMENT FOR PATIENT CARE

S. W. Booyens

CONTENTS

INTRODUCTION

The nurse manager is responsible for determining the staffing requirements of nursing personnel for her institution and has to decide on the methods of personnel assignment which will prevail. The methods chosen will affect the number of nursing posts to be established and the number of posts for the different categories of nurses because the different methods require different staff mixes. Each method has its advantages and disadvantages, so a particular method may be more applicable to a particular situation or set-up than another (eg a large medical ward may have different requirements from an intensive care unit). When choosing a method or methods, the needs of both patients and staff members should ideally be considered.

FUNCTIONAL METHOD

The functional method of assignment originated during the Second World War. Large numbers of patients had to be cared for by a limited number of nurses.

In this method the different nursing tasks are separated and each nurse in a unit is assigned one or more nursing functions for a number of patients or for all the patients in a ward. Thus, for example, some nurses are responsible for making beds and washing patients, others are responsible for treating bedridden patients' backs and pressure parts, others are responsible for the administration of medications, others for the measuring and charting of patients' temperatures and their pulse and respiration rates, and others are responsible for measuring patients' blood pressure and recording intake and output.

The functional assignment method is sometimes also used for district care visits. A more senior member of staff visits a patient's home to do health teaching, counselling, and carry out complex care techniques — eg dressings — while a junior member of staff would visit the same patient to assist with bathing and personal care (Tappen 1983: 359).

The functional method implements classical scientific management principles (Marriner-Tomey 1988: 146), for example:

- efficiency is emphasized;

- division of labour according to abilities;

- rigid control measures;

- procedure manuals are used to describe standards of care.

All the responsibilities and authority flow from the charge person downwards to the staff members working in a unit. The sister in charge is thus saddled with a wide span of control. This makes her controlling function difficult (Bernhard and Walsh 1990: 44).

Advantages

The main advantage of this method is its efficiency. A heavy workload can be completed in a relatively short period of time. It is thus the method of choice when staffing is poor, and in emergency and disaster situations.

Another advantage is the fact that each staff member has an opportunity to become extremely competent in the one or two tasks in which she specializes — eg a nursing auxilliary who decks a 'shaving trolley' might become a favourite among the male patients when doing her shaving round. Certain staff members tend to derive satisfaction from the outstanding performance of some of these smaller repetitive tasks.

When a number of patients need only routine care, this is the preferred method.

Disadvantages

The main disadvantage of this method is that it uses the assembly line type of division of labour, with the result that it is mechanistic and impersonal, and it emphasizes the more technical aspects of nursing care (Tappen 1983: 359).

The staff experience their work as repetitive and boring, and they often fail to interpret the significance of a particular reaction of a patient to his treatment because they do not really nurse the patient holistically. This is especially true if the documentation of patient care is of a low standard.

The patient experiences care as being divided among many people; each does one or two tasks but they often neglect to communicate the problems he is experiencing to the correct nurse who is willing — or who has the power — to attend to them timeously.

From the manager's point of view it is difficult to fix responsibility for errors in patient care. When the responsibility for patient care is divided among several nurses it is easy for each nurse to shrug off responsibility for omissions or neglect (Gillies 1982: 173).

CASE METHOD

In the case method of assignment one nurse is accountable for the total care of one or more patients for the period of her work shift. Private duty nursing is a good example of this method. The case method is also used extensively in intensive care units. When there is a patient who is seriously or critically ill in a general ward, this method is often used to care for all the needs of this specific patient. It is often termed 'specialing a patient'.

Advantages

The organization of work and the assignment of nurses to patients is relatively easy for the sister-in-charge, provided she has sufficient staff members on the ward.

The co-ordination of the different services to provide the care for one or two patients is done by the nurse assigned to them, and thus visits of other health team members are well spaced.

It is easy to fix the responsibility for care, because a specific nurse assumes accountability for a reasonable length of time for a specific patient or patients (Tappen 1983: 358).

The patient–nurse relationship should be good, because the one assigned nurse is responsible for seeing that all the nursing care needs of the patient are being met.

A high level of work satisfaction is experienced by the nurse because she cares for the patient holistically and is able to follow the patient's path to recovery closely. When a patient's condition deteriorates all the time, she has the satisfaction of having given all the nursing care possible to ease his suffering.

Disadvantages

One of the major disadvantages of this method is the large number of registered nurses or senior nursing students required per shift. The number required is usually not available. A second problem with this system is that the staff members available can be utilized more efficiently — ie junior nurse students and nursing auxilliaries could be used for giving technical care, while the few senior members of staff could do the nursing care planning for many patients.

Although one or more patients are assigned to one nurse per shift, the patient will be nursed by at least three different nurses during a 24-hour period when the 8-hour shift system operates. The patient–nurse relationship is thus divided between three people, but often the patient is exposed to more than three nurses because of nurses taking their off-duty days, or becoming ill, or being absent from work for other reasons.

Confusion may result when each nurse who is responsible for a patient or two orders the supplies and services necessary for the care of her patients from the supportive services (eg meals, drugs) and from paramedical services (eg x-rays, laboratory, physiotherapy, etc.).

TEAM NURSING

Team nursing was designed to overcome the problems created by the functional method and to make the best use of the abilities of the available staff members (Tappen 1983: 360).

The patients in a unit are divided into different groups. Each group of patients is nursed by a specific team of nurses. The number of patients in a group varies according to the types of diseases they are suffering from and the acuity levels, as well as the number and categories of nursing staff which are available.

Each team is led by a registered nurse. The other members included in the team are usually student and auxilliary nurses. The team leader is accountable for the total care of all the patients in her group and is responsible for delegating patient care to the members of her team.

Each team member is usually responsible for the total care of one or more patients. The team leader assigns the care of certain patients to a specific team member on the basis of the member's abilities and experience and the needs of the patient. The team leader assists the various team members with the patient care where needed.

The team leader supervises her team members and reports to the sister-in-charge. This reduces the charge sister's span of control.

Underlying principles

1. Individualized nursing care plans, personalized care, and nursing care objectives for each patient are emphasized, rather than the completion of nursing care tasks (Price, Franck and Veith 1974: 67).

2. The team leader should be a registered nurse.

3. The team leader should use a democratic or participative leadership style (Tappen 1983: 360).

4. Frequent and effective communication between team members is necessary. Team conferences should be held regularly. The aim of these is to discuss the care given to each patient in the team and the effects thereof, and to utilize the experience and abilities of all team members to do the initial or further nursing care plans for specific patients (Bernhard and Walsh 1990: 45).

Advantages

When team nursing is carried out according to the correct principles, a number of positive outcomes are observed.

- The professional nurses who function regularly as team leaders develop valuable leadership skills.

- The individual skills and knowledge of each team member are emphasized because each member must contribute to nursing care planning during team conferences.

- The increased amount of communication and co-operation between members of the team, and the full utilization of each one's abilities, raise staff morale (Tappen 1983: 361). The job satisfaction of the nursing staff is thus increased.

- The patients are, on the whole, more satisfied with their care because of the more personalized holistic nursing care approach.

Disadvantages

Registered nurses who are assigned as team leaders often do not possess the necessary interpersonal, leadership, or clinical skills for their role (Tappen 1983: 361).

Teams are often constructed poorly, with the result that they are ineffective. A team consisting of only two or three members and catering for the needs of a large number of patients, for example, has to use the functional method to do the work (Gillies 1982: 174–5).

When the composition of a team must be changed too regularly and too drastically from day to day because of nurses' off-duty days, some of the necessary co-operation and team spirit may be lost (Bernhard and Walsh 1990: 45).

PRIMARY NURSING

The underlying philosophy of primary nursing is that comprehensive, continuous, co-ordinated and individualized nursing care is delivered to a patient by a registered nurse who has the autonomy and authority to assume the overall and final accountability for the planning, delivery, and outcome of that care.

Primary nursing works best in an organization with mainly registered nurses as nursing staff members. Primary nurses are usually given a case-load of four to five patients for whom the planning, implementation, and evaluation of nursing care must be shouldered (Gillies 1982: 175).

It is the responsibility of the primary nurse to do the clinical assessment of the health care needs of the patients in her care, to spell out their nursing care needs, to draw up their nursing care plans, to implement the nursing care, and to co-ordinate the care with the other members of the health care team — ie doctors, physiotherapists, social workers, and others. She must also evaluate each patient's response to the care given, and change and adapt the nursing care plan accordingly.

Ideally the primary nurse chooses the patients for whom she will assume responsibility according to her specific capabilities and their health care needs. In many hospitals, however, the sister-in-charge assumes the responsibility of matching patients and their needs to suitable primary nurses.

The primary nurse who assumes responsibility for a patient is accountable for that patient throughout his stay in the hospital, for his follow-up care after discharge if necessary, and for his care when the patient is readmitted into the same hospital (Gillies 1982: 175).

The registered nurse who is doing primary nursing is responsible for the care of her patients on a 24-hour basis. She is assisted by a second registered or senior nurse to whom she can delegate the care of her patients when she goes off duty. She is, however, not relieved of the responsibility for the patients under her care when she is not on duty because she takes the final responsibility for ensuring that the nurses who assist her in her task for caring for her case load of patients render the nursing care strictly according to her prescriptions. She must be prepared to be contacted during her off-duty days when urgent changes in nursing care plans are called for.

The primary nurse must preferably be a registered nurse because nurses with less experience and training usually do not possess the necessary clinical knowledge and problem-solving skills to assume such a big responsibility for the total, comprehensive care of a number of patients (Gillies 1982: 175).

In the primary nursing care system the role of the sister-in-charge of a unit is different. She need not be, and actually should not be, an authoritarian control person who actively monitors the care of her patients. It is the primary nurse who is the real authority on the patients under her care and who is responsible for planning, bringing about, and evaluating the outcome of the care given. The role of the person-in-charge thus changes to that of a 'coach, resource person and quality control advocate' (Gillies 1982: 175–6). The sister-in-charge is, however, still responsible for co-ordinating the basic running of the ward — ie for ensuring that adequate equipment, supplies, drugs, linen, etc. are available.

Primary nursing grew from the nursing profession's desire for autonomy and with the evolution of the nursing profession itself. The primary nurse functions on par with other health professionals such as doctors, occupational therapists, and physiotherapists (Marram et al. 1976: 3).

Primary nursing must not be confused with primary care. Primary care refers to the first health worker who comes into contact with a patient and who does the initial assessment, diagnosis, and treatment of that patient. Primary nursing is done by a nurse who assumes the responsibility for the total care of a small group of patients throughout their hospitalization on a 24-hour basis (Marram et al. 1976: 2).

Advantages

The primary nurse has detailed knowledge of a small group of patients and is personally accountable for their care in a holistic sense; one may thus expect that the quality of nursing care given will be good (Bernhard and Walsh 1990: 47).

Primary nurses, once accustomed to this mode of work, generally feel that they are functioning more effectively under this system than under others. They also derive more job satisfaction from being involved in the entire care of a patient (Tappen 1985: 362).

Patients are more satisfied with their care and feel that they are treated as special human beings whose emotional needs are met together with their physical needs (Marram et al. 1976: 4).

A number of researchers found primary nursing more cost-effective than other modalities because patients are able to leave the hospital sooner and medical legal risks are restricted to the absolute minimum.

Disadvantages

With this system a much higher proportion of professional nurses to ancillary personnel are required (Tappen 1985: 362).

Not all registered nurses feel themselves adequately prepared to take on the entire responsibility for a group of patients as is expected in this type of nursing. They are often accustomed to working in the routinized setting of functional nursing care and feel that they need additional education to take on the role of a primary nurse (Tappen 1985: 363).

The role of ancillary personnel — ie auxilliary nurses — is ill-defined under this system and thus these personnel may not always be utilized to their full capacity (Tappen 1985: 363).

MODULAR NURSING

Modular nursing is a modification of team and primary nursing. It is sometimes used when there are not enough registered nurses available.

The patients in a unit are divided according to the layout of the ward. For example, patients in room numbers 1–6 which are situated near each other, or the patients in beds 1–10 and 10–20 in a Florence Nightingale-type ward may be grouped together and be nursed by a team. Each group of patients (usually eight to twelve) is nursed by a small team of nurses consisting of two to three staff members. Each team must be led by a senior nurse or registered nurse, if available. The leader's responsibilities include giving and receiving shift reports, and offering and asking for help from the leader of another team (Bernhard and Walsh 1990: 48).

Each pair or team of nurses is responsible for the patients in their group, from admission to discharge, for any follow-up care, and throughout any subsequent readmissions to the same hospital (Gillies 1982: 176). Each team of nurses must arrange for another group of nurses to care for their patients during their off-duty hours and days (Gillies 1982: 176).

The sister-in-charge assumes an important role in this system. She is responsible for supervising the nursing care of all the patients in her unit and has to co-ordinate the work. She will assign an additional nurse auxilliary or other category of nurse to a team when the need arises. She also ensures that the different team leaders stay in contact with one another, although indirectly, regarding all the patients and their needs in the unit (Bernhard and Walsh 1990: 48).

Advantages

Some researchers suggest that nursing care productivity under this system is better than with either team or primary nursing. There appears to be more communication and co-operation between the different staff members on a unit than with either primary or team nursing (Bernhard and Walsh 1990: 48).

Disadvantages

When a patient moves from one bed or room to another he might fall in a different patient-group and thus will have to get accustomed to a new set of nurses (Bernhard and Walsh 1990: 48).

There is a division of the final accountability for patient care between the sister in charge of the unit and the leader of each team.

CONCLUSION

Each method of nurse-patient assignment is of value in a given set of circumstances. The nurse manager should thus possess a thorough knowledge of the advantages and disadvantages of each in order to decide which method or combination of methods should be utilized in her institution. She will probably base her decision on the number and type of patients to be nursed, the number and categories of nurses available, the amount of job satisfaction and professional growth she wants her staff members to achieve, the institution's policy regarding the combatting of medico-legal risks, and her own views regarding improvement of quality nursing care.

References

Berry, A. J. and Metcalf, C. L. (1986). Paradigms and practices: the organisation of the delivery of nursing care. *Journal of Advanced Nursing,* volume 11, pp. 589–97.

Bernhard, L. A. and Walsh, M. (1990). *Leadership. The Key to Professionalization of Nursing.* Second edition. Mosby: St Louis.

Gillies, D. A. (1982). *Nursing Management: A Systems Approach.* Saunders: Philadelphia.

Marram, G. (1983). The evolution of nursing care modalities: primary nursing. *International Nursing Review,* volume 31, number 2, pp. 50–2.

Marram, G., Flynn, K., Abaravich, W. and Carey, S. (1976). *Cost-Effectiveness of Primary and Team Nursing.* Contemporary Publishing: Wakefield.

Marriner-Tomey, A. (1988). *Guide to Nursing Management.* Mosby: St Louis.

Metcalf, C. Job satisfaction and organizational change in a maternity hospital. *International Journal of Nursing Studies,* volume 23, number 4, pp. 285–98.

Parasuraman, S., Drake, B. H., and Jammuto, R. F. (1982). The effect of nursing care modalities and shift assignments on nurses' work experiences and job attitudes. *Nursing Research,* volume 31, number 6, pp. 364–7.

Sherman, R. O. (1990). Team nursing revisited. *JONA,* volume 20, number 11, pp. 43–6.

Tappen, R. M. (1983). *Nursing Leadership: Concepts and Practice.* F. A. Davis: Philadelphia.

Wright, S. (1985). Special assignment. *Nursing Times,* volume 81, number 35, pp. 36–7.

CHAPTER 13

RECRUITMENT AND SELECTION

S. W. Booyens

CONTENTS

INTRODUCTION

In a service organization, it is important that the people who are appointed are selected wisely from the outset. No amount of training and motivation can really offset the error of appointing the wrong person for a job (Stanton 1977: 2).

> Recruiting is that set of activities an organization uses to attract job candidates who have the abilities and attitudes needed to help the organization achieve its objectives. (Ivancevich and Glueck 1986: 190)

Ideally, a professional nurse with the necessary seniority should not only do recruiting herself, but she should be in charge of the whole recruitment programme for nursing personnel in a big institution. Recruitment should not only be an intense short-term effort to fill a number of vacant posts; it should be an ongoing effort to build the image of the organization so as to ensure a steady supply of applicants. Nursing posts become available almost continuously because nurses are seen as an extremely mobile group of professionals.

PLANNING A RECRUITMENT PROGRAMME

Before embarking on recruitment activities, the person in charge of recruitment efforts must first gather some pertinent information in order to make a worthwhile plan of action. Information should be collected regarding the following:

1. The total number of nursing posts available in the organization, and the numbers for each category of nurse.

2. The number of posts in each category which are filled, and the number of vacant ones.

3. The percentage of personnel in each category who are 20–35 years and 50–65 years old (Gillies 1982: 191).

4. The annual turnover rate for all the nursing personnel in the organization, and the annual turnover rate for each category.

5. The percentage of nursing staff living within the immediate vicinity of the hospital, the percentage living within the same community, and the percentage of staff who commute daily from nearby towns (Gillies 1982: 192).

6. The the number of registered nurses employed in the community, excluding those in one's own institution, and their places of employment.

7. The number of nurses completing the basic course each year from the training colleges where most of the job applicants are drawn (Gillies 1982: 193).

8. The salaries and fringe benefits of nursing personnel in one's own institution, as well as those of every other institution/organization which employs nursing personnel in the same community.

9. The sources of job dissatisfaction, frustrations encountered with administrative policies, unacceptable work practices or expectations, and other areas of discontent discovered during exit interviews.

10. The types of recruitment activities which yielded the best results in the past for the particular institution.

11. What image of the institution must be communicated via the recruitment campaign during the year?

12. The budget available for the year for recruitment purposes.

13. The objectives which must be reached with the recruitment programme.

FACTORS INFLUENCING RECRUITMENT

Both external and internal factors play a role in the efficacy of a recruitment programme. External factors include:

1. Government or statutory body restrictions. The requirements of the nursing council regarding who may practise nursing must be taken into account.

2. Conditions in the labour market. This is an important factor to consider (Gerber, Nel, and van Dyk 1987: 146). If there are more qualified personnel than vacant posts, then informal recruiting can be used. If, on the other hand, the number of vacant posts far outweighs the number of professionals who are available, then an intensive recruitment programme must be launched (Gerber, Nel, and van Dyk 1987: 46).

Internal factors include:

1. Organizational policy. The policy of an organization regarding the filling of vacant posts either mainly from within its own ranks (ie through the promotion of employees) or mainly from the outside, will influence a recruitment effort. If an organization's policy is to fill vacant posts from its own employees, the new employees will only be recruited for entry level posts. Recruitment in nursing is, however, usually aimed at school leavers and at registered nurses.

2. The image of the institution. The image that the public has of a particular institution will make the recruitment effort easy or difficult. If the image is a negative one, the recruiter will have to try and counter this image during the recruitment programme by emphasizing the particular institution's positive points.

3. The requirements set before the potential job seekers. If an organization sets unnecessarily high requirements, the recruitment effort will not succeed in getting enough applicants who are interested in the available jobs. It is therefore very important that realistic requirements must be set. These can only be arrived at after a thorough investigation of job analyses, job descriptions, and job specifications in the organization (Gerber, Nel and van Dyk 1987: 146). Requirements must be job-related.

RECRUITMENT STRATEGIES

More than one method or strategy is usually used to recruit the necessary number of applicants.

Employee referrals

Before going outside to recruit it is customary to ask present employees whether they know of suitable individuals who could be encouraged by them to apply for a job. Employee morale can be improved using this method, and turnover could be reduced. Caution must be exercised here, however, because not every person who an employee has suggested can be appointed.

Advertisements

Newspaper advertising generates the greatest number of experienced nurses as applicants. This was found in a study regarding the effectiveness of recruiting sources for staff nurses which was carried out during February to April, 1987, in which 32 hospitals in Oklahoma, USA, particpated.

When writing an advertisement, it should be aimed at one person in order to personalize it. The use of the words 'you' and 'we' are effective because the reader gets the impression that someone is talking to her specifically.

Organize your thoughts first. Think of all the advantages of applying for the job you have to offer. Try to anticipate the needs and desires of the applicant you want to attract. Limit each sentence to one idea or one important aspect of the offer. Make your advertisement easy to read. Avoid abbreviations and slang (Pretoria News 1992).

The greatest attraction in an advertisement is the benefits which are offered to the prospective employee. The description of what the work entails is of secondary interest and the requirements which are specified for the successful applicant are of minimum interest (Jackson 1972: 32).

An advertisement must thus first tell the prospective applicant about the rewards, benefits, and opportunities of the job, eg:

- the prestige of the hospital (or its mission statement);

- the opportunities associated with the job;

- the intrinsic satisfaction which can be derived from the job;

- fringe benefits.

Secondly, the main aspects of the job description must be given. The third section must state the requirements necessary to do the job, eg experience, qualifications, etc. (Jackson 1972: 32–3).

Advertisements are usually placed in local newspapers, in the magazine or newspaper of the nursing association, and in nursing journals. Advertising in trade journals is sometimes used because it is a cost-effective way of building an identity and generating a response.

Career days

When a recruitment officer is given the chance to address a gathering of senior school students, this opportunity should be used wholeheartedly because it is a very cost-effective way of recruiting. The recruiter would do well to show a neatly-made video programme at such an opportunity, and then answer questions from the audience on salaries, fringe benefits, job responsibilities, promotional opportunities, and the like. It must be borne in mind that sketching an excessively rosy picture of the profession might cast doubt in the students' minds about not only the credibility of the recruiter but also about the profession. Each type of work has its difficult and unattractive aspects, and while the recruiter will not attempt to present these in an unduly lurid or negative manner, she must always be truthful when questions are asked about such aspects.

Open house

Another method which is used to recruit nursing personnel is to hold an 'open day'. Invitations to attend such a day are usually sent to secondary schools, employment agencies, the nursing profession at large, and any other local interest groups such as women's organizations. When a hospital is an acute care institution, a display of the different sections and the activities which take place within them is usually presented in a foyer or other suitable exhibition space. Conducted tours to preselected units/sections are usually also undertaken. The display and tours can and should be supplemented with a short welcoming address by the hospital's superintendent or matron-in-charge. There should be relevant literature and brochures, and enough knowledgeable nursing personnel to answer questions.

Vacation work

There are a number of advantages in hiring pupils from high schools to do vacation work in a hospital. The pupils are placed in a real-life work set-up, and experience it first-hand. The institution gets some staff when there is usually a shortage. The pupils may go back to school and act as recruiters for an institution if they experience their stay as worthwhile and if they perceive the institution favourably.

The disadvantages are that these staff members are not trained at all, so they need extra supervision. In a hospital, where life and death are always at stake, a mistake by these untrained people could have serious repercussions. Students usually do not have experience of a work set-up and often expect things to be better organized than they are during their brief work period. They are thus not drawn to the organization and may discourage other interested senior school pupils from entering nursing (Ivancevich and Glueck 1986: 211–2).

Recruitment literature

Literature for recruitment must be planned and produced thoughtfully so as to facilitate the recruiting effort. Cost-effectiveness must be taken into account. Such literature must conform to certain standards to be effective:

- Information must be up-to-date.

- Information must be portrayed creatively.

- It must contain all the information which interested individuals would like to know — eg salary scales, training periods, promotional opportunities, etc.

- Bright colours, dramatic pictures, and a brisk narrative style will give the impression of an exciting, modern profession (Gillies 1986: 195).

Other strategies

When recruiting is done in the local market, the use of non-traditional media may be of help — eg radio, television, billboards, direct mail, and innovative strategies such as displays of the nursing professional at work in interesting settings.

THE RECRUITER

The recruiter is viewed by prospective employees as a representative of the hospital or nursing profession. She is seen as an example of the kind of person the profession would like to employ. It is therefore important that the recruiter should possess such personal characteristics as poise, friendliness, and enthusiasm for her profession. Some of the more common complaints against recruiters, according to Ivancevich and Glueck (1986: 213–6), are:

- Lack of interest in the applicant.

- Lack of enthusiasm.

- The recruiter asks too many personal questions about the applicant's social class, parents, and so forth.

- The recruiter gives a speech and then, almost as an afterthought, asks if there are any questions. The interested applicants would like to have enough time to ask questions about the job itself and the work climate.

It is thus important that recruiters should be trained. They should be trained so that they can project a clear picture of the benefits of a career with a particular organization to prospective applicants. Ideally they should also be able to help with interviewing.

PROCESSING RESPONDENTS

When the recruiting process is successful, many candidates may want to apply for a job. The person who is concerned with preselection interviewing (usually a nursing service officer) and the secretary or receptionist who answers the telephone and has to handle queries regarding vacancies, must be chosen well. These people must be friendly, and must have the necessary basic facts about the job such as nominal salary scale, duty hours per week, etc. at their fingertips. They must be prepared to listen carefully to each job-seeker's queries and see that the necessary application forms are sent out or are completed at their offices. A rude, short-tempered, abrupt attitude will not attract any applicant, because the applicant will immediately perceive this type of behaviour as typical of the rest of the organization and will thus look elsewhere for a job. It is also important to be as expedient as possible in processing applications for a job in order not to lose candidates who might lose interest when they have to wait too long for a reply.

The next step in the employment process is the initial selection of suitable candidates from their completed application forms or from preliminary job interviews. Before studying the list of application forms, it is essential to reread the job descriptions as well as the job specifications. These two documents should provide the necessary knowledge about the job which will form the basis for the assessment of all the applicants. In reviewing the application forms, one has to look at the following aspects:

- Age, sex, nationality, health status.

- Education — eg school, professional.

- Employment history.

- Referrals.

- Relevant experience.

According to Einhorn et al. (1982: 119) there are also other things one should specifically look for in application forms, eg:

- Time gaps — are there periods of time between different appointments which are not accounted for?

- Education — has this individual had the necessary educational preparation for this specific job?

- Incomplete information — are there areas where the information given is vague and incomplete?

- Employment history — does the applicant's employment history show stability and success?

- Salary — what is the applicant's salary history? What can you infer from the information given?

- References — are the right people given as references? Are important people, such as immediate supervisors, omitted?

All applications should be acknowledged by a short note, or even a postcard, containing a statement of thanks for applying and stating that the application is receiving attention. The candidates whose applications are rejected from the start should receive letters of rejection as soon as possible. It is necessary to convey to the applicant that his application was examined in depth and that he is being treated fairly. Although the letter itself is formal, the informal 'Dear Mrs/Miss' and 'yours sincerely' are used at the beginning and end (Goodworth 1979: 19). Those applicants whom the employer wishes to interview in order to do the final selection should receive an invitation to the interview. This letter should clearly give the date, time, venue, and the approximate duration of the interview.

Preparing for the interview

The interviewing process can only be an effective method of selection if it is done in a structured, systematic way and is designed beforehand. When preparing interviews, the nurse manager should see to the following aspects:

1. Preparation of the shortlist. The manager must decide on the number of candidates that can be interviewed for possible appointment, depending on the number of available vacant posts. Once the number has been decided on, all the application forms are reviewed. The best candidates, as they appear on paper, are then selected. It must be remembered that the job specification will serve as a blue-print for selection purposes during this elimination phase. It is also important to remember that the data on the application forms should be interpreted correctly. The aspects mentioned under 'processing of respondents' should be taken into account.

2. Preparation of interviewer(s). The interviewer must study the application forms of the candidates with whom interviews will be conducted carefully. The job description must also be studied in detail. The interviewer must then develop a structured format for the questions or aspects to be covered in the interview. The questions must be formulated in a chronological order.

3. Preparation of a venue. The office where the interview will take place should be quiet. The recommended seating is two comfortable chairs placed alongside two edges of a table or desk — not opposite each other. Care must be taken that the room is not too cold or too hot, that clutter is removed, and that the physical atmosphere appears comfortable. The environment should be a welcoming one, preferably with plants, adequate lighting, appropriate wall decorations, and appropriate reading material (eg *Curationis,* or *Nursing RSA*) supplied in the waiting area.

4. Other preparations:

   • The secretary must have a list of the candidates to be interviewed.

   • The interviewer should schedule at least 15 minutes before and after each interview to allow enough time for writing up his/her conclusions concerning the interview and to be able to attend to other urgent matters which develop during the period of the interview.

   • A tea break should be placed in the programme, so that the interviewer is not forced to squeeze this in.

- The secretary should be told not to put calls through.

- Allow for at least 20–30 minutes per interview.

- Do not interview more than six to eight candidates per day.

- Waiting facilities must be organized.

Conducting the interview

The following must be considered when conducting an interview for selection purposes:

- The applicant must be greeted in a friendly manner and made to feel as comfortable as possible.

- An interview is a purposeful conversation between the employer and the applicant. The employer seeks information regarding the applicant's knowledge, skills, and abilities for a particular job, and the candidate seeks information regarding the requirements and nature of the job and the philosophy and characteristics of the employing organization in general.

- Both the positive and the negative aspects of the job must be described to the prospective employee in sufficient detail (Gillies 1982: 198).

- The primary skill which should be used in interviewing is active listening. This is demonstrated by looking at the interviewee, by sitting in an alert manner, and by responding with a word or phrase where necessary (Shouksmith 1978: 42).

- The interviewer should enhance an applicant's openness towards him/her by showing a relaxed demeanour, by leaning slightly towards the candidate, and by maintaining eye contact.

- The interviewee should be encouraged to talk freely and to reveal his/her thoughts and feelings. Open-ended, non-directive questions should thus be asked most of the time.

- The talk must deal with the topics decided beforehand.

- Paraphrasing and summarizing are useful techniques for encouraging an interviewee to talk (Shouksmith 1978: 43).

- The interviewer must be aware of his/her own prejudices so that these are avoided as far as possible during the interview and the assessment of the applicant.

- Keep control over the interview. The interviewer must not appear dominating, but must steer the interview back on track when the interviewee tends to digress from the matter under discussion (Gerber, Nel and van Dyk 1987: 173).

- Opinions about an applicant's ability to fill a position must not be given during the interview (Gillies 1982: 198).

- Avoid giving advice or moralizing during an interview.

- When an applicant's answer is vague, inaccurate, or incomplete, probe to find the truth.

- The interviewee must be given a chance to ask for any additional information.

- End the interview by telling the applicant when the final selection will take place and how and when she will be informed of the decision.

- Notes must be made during or directly after the interview. The notes, however, must be made on a standardized interview outline, so that a comparison of the candidates who were interviewed is possible.

Shouksmith (1978: 36) quotes the following 'Hawthorne rules' for conducting an interview:

Rule 1. The interviewer should listen to the speaker in a patient and friendly, but intelligently critical, manner.

Rule 2. The interviewer should not display any kind of authority.

Rule 3. The interviewer should not give advice or moral admonition.

Rule 4. The interviewer should not argue with the speaker.

Rule 5. The interviewer should talk or ask questions only under the following conditions:

- to help the person talk;

- to relieve fears and anxieties which are inhibiting the speaker from relating to the interviewer;

- to steer the discussion onto a topic which has been omitted or neglected;

- to discuss implicit assumptions if this is advisable.

SELECTION

The first step is to compute a valid and comprehensive list of items to be measured, eg:

- basic educational qualifications;

- post-basic qualifications;

- employment history;

- career goals;
- reaction to policies such as shift-work, night duty;
- general appearance;
- language ability;
- general impression.

The best way to compare candidates is to use the above or any other valid assessment aspects as headings on a sheet of paper and then to fill in under each heading each applicant's characteristics regarding the heading as assessed during the interview.

Considerable effort and time has been spent by a number of nursing institutions in developing an effective interviewing tool which can be used repeatedly and which makes for a relatively easy evaluation of the responses obtained after the interviewing process. The following is a list of recommended characteristics for the interviewer to assess before and while interviewing candidates for a professional nurse's post and higher posts, excluding nurse managers (adapted from Battle et al. 1985):

1. Characteristics documented in application forms: references, copies of certificates, testimonials:

   - Additional post-basic courses — nursing and other.
   - Reference to special proficiencies.
   - Special accomplishments in nursing — eg publications, awards, etc.

2. Clinical proficiency (obtained from the interview and available records). Note experience: what type of experience, recency of experience, complexity of performance, and whether it was in a relevant clinical area. Also note knowledge and skills such as patient-teaching skills.

3. Administrative abilities (obtained from the interview and from available records). Note experience: what type of experience, recency of experience, and complexity of experience. Also note knowledge and skills.

4. Research (information obtained from the interview, records, resumés, etc.). Again note experience: what type of experience, and whether it includes initiation of projects and participation in projects. Also note the use of this experience. Does the candidate communicate findings to others? What use do these findings have in practice?

5. Education (obtained from interview and available records). Note experience in teaching staff, the recency of experience, and the

complexity of performance that was required. Also note knowledge/skills.

6. Note other significant factors (obtained from the interview and application letter). These might include the candidate's philosophy, communication skills (verbal, non-verbal, and written), her interpersonal skills, leadership skills, her goals in relation to her position, her participation on committees, and her general professional image including grooming, composure/poise, her ability to sell herself, her attitude towards responsibility, and her willingness to take action. Also note her willingness to undertake additional job responsibility, whether she has sufficient confidence to discuss shortcomings, whether she shows evidence of being a self-starter, whether she follows through on projects that have been assigned and initiated, and whether she is willing to share credit for accomplishments with others.

Selecting nurse managers

The selection and interviewing of candidates to fill nurse manager positions poses specific problems. Managers cannot be selected using the same guidelines as those used for the professional nursing personnel lower down in the hierarchy. A number of tools for the effective selection of this category of nurse have been developed in the USA.

Research suggests that the types of competencies which the nurse manager should have in order to be a successful manager, and which should thus be assessed during the selection phase, are the following:

- Ability to get the job done. This would be assessed by evaluating the initiative that the person shows: taking action before being asked, seizing opportunities, and doing significantly more than is required.

- The person's achievement orientation — commitment to accomplishing challenging objectives.

- Management — ie working through others. This would be assessed by evaluating an individual's ability to direct others: to use the power of one's position in an appropriate way, to set standards of behaviour, and to tell others what is expected of them. The selectors would also consider the individual's group management skills such as the promotion of teamwork, keeping the group informed, reducing internal conflict, and finding solutions which satisfy all the parties involved (Dubricki and Sloan 1991).

- Interpersonal relationships — ie working with others. Assessment of this would focus upon:

  (a) use of influence strategies, eg development of planned sequences of actions to influence others;

  (b) interpersonal sensitivity, eg ability to understand other people's motives, concerns, feelings, strengths, and weaknesses;

  (c) direct persuasion, eg ability to present a logical, compelling case.

- Problem-solving — ie thinking issues through. An individual's analytical thinking abilities are assessed, eg whether she is able to break a complex problem into its component parts, to think about the parts systematically, and to make systematic comparisons of different aspects of an issue.

- Personal performance — ie managing oneself. The applicant's self-confidence is evaluated. This is a belief in one's own capability to accomplish a task and one's willingness to exercise independent judgement (Dubricki and Sloan 1991).

In some institutions, in addition to the interviewing process, candidates are presented with a number of complicated nursing management problems which they have to solve. These problems are in a written form and the candidates must provide written answers to them in a period of seven days. Outside reviewers are then asked to evaluate the responses according to the following criteria:

- identification of the problem;

- use of a systematic problem-solving method;

- rationale for action;

- adequate follow-up of the action taken, and

- the appropriate use of a management theory (Johnson et al. 1984: 27).

In another health centre, in the USA, the selection of the appropriate candidate for a nurse manager's post also consisted of an interview as well as written answers to questions. An example of such a written-response question is the following (Ertl 1984: 31):

> Rank the following activities in their order of importance as they relate to the manager's function and explain in writing your top three choices
>
> - Budget preparation and monitoring.
> - Patient care assignments.
> - Quality assurance activities.
> - Attendance at management meetings.

- Performance appraisal of personnel.
- Staff development activities.
- Self development activities.
- Patient rounds.
- Physician interactions.
- Staff meetings.
- Staff interactions.

The following interview questions could be useful when selecting a nurse manager (Ertl 1984: 30–1):

1. What motivated you to apply for this post and what do you hope to gain from it?

2. Describe the goals you would like to attain in your professional life in the coming five years.

3 What do you feel would make you an asset for this organization and for your co-workers?

4. Identify the strengths which you think make you the most suitable candidate for the post.

5. Identify and discuss your limitations.

6. Describe the methods that you would use to evaluate the competencies of your staff.

7. How would you divide your time between your clinical and managerial responsibilities?

8. How do you see this position in relation to the medical staff, nurse managers, other managers, the superintendent, nursing students, and clinical instructors?

9. We are somewhat concerned about the depth of your management and/or clinical experience. How would you overcome this?

CONCLUSION

The recruitment of nursing personnel who will be an asset to the particular health organization is fairly easy during times of economic depression, but it has often been a taxing and sometimes unsatisfactory task in the past when it was difficult to lure sufficient numbers of professional nurses to work in health care institutions. The selection process is equally taxing and time-consuming, and needs to be executed with care and commitment if an organization wants to have an effective and efficient personnel force which guarantees quality care to patients.

References

Battle, E. H., Bragg, S., Delaney, J., Gilbert, S., Roesler, D. (1985). Developing a rating interview guide. *JONA,* volume 15, number 10, pp. 39–45.

Courtis, J. (1976). *Cost-effective Recruitment.* Institute of Personnel Management: London.

Dubricki, C. and Sloan, S. (1991). Excellence in Nursing Management. *JONA,* volume 21, number 6, pp. 40–4.

Einhorn, L. J., Bradley P. H. and Baird, J. E. (1982). *Effective Employment Interviewing.* Scott, Foresman and Co.: Illinois.

Ertl, N. (1984). Choosing successful managers. *JONA,* April 1984, pp. 27–33.

Genua, R. L. (1979). *The Employer's Guide to Interviewing.* Prentice Hall: New Jersey.

Gerber, P. D., Nel, P. S. and van Dyk, P. S. (1987). *Human Resources Management.* Southern: Johannesburg.

Gillies, D. A. (1982). *Nursing Management: A Systems Approach.* Saunders: Philadelphia.

Goodworth, C. T. (1979). *Effective Interviewing for Employment Selection.* Communica: Europe.

Henderson, P. E. (1989). Communication without words. *Personnel Journal,* January 1989. pp. 22–9.

Herriot, P. (1989). *Recruitment in the 90s.* Institute of Personnel Management: London.

Jackson, M. (1972). *Recruiting, Interviewing and Selecting.* McGraw Hill: London.

Johnson, E. P., Wagner, D. H., Sweeney, J. P. (1984). Identifying the right nurse manager. *JONA,* November 1984, pp. 24–9.

Jolma, D. J. and Weller, D. E. (1989). An evaluation of nurse recruitment methods. *Journal of Nursing Administration,* volume 19, number 4, April 1989, pp. 20–3.

Labig, C. E. (1990). Effectiveness of recruiting sources for staff nurses. *Journal of Nursing Administration,* volume 20, number 7/8, July/August 1990, pp. 12–17.

Pretoria News, 7 May, 1992.

Shouksmith, G. (1978). *Assessment through Interviewing.* Massey University: New Zealand.

Smeltzer, C. H., Tseng, S. and Harty, L. M. (1971) Implementing a Strategic Recruitment and Retention Plan. *JONA,* volume 21, number 6. June 1971, pp. 20–7.

Stoops, R. (1982). Recruitment. *Personnel Journal,* February 1982, p. 102.

Wall, L. L. (1988). Plan development for a nurse recruitment–retention programme. *JONA,* volume 18, number 2, February 1988, pp. 21–5.

CHAPTER 14
ASSIGNMENT OF STAFF

S. W. Booyens

CONTENTS

INTRODUCTION

Planning for human resources in general, and for a nursing service in particular, is one of the management tasks which demands the most time and money (Kruger 1984: 31). Planning for the provision of staff is a complex task which is never completed because of the dynamic nature of patients' problems, the preferences of nursing personnel, their availability patterns, and the changes which occur in the technological, social, political, and economic spheres of society (Kruger 1984: 37).

The provision of nursing personnel accounts for a large portion of the budget of an institution, so it must be done as accurately as possible. The most accurate and acceptable method of calculating the number of nursing posts needed for a unit and for an institution as a whole is the use of a patient classification system (Kruger 1984: 33).

PATIENT CLASSIFICATION

For nurses, the term 'patient classification' means the 'categorization of patients according to an assessment of their nursing care requirements over a specified period of time' (Giovanetti 1979: 4). Patients are usually classified to determine the total number of staff needed and to assign them.

The patient classification method rests on the following principles:

- The identification of patients, and the classification of patients into groups or categories according to their nursing care requirements.

- The quantification of the nursing care requirements of each category.

- The establishment of a ratio for professional nurses to sub-professional nurses.

Patient classification systems developed in response to the variable nature of nursing care demands. The number of patients in a unit may stay the same, but the nursing care demands of the patients may fluctuate from shift to shift and from day to day. The number of patients in a unit may thus not be an adequate indication of what the nursing care demands are. By grouping patients into categories which reflect the nursing care requirements for a particular group, a more rational and sensitive approach is followed to determine the need for nursing manpower (Giovanetti 1979: 4).

A wide variety of patient classification systems exist at present. According to Abdellah and Levine, there are two common types of patient classification systems: the *prototype evaluation system* and the *factor evaluation system.* In the prototype evaluation system the characteristics of patients who would be classified into a particular group are described. In the factor evaluation system a number of critical direct nursing care indicators are separately rated and then combined to indicate a patient's category (Giovanetti 1979: 5).

DETERMINATION OF NURSING CARE TIME

In a patient classification system it is necessary to arrive at a quantification of effort or time. In the prototype evaluation system the time required to care for a typical patient in each category is determined. This is done by timing different nurses as they care for a number of characteristic patients in each category. The times taken to care for each category are then averaged (Gillies 1979: 221).

With the factor evaluation system the average time required to perform each nursing care task in each category must be determined. This is done by timing the actual performance of these tasks by a number of nurses (Gillies 1979: 221).

It is not important whether an institution uses average care times for a category, or average care times for procedures, or a combination of both. The techniques which are used to collect data and the manner in which observational studies are conducted are, however, important (Giovanetti 1979: 6).

A particular classification system may be applicable to a variety of settings, but the quantification of procedures or care times cannot be transferred from one hospital to another or from one unit to another. There are a number of factors which affect the determination of care times, such as the attitudes of staff members, their abilities and skills, the available physical facilities, the practices of physicians, the architectural layout of the unit, and the nurse–patient assignment method used in the hospital (Giovanetti 1979: 6).

FACTOR EVALUATION SYSTEM

In the factor evaluation system a number of nursing care elements or nursing care descriptors are identified. These descriptors of nursing care are then broken down into sub-elements. Standard nursing care times must be computed for these sub-elements, so the sub-elements must relate to observable, measurable tasks (Gillies 1979: 221).

Nursing care descriptors

Nursing care descriptors, or categories of nursing care activities, are determined by the nursing staff of the hospital. Examples of nursing care descriptors are the following:

1. ● activity

   ● positioning

   ● diet

   ● intravenous fluids

   ● observations (Gillies 1979: 222)

2. ● personal care

   ● feeding

   ● observation

   ● ambulation (Gillies 1979: 222)

3. ● physical activities

   ● observation

   ● medication

   ● treatment

   ● psycho-social

   ● rehabilitation and teaching (Kruger 1984: 33)

In the ARIC computer-based patient classification system, patients are classified according to what are known as *dependent* and *independent* descriptors.

The dependent descriptors include the following:

● intake/output

● vital signs

● routine medications

● mouth care

● positioning/activity

The independent descriptors include an analysis of the patient's support system and his need for nursing intervention, as well as of the extent of co-ordination of nursing care that must be carried out and the referral activity involved in his care (Giovanetti and Johnson 1990: 35).

Each nursing care descriptor is explained and divided into different levels ranging from low intensity to very high intensity. These are used to classify each patient at a given moment in time.

An example of the different care levels set forth for the descriptor of *rehabilitation and teaching* might be the following:

1. Light care. Ten minutes or less need to be spent by the nursing personnel per 24 hours to teach the patient and/or his relatives about his treatment, diet, medications, ward care, etc.

2. Moderate care. Fifteen minutes per 12 hours need to be spent on teaching.

3. High care. About 30 minutes per eight-hour shift need to be spent on teaching.

4. Intense care. One hour or more per eight-hour shift needs to be spent on teaching (Kruger 1984: 34).

Validity and reliability of the classification instrument

The measuring device which is used to classify patients according to their nursing care requirements must conform to the normal standards for reliability and validity before it can be used with confidence. *Validity* is the extent to which an instrument actually measures what it sets out to measure. Remember that a patient classification instrument does not measure a patient's actual needs for nursing care. A patient classification system only groups patients in terms of the amount of nursing care time to be received according to perceived nursing care requirements (Giovanetti 1979: 7).

Content and face validity are usually sought for such an instrument. Content validity is established by presenting the criteria for classification to a panel of nurse experts who examine them to ensure that they are relevant and useful for the purpose of classifying according to nursing care time. Face validity simply involves agreement among the developers and the users of the instrument that the criteria for classification seem reasonably correct and will provide reasonably correct classifications (Giovanetti 1979: 7).

Reliability refers to the fact that it is important that the instrument is clear and easy to use to the extent that different nurses classifying the same patient at the same time will obtain very similar results (Giovanetti 1979: 7). The inter-rater reliability of a patient classification instrument can be maximized by training nursing staff members carefully in the proper interpretation and application of the tool (Gillies 1979: 225).

STEPS IN THE CLASSIFICATION PROCESS

Step 1

The development of a valid and reliable classification instrument.

Step 2

The determination of the average number of nursing care hours for each category into which patients will be classified. (This is usually done by time and motion studies which are undertaken in a specific institution.)

Step 3

A well-planned in-service education programme must be presented in order to train all the nursing staff members who will be classifying patients. It is essential that staff members interpret the criteria set for classification similarly and that they be given practice sessions during the in-service education phase.

Step 4

Trained nursing staff members classify the patients in their units using the classification instrument. Each patient in the unit must be evaluated each day at the same time for a representative period (eg one to three months). An evaluation form is completed for each patient when he is evaluated.

The evaluation form contains a column with the nursing care descriptors. The patient being evaluated is given a rating — eg 1, 2, 3 or 4 — according to the level of activity or the required nursing care time which is to be used for each descriptor. For example, 'medication = 4' involves complex and delicate procedures, often carried out by two staff members on a two- to four-hourly basis; 'physical activities = 1' means that the patient cares for himself and does not need assistance (Kruger 1984: 34). Apart from the in-service education programme which must be attended by the personnel members doing the classifications, it is also necessary for them to have a written reference at hand spelling out what is meant by the different levels of activity and nursing care requirements for each descriptor.

Step 5

The rating results for each descriptor are now added and one thus arrives at a total score for each patient on each day that the classification forms were completed. Depending on the total score, the patient is now placed into a predetermined category — eg 6 to 9 points = group 1, self care, 1.5 hours/per day; 10 to 14 points = group 2, minimal care, 2.5 hours/per day (Kruger 1984: 33). The number of hours of nursing care for each group has been established beforehand.

Step 6

The average number of patients per group who were nursed during the month in the unit is calculated as follows. The number of patients per group is counted for each day of the month. At the end of the month the average bed occupancy rate for each group is determined: the number of patients per group per day is added up and then divided by the number of days of the month. When the classification of patients is done over a period of 3 or 6 months, the monthly totals for each group are added and divided by the number of months. An average census figure is thus derived for each patient group.

Step 7

The number of nurses necessary for a unit can now be determined and will depend on the grouping of the different patients according to the classification system. This is usually done using the following formula:

A. Patient group 1 — average daily census × average hours of nursing care/day = daily total average nursing care hours for unit.
Patient group 2 — average daily census × average hours of nursing care/day = daily total average nursing care hours for unit.
Patient group 3 — average daily census × average hours of nursing care/day = daily total average of nursing care hours for unit.
Patient group 4 — average daily census × average hours of nursing care/day = daily total average nursing care hours for unit.

B. Daily average nursing care hours per unit × 7 days over hours worked by each nurse per week (day duty) = number of nurses needed per week, eg:
patient group 1 — 7 × 1.5 = 10.5
patient group 2 — 6 × 2.5 = 14.0
patient group 3 — 8 × 4.0 = 32.0
patient group 4 — 9 × 6.0 = 54.0
                            ─────
                            110.5

$$\frac{110.5 \times 7}{40} \times \frac{773.5}{40} = 19 \; nurses$$

Step 8

The number of professional nurses versus sub-professional nurses must now be calculated. The number of nurses determined in step 7 is thus divided into two groups: professional and sub-professional nurses. This subdivision is made according to a predetermined formula which is usually taken from time and motion studies carried out in a particular hospital. An example of such a subdivision is the following (Kruger 1984: 35):

	% professional nurses	% sub-professional nurses
Patient group 4	60%	40%
Patient group 1	20%	80%

Step 9

Apart from the calculated number of nurses per unit, additional posts must be calculated for the following:

- the number of relief posts for night duty;
- the number of relief posts for annual leave and for sick leave;
- the number of relief posts needed for college attendance of student nurses;
- the number of posts for the training of nurses who want to follow a post-registration nursing course.

SCHEDULING

Scheduling, as part of the staffing function, is an important managerial task. Without proper scheduling there will not be sufficient numbers of staff, or the correct mix of staff, to care for the patients. The aim of scheduling nursing staff members should be to provide adequate nursing care throughout each day for seven days a week while providing a simple, predictable work schedule with stable work groups that reduce employee fatigue and enable nursing personnel to pursue other interests and activities (Fraser 1972: 12)

Principles

There are some general principles which apply to the scheduling of nursing personnel irrespective of the institution in which it is carried out. These are the following:

1. Nursing staff members are not freely interchangeable. It should not be expected of a 'float' nurse to function at the same high level of efficiency as the nurse who is regularly working in the unit to which the 'float' nurse was assigned (Gillies 1982: 228).

2. When all personnel on a unit work a shift of eight hours per day and a five-day week, each employee will have to work two

weekends out of every three to ensure an equal distribution of staff throughout the seven days of the week (Gillies 1982: 228).

3. Overstaffing is just as unsatisfactory as understaffing. When overstaffing occurs in a unit, a staff member is often sent to another unit which is understaffed. Staff members resent this and experience high stress and frustration levels when they are subjected to this practice. When marked overstaffing occurs the quality of nursing care is lowered because staff members tend to socialize more, with the result that standards of nursing care are lowered (Gillies 1982: 219).

4. Fairness should be demonstrated when favourite holidays, vacation time, and days off are distributed.

5. Duty schedules should be displayed well in advance so that staff members are able to plan their social and other activities around their duty hours.

6. The scheduling system must provide a means for making quick staffing adjustments in cases of unforeseen absenteeism, illnesses and other emergencies (Gillies 1982: 228).

7. If a system of cyclical scheduling (a fixed type of schedule) is used, all employees should be scheduled according to the master staffing plan, with no exceptions being made for certain individuals (Gillies 1982: 228).

8. If part-time personnel are not willing to rotate their shifts from one week to the next, and do not work some weekends, the full-time personnel will have to work more late and evening shifts and weekends than when no part-time staff were used.

9. Projections of nursing care requirements beyond one day in the future are extremely difficult to make because of the variable nature of patient numbers and patient conditions (Gillies 1982: 228).

10. When employees must change from one shift to another there must be sufficient time off between the two shifts to enable the employee to travel back and forth between home and work and enjoy at least eight hours of sleep (Gillies 1982: 229).

11. A balance must be struck between the needs of the employer for predictable and adequate staffing and the needs of the employee for personal and job satisfaction (Gillies 1982: 229).

12. Staff members who have had an input into the planning of the duty schedules will accept them more readily than those who did not have an input.

Policy decisions regarding scheduling

Although one institution may have a variety of scheduling systems operating in it, it is necessary to have policy guidelines on a number of issues regarding scheduling. These are, among others, as follows:

1. The monthly changeover dates for the current year.

2. The official definition of a 'weekend' for day staff and night staff — eg from 16:00 on Friday to 07:00 on Monday.

3. The number of hours to be worked by the full-time employee per day, per week, and per month.

4. The day on which a week is started — eg Sundays.

5. The policy regarding the rotation of shifts by part-time personnel and how often, and for how long, they must work on weekends.

6. The number of hours that must elapse between the end of one shift of duty and the beginning of the next one — eg the time elapsing after the shift 07:00 – 15:00 on Wednesday, and the beginning of the next shift of 15:00 – 11:00 on Thursday, is 24 hours.

7. Whether the two days off per week must be consecutive.

8. The procedure that must be followed when nurses want to request specific holiday and vacation time.

9. The procedure to be followed in granting holidays and vacation time.

10. The procedure to be followed when resolving a conflict between nurses requesting the same days or holiday time off (Gillies 1982: 229).

11. How far in advance the duty rosters must be displayed for personnel members to be able to plan their outside activities.

12. The number of weekends to be worked by each employee per month, as well as the number of duty hours which constitute a weekend.

13. The maximum number of days which may be worked between off-duty days.

14. The length of tea, lunch, and dinner breaks.

15. The definition of overtime work.

16. The pay rates for overtime work.

17. The maximum and minimum hours of overtime work.

Flexitime work schedules

The shortage of registered nurses which many hospitals experienced during recent years has spurred a variety of experiments with flexitime schedules.

> A flexitime system is a system in which the workday is divided into care time and choice time. The worker is able, within certain predetermined limits, to begin and end his work-day as it suits him. (Searle 1988: 123)

Some directors of hospital services advocate flexible scheduling systems which respect the personal needs of the staff, varying from unit to unit. For example, some staff members work from 10:00 to 15:00 each day, others from 19:00 to 24:00. Still others work 10-hour or 12-hour shifts. Although such a variety of schedules could be more difficult for the manager to contend with than the more traditional types of schedules, the benefit of attracting and retaining more registered staff, who work diligently because the hours really suit them, would offset the disadvantage of more administration regarding scheduling.

The manager must, however, be careful when instituting flexitime schedules. If the nurses working flexitime appear to be standing out as an élite group to whom special concessions have been made, the morale of the staff may be seriously affected. It is thus advisable to offer flexitime schedules to all the registered nurses on all the units, and then try to mesh the traditional hours with the flexitime base (Laviolette 1981: 42).

JOB SHARING

Job sharing describes the situation where two or more employees share the responsibilities and benefits of a single full-time post (Buchan 1991: 32). Only a small proportion of all the part-time employment posts in an institution are usually used for job sharing. Job sharing is nevertheless seen as a worthwhile staffing strategy and displays the following characteristics:

1. Job share posts often require more complex skills — and the job content is more demanding — than that of traditional part-time posts.

2. Job sharing is a way of opening career opportunities to women.

3. Recruitment and retention of staff, especially in a 'tight' labour market, is facilitated by job sharing.

4. Re-entry into the job market by career-orientated employees who cannot work full-time is stimulated.

5. A reduction is usually achieved in labour costs: job sharers tend to be more productive than full-time workers.

6. The job sharers must be compatible with each other.

7. The effective sharing of one job will depend largely on good communication between the different job sharers, between job sharers and patients, and between job sharers and management.

8. Job sharing may provide equal opportunities in the job market by opening up posts for part-time work (Buchan 1991: 32–3).

SHIFT PATTERNS

A large variety of shift patterns are worked by nurses. Some of these are the following:

1. Five days per week with eight-hour shifts, working two weekends in every three.

2. The eight-hour shift pattern in which the nurse works for a specified period during the morning shift, and is then changed to the night or late afternoon shift (shift hours: 07:00–15:00, 15:00–23:00, and 23:00–07:00).

3. Non-traditional shifts covering day and night duty: eg 07:00–17:00, 17:00–22:00, and 21:00–07:00.

4. Twelve-hour and six-hour day shifts, eg 07:00–19:00, 07:00–13:00, 07:00–19:00, 13:00–19:00, etc.

5. The twelve-hour night shifts, eg seven nights on duty and seven nights off, with duty hours of 19:00–07:00.

6. The system of internal rotation where a mixture of early day and late afternoon shifts and at least four nights are worked per month, with the proviso that a total of 160 hours must be worked at the end of four weeks.

7. Cyclical scheduling, where shifts and work days are assigned to staff members according to a predictable and repeating pattern.

An example of a cyclical scheduling pattern where nurses are working ten-hour shifts is the following one, where nursing personnel are working the following shift hours:

— 06:00–17:30
— 09:00–18:30
— 12:00–22:30
— 14:00–00:30
— 19:30–06:00
— 22:30–09:00

When a cyclical pattern of ten-hour shifts is worked, the nurse works four days per week with three days off, including every second weekend. This type of pattern, however, needs a considerable number of nurses per unit — ie a minimum of 17.

Shift rotation and the body clock

Little research, if any, has been done on the effects that the different shifts and the rotation of these shifts have on the nurses' bodies. It is believed that night shifts reduce the quality and quantity of a nurse's sleep causing chronic fatigue and a disturbance of the body's own daily clock (Brown, 1988: 28). These disturbances are, however, not so significant in people working on night duty permanently.

Research suggests that the body's response to rapid shift changes is to run 'free'. It follows its own clock in these circumstances and runs an hour or so 'slow' each day. The margin for error is thus increased (Brown 1988: 28).

An Australian scientist, Professor George Singer, studied behaviour in people working on different rota systems. He found a very high error and accident rate among people working an early morning shift which followed a late afternoon/evening shift. He recommended that this combination should be avoided at all costs, yet this combination is frequently found in nursing schedules (Brown 1988: 28).

Singer made the following recommendations on rotation systems in order to reduce the chance of errors:

1. An employee should not work more than three consecutive nights.

2. The morning shift should not begin earlier than 08:00.

3. Changing from one shift to another should be flexible.

4. The length of shift to be worked should depend on the job's physical and mental workload. The night shift should be shorter than the day shift.

5. Short intervals of time off between shifts should be avoided.

6. There should be some free weekends, including at least two consecutive days.

7. The rotation of shifts should follow a regular pattern.

8. The shift rotation pattern should move forwards — eg early day duty, late afternoon shift, night duty, followed by off-duty days, and not the other way round. This arrangement is sympathetic to the body's internal clock.

9. Twelve-hour shifts cause the least amount of erosion of the quality and quantity of sleep (Brown 1988: 28).

10. The older the worker, the less will be her tolerance for shift work. Older workers have an increased risk of getting insufficient sleep.

11. Shift work may exacerbate existing health problems — eg asthma, diabetes, and epilepsy.

12. Workers on permanent night shift are often more satisfied than those working rotating schedules because they can plan their social life more easily.

13. The worker with shift maladaptation syndrome shows the following symptoms: sleep disturbances with chronic fatigue, heartburn, constipation or diarrhea, alcohol or drug abuse usually related to self-treatment of insomnia, depression, malaise, personality changes, and interpersonal conflicts.

14. Nurses who work on rotating shifts which include night duty experience the most job-related stress.

15. The night shift should be shorter than the morning or evening shift.

16. Nurses should have days off after night shifts so that sleep shortages can be remedied.

17. Factors in the night-time physical work environment which may contribute to fatigue and tiredness should be identified and remedied — eg adequacy of lighting, ventilation, temperature, noise.

18. The availability of nutritious food is of special importance for night duty nurses because gastrointestinal upsets are often encountered among night workers.

19. Accurate records should be kept about absenteeism, sickness, turnover, and injuries in order to identify problem areas regarding shift work.

CONCLUSION

It is clear that in order to assign nursing personnel scientifically, according to the needs of the patients, and to schedule the assigned nurses according to the care activities and the nurses' preferences as far as possible, is a task that nursing management should tackle with care and dedication. As managers become better in this area they will be rewarded by experiencing less staff turnover and absenteeism, and more general job satisfaction among nursing personnel.

References

Brown, P. (1988). Punching the body clock. *Nursing Times,* volume 84, number 44, November 2, pp. 26–8.

Buchan, J. (1991). A share in the future. *Nursing Times,* volume 87, number 23, June 5, pp. 32–3.

Fraser, L. (1972). The reconstructed work week. *Journal of Nursing Administration.* September–October 1972, pp. 12–16.

Gillies, D. A. (1982). *Nursing Management. A Systems Approach.* Saunders: Philadelphia.

Giovanetti, P. (1979). Understanding patient classification systems. *Journal of Nursing Administration,* February 1979, pp. 4–9.

Giovanetti, P. and Johnson, J. M. (1990). A new generation patient classification system. *Journal of Nursing Administration,* volume 20, number 5, pp. 33–40.

Hung, R. 1991. A cyclical schedule of 10-hour, four-day work weeks. *Nursing Management,* volume 22, number 9, pp. 30–3.

Kruger, A. (1984). Verpleegmannekragbeplanning volgens die pasiëntklassifikasiesisteem. *Curationis,* volume 7, number 1, pp. 31–6.

Laviolette, S. 1981. Shortage spurs flurry of flexitime experiments. *Modern Healthcare,* March 1981, pp. 42–5.

Siebenaler, M. J. (1991). Shiftwork. Consequences and considerations. *AAOHN Journal,* December 1991, volume 39, number 2, pp. 558–67.

Velianoff, G. D. (1991). Establishing a 10-hour schedule. *Nursing Management,* volume 22, number 9, pp. 36–8.

CHAPTER 15

ABSENTEEISM

J. H. Roos

CONTENTS

INTRODUCTION

Absenteeism in a workforce is a costly and complex problem for management — especially in nursing — because attending to patients' needs cannot be postponed (Lee and Eriksen 1990: 37). Absenteeism is often associated with turnover but, because of it's unpredictability, it is more disruptive to the work environment than turnover (Taunton, Krampitz and Woods 1989: 13).

Absenteeism problems are usually more tied to an organization's culture than employee behaviour. In other words, those organizations which do not have control regarding absenteeism, where absences go fairly unnoticed until they become extreme, or where the monitoring of absenteeism is only done sporadically, will experience higher levels of absenteeism than those organizations that have strict and regular control of absenteeism patterns (Levesque 1992).

DEFINITION OF ABSENTEEISM

Absenteeism can be broadly defined as any time away from scheduled work (Gillies 1989: 318). Often it is viewed as a form of 'withdrawal' from unsatisfactory conditions of work (Price and Mueller 1986: 2). While most authors view absenteeism as totally negative, Price and Mueller (1986: 6) maintain that an absence every now and then may help to relieve work-generated tensions and thus maintain the motivation to work.

PATTERNS OF ABSENTEEISM

Gillies (1989: 319) classifies absenteeism in terms of amount, frequency, and pattern of work time lost. Some workers are absent from work sporadically, unpredictably, and casually, while others show a predictably higher rate of absenteeism on weekends, holidays, vacation periods, or paydays. Variables like sex, age, and the distance employees must travel between work and home also have an influence on absenteeism.

The professional status of the employee may influence the rate of absenteeism. The rate of absenteeism appears to be higher among non-professionals than among professionals (Lee and Eriksen 1990: 37). This could be ascribed to the fact that professional people have more flexibility in their working time than hourly-paid workers (Chadwick-Jones, Nicholson, and Brown 1982: 3).

Individuals with personality problems tend to be absent from work more frequently than those with more stable characters, eg:

- the hypochondriac and the immature personality;

- the person with problems related to alcoholism and drug abuse;

- the person who tends to clash easily with other members of the work group (McDonald and Shaver 1981: 14).

Unemployment is also related to absenteeism. Studies found that during economic recessions the average absence rate drops remarkably. Two factors that may influence the absence rate are:

- employees laid off during a recession are more likely to be those with high absence rates;

- the remaining employees' fear of job loss will motivate them to attend work regularly (Rhodes and Steers 1990: 5).

MEASUREMENTS OF ABSENTEEISM

The following are the five measurements according to which absenteeism is expressed: single days, frequency, paid, unpaid, and total number of days (Price and Mueller 1986: 45).

Single-day absence

Some authors regard the total number of single-day absences per employee per month/year as giving the most accurate figure (Chadwick-Jones et al. 1982: 58). Some single-day absences may be involuntary (due, for instance, to bad weather conditions) but most will be the result of a choice made by the employee.

Frequency of absence

The frequency of absence is indicated by the average number of times absent per month for each employee (Price and Mueller 1986: 45). The frequency of periods absent (eg days, weeks) is counted, not the number of days absent.

Paid and unpaid absence

Paid absence is the average number of days absent per month for which an employee is compensated, while unpaid absence refers to uncompensated days away from work per month.

Number of days' absence

Days absent are measured in terms of the average number of days absent monthly per employee including paid and unpaid days (Price and Mueller 1986: 46).

Rhodes and Steers (1990: 48) use another method to measure absenteeism. This measure has two main components: the *category of absence* and *absence metrics*.

The category of absence is based on policies and employer-employee contractual arrangements. The following categories may be included:

1. certified medical illness;

2. certified accident, which could be:
   - a work related accident
   - a domestic related accident
   - contractual absence (eg jury duty, bereavement, union activities, disciplinary suspension)
   - other

Absence metrics indicate how absence is measured. Absence can be measured as follows:

1. Measure of magnitude, measuring total time lost per employee during a given period of time (it may be hours or days). Example:

$$hours\ lost\ per\ employee = \frac{no.\ of\ hours\ absent\ during\ period}{total\ number\ of\ employees}$$

2. Measure of occurrence. This indicates the number of episodes of absence within a particular time period, regardless of their duration.

3. Measure of duration. This may be measured as the average length of absence. Example:

$$average\ length\ of\ absence = \frac{total\ days\ absent}{scheduled\ workdays}$$

(Rhodes and Steers 1990: 19–22).

WHY MEASURE ABSENTEEISM?

Absenteeism should be measured for several reasons. These include management of the payroll and benefits, planning human resource requirements for scheduling, identification of absenteeism problems, and measuring and controlling personnel costs.

Managing the payroll and benefits

Information regarding each absentee is necessary, including the reason for, and duration of, absence to determine if the absence is compensable. Most employers give employees only a limited number of days leave per annum, or for a three year cycle, for which they may claim compensation.

Planning human resource requirements for scheduling

Historical data on absenteeism may be used by managers to forecast attendance. This may prove to be very helpful when scheduling. In this way, overstaffing or human resource shortfalls may be avoided.

Identification of absenteeism problems

A degree of absenteeism is inevitable and unavoidable, and the existence of absenteeism does not necessarily indicate a problem. It is therefore necessary to compare absence rates in various organizations and/or in the different departments of one organization to determine whether a problem exists or not.

Measuring and controlling personnel costs

The organization may be able to calculate the cost of absenteeism. This will assist in the development of policies and programmes to control absenteeism (Rhodes and Steers 1990: 16).

FACTORS CAUSING ABSENTEEISM

Factors that influence attendance at work can be classified under two headings, namely the *ability* to come to work, and the *motivation* to attend work.

The ability to attend work

These factors are usually unavoidable, external to the work environment, and related to family responsibilities. Because nursing is mainly a female profession, it is highly vulnerable to problems associated with ill children. Employees may become ill themselves, or may be involved in accidents. Another factor may be transportation problems (the distance from work, the weather, and the availability of public transport) (Chadwick-Jones et al. 1982: 53).

The motivation to attend work

This affects voluntary absence. Management has difficulty in deciding which types of absences are excusable (Chadwick-Jones et al. 1982: 53). Studies show that job satisfaction is inversely related to absenteeism. Working conditions and supervision are identified as organizational variables influencing job satisfaction (Lee and Eriksen 1990: 37).

A participative leadership style of management, an adequate number of qualified personnel on duty, and the decentralization of power and decisions contribute to job satisfaction (Lee and Eriksen 1990: 38; Taunton, Krampitz and Woods 1989: 13).

Dissatisfaction with the job itself, boredom, and a belief that a particular activity is not necessary, as well as ineffective supervision, and poor intragroup and intergroup work relations often lead to absenteeism (McDonald and Shaver 1981: 13). Lack of control over decisions affecting one's work, overworking, and physical exhaustion are contributing factors (McDonald and Shaver 1981: 13).

Personnel policies with liberal sick-leave benefits, lack of attendance policies or failure to consistently enforce them, lack of communication channels to upper management, ineffective grievance procedures, low pay, unpleasant working conditions, and lack of effective employee selection, placement, orientation, and training may contribute to a high rate of absenteeism (McDonald and Shaver 1981: 14).

The size of a unit (the number of employees per unit) may also give rise to absenteeism. An increased unit size is directly and strongly related to absenteeism (Gardner 1986: 27). In large departments, the presence and contribution of each worker is less apparent (Hoverstad and Kjolstad 1991: 1048). In general, employees working in a larger unit feel a lack of belonging and cohesiveness.

EFFECTS OF ABSENTEEISM

It is costly. The hospital has to pay the absent nurse and pay overtime to the person who replaces the absent nurse. The nurse who must replace the absent one may not be available and, in most cases, needs more supervision and orientation to the work situation.

The morale of the staff may be lowered because of overtime work, substitute nurses, and working with fewer staff than required (Lee and Eriksen 1990: 37). The continuity and quality of patient care may be seriously affected (Taunton, Krampitz and Woods 1989: 13).

STRATEGIES FOR REDUCING THE RATE OF ABSENTEEISM

Several strategies can be used to reduce the rate of absenteeism. These include the recording of absence data, formulating an attendance policy, reconciling the needs of employees' families with the needs of the workplace, managing transport needs, promoting health care needs, promotion of safety in the workplace, applying appropriate employee selection and orientation procedures, following up absences, applying disciplinary measures where necessary, and undertaking a variety of organizational measures.

Recording absence data

The most critical link in gathering and recording absence data is the supervisor to whom the employee reports. Maintenance of comprehensive and reliable data to pinpoint the problem is necessary (McDonald and Shaver 1981: 14). Monitoring will let managers know what is going on so they can take the necessary action.

It is important for uniform standards to be established so comparable records can be kept throughout the organization. The records should include the type of absence, the reason given, date, and duration (Schappi 1988: 7).

There are various examples of forms that can be used to record absence. The most practical form seems to be a year-planner format. Every year a new form is attached to the employee's file. This form makes provision for recording absence and reasons for absence. It will enable the personnel department to establish absenteeism patterns in the organization, as well as for the individual.

Formulating an attendance policy

Establish an easily-understood attendance policy under the aegis of top management. It should be clearly explained and communicated so that both employees and supervisors understand its provisions, standards, procedures, and guidelines (Schappi 1988: 3). This policy must make provision for specific types of leave — eg maternity, military, funeral, or study leave. The institution's rules must also include notification requirements or a doctors' certificate for sick leave (Schappi 1988: 26). McDonald and Shaver (1981: 15) suggest that group meetings should be held to make sure that everyone understands the set policy. It is also important that this policy is not permissive. Permissiveness in such a policy increases absenteeism because it is easier to be absent when there is little fear of punishment for excessive absenteeism (Price and Mueller 1986: 231).

Reconciling family and work needs

The employer must try to reconcile employees' family needs with work needs. This may lead to the development of child care centers at the hospital or institution, or the use of flexitime schedules (Schappi 1988: 56). The establishment of an on-site sick child bay could also enhance work attendance (Miller and Norton 1986: 42).

Management of transport problems

Arranging transport for employees by co-ordinating work hours with public transport, or investing in hospital transport for employees, should serve to reduce absenteeism considerably.

Promotion of health care

Schappi (1988: 70) maintains that most illness-related job absences in the workplace result from potentially controllable problems such as alcoholism, smoking, high cholesterol, hypertension, and obesity. It is also important to control stress and to implement physical fitness programs. The workplace is the prime location from which to promote health care and disease prevention. Research carried out by Jones, Bly and Richardson (1990: 98) supports the positive impact of a health promotion program.

Provision of free health care

Free health care for employees may be another method to reduce illness and absence because employees are sometimes unable to pay for a doctor's visit, or have to wait several days for a doctor's appointment (Gillies 1989: 322).

Safety at work

Accidents that occur while the person is on duty — ie on-the-job accidents — are a major cause of job absences and should be eliminated. Steps should be taken to identify and eliminate workplace hazards and to train and educate workers in job safety and health (Schappi 1988: 93).

Selection/orientation of employees

The applicant must receive an accurate picture of the job and the organization at the job interview (Rhodes and Steers 1990: 100).

When conducting a selection interview, the interviewer must try to assess the 'work ethic' of the applicant. Supervisors should also emphasize good work-attendance to a new employee during the orientation phase (Schappi 1988: 116).

Establishment of a reward system

Price and Mueller (1986: 211) believe that hospitals should reward attendance rather than punishing non-attendance. These rewards may be in the form of posting names on bulletin boards, announcing the names of employees in notices, or giving monetary rewards. Some hospitals allow employees to bank portions of unused sick leave for future reward, but such a system can be very expensive (Lee and Eriksen 1990: 40).

This does not eliminate the need for punishment for non-attendance. Striving for perfect attendance, however, can be harmful since it may encourage sick employees to come to work and in this way diseases may be transmitted to other employees and patients.

Discipline

Some form of discipline regarding absenteeism is essential. A progressive disciplinary system which imposes penalties increasing in severity for unexcused or, in some cases, even excused absences is often used. A policy where the employees are penalized for absenteeism without consideration of the reasons for the absence seldom works. McDonald and Shaver (1981: 17) warn that legal difficulties may evolve, so consistency and careful documentation of each incident of absenteeism is essential.

Follow-up of chronic absentees

Chronic absentees should be identified and followed-up. The measures to be taken for each type of absentee should be in accordance with their specific personality problems. McDonald and Shaver (1981: 17–18) describe the types of absentees and suggest the following steps to be taken:

- The hypochondriac absentee will use her maximum sick leave and is always complaining about aches and pains. The supervisor should avoid a discussion of symptoms but make it clear that she causes problems for the rest of the nursing team.

- The immature absentee lacks self-discipline and is influenced by other nursing staff who take time off. The supervisor should assume a parent role and teach her more effective work habits.

- The escapist absentee stays away from work because she is bored. Counselling or a transfer may rectify this problem.

- The abusive absentee takes time off to get back at the supervisor for real or imagined wrong-doing on the part of the supervisor. She may be hostile and resentful and will challenge the right of the supervisor to discipline her.

- The poorly motivated absentee seldom does more than the minimum required to keep her from getting fired. The supervisor should try to appeal to the employee's sense of self-respect and pride.

- The burnt-out absentee is probably exhausted from overwork, but her real problem is psychological. The supervisor should be understanding and should try to restore the person to her former level of personal and professional well-being.

Organizational aspects

Tyani (1990: 125) recommended the following organizational measures to combat absenteeism: conditions of service should be set down in writing; a fair distribution of workload should be practised; there should be a complete grievance procedure; free and open communication should exist between management and professional nurses; supervisors should make regular ward rounds and should be educated to raise the quality of supervision.

CONTROL OF SICK LEAVE ABUSE

The sick leave patterns of all employees should be monitored, but particular attention must be paid to high frequencies of single days off and the use of first or last work days for sick leave, as well as days before or after holidays and pay days. Supervisors should be allowed to use their discretion in asking for a medical certificate as proof of illness or in paying an unexpected visit to the home of the sick employee when they become suspicious. Employees should also indicate their reason for absence on a leave form when returning to work. Managers should seriously consider disciplinary steps when an employee's number of sick leave incidents (not days) exceed five per year (Levesque 1992).

CONCLUSION

The nurse administrator should regard absenteeism as a challenge. If she is able to identify the predisposing factors causing absenteeism in the service and make use of strategies for reducing the rate of absenteeism, she might be able to combat this problem successfully.

References

Chadwick-Jones, J. K., Nicholson, N., and Brown, C. (1982). *Social Psychology of Absenteeism*. Praeger: New York.

Firth, H. and Britton, P. (1989). 'Burnout', absence and turnover amongst British nursing staff. *Journal of Occupational Psychology*, volume 62, pp. 55–9.

Gardner, J. E. (1986). *Stabilizing the workforce*. Quorum: Westport.

Gillies. D. A. (1989). *Nursing Management — A Systems Approach*. Saunders: Philadelphia.

Hoverstad, T. and Kjolstad, S. (1991). Use of focus groups to study absenteeism due to illness. *Journal of Occupational Medicine*, volume 33, number 10, pp. 1046–9.

Jones, R. C., Bly, J. L. and Richardson, J. E. (1990). A study of a worksite health promotion program and absenteeism. *Journal of Occupational Medicine,* volume 32, number 2, pp. 95–9.

Lee, J. B. and Eriksen, L. R. (1990). The effects of a policy change on three types of absence. *Journal of Nursing Administration,* volume 20, numbers 7/8, pp. 37–40.

Levesque, J. D. (1992). *The Human Resource Problem Solver's Handbook.* McGraw-Hill: New York.

McDonald, J. M. and Shaver, A. V. (1981). An absenteeism control program. *Journal of Nursing Administration,* volume 11, number 5, 13–18.

Miller, D. S. and Norton, V. M. (1986). Absenteeism. Nursing service's albatross. *Journal of Nursing Administration,* volume 16, number 3, 38–42.

Price, J. L. and Mueller, C. W. (1986). *Absenteeism and Turnover of Hospital Employees.* Jai Press: Greenwich.

Rhodes, S. R. and Steers, R. M. (1990). *Managing Employee Absenteeism.* Addison-Wesley: New York.

Schappi, J. V. (1988). *Improving Job Attendance.* BNA: Washington.

Taunton, R. L. Krampitz, S. D and Woods, C. Q. (1989). Absenteeism–retention links. *Journal of Nursing Administration*, volume 19, number 6, 13–20.

Tyani, B. I. N. (1990). *Absenteeism — A Nursing Service Problem in the Republic of Transkei.* MA (Cur) dissertation, University of South Africa, Pretoria.

CHAPTER 16

TURNOVER

S. W. Booyens

CONTENTS

INTRODUCTION

The constant heavy losses of recruited neophytes and qualified nurses from the profession constitute one of the biggest headaches for nursing service managers. It is a laborious and time-consuming task to recruit enough nurses into the profession, and the retention of staff is even more difficult. Reducing the turnover rate among personnel is one of the best moves management can take in the cost-effective management of an institution.

COMPUTATION OF THE TURNOVER RATE

The formula for computing the turnover rate is as follows:

$$annual\ turnover\ rate = \frac{number\ of\ voluntary\ terminations\ per\ year}{average\ number\ of\ employees} \times \frac{100}{1}$$

The nurse manager should apply this formula for each category of nursing personnel in the hospital, for each year, ie:

$$annual\ turnover = \frac{number\ of\ professional\ nurses\ terminating}{average\ number\ professional\ nurses\ on\ payroll} \times \frac{100}{1}$$

The number of nurses (part-time or full-time) who left the service, and the number of posts filled during a year, should be counted.

The nurse manager should see that the turnover rate is computed for each category of nurse for each year — ie first year student nurses, second year student nurses, third year student nurses, fourth year student nurses, professional nurses, senior professional nurses, all professional nurses, staff nurses, and auxilliary nurses. When these rates are computed and compared over a period of three to five years it is easy for nurse managers to see where the biggest turnover problem lies, whether it is a problem that is worse at some times than at other times, and whether the turnover rate is increasing steadily or alarmingly among certain categories of personnel.

The optimum turnover rate is 5–10% per annum. It is not necessary to have a 0% turnover rate. An organization needs the ideas and innovation that newcomers can bring with them.

CAUSES OF TURNOVER

Turnover among nursing personnel is either avoidable or unavoidable. Unavoidable turnover is associated with marriage, pregnancy, and transfer of the husband. Avoidable turnover results from failure of the job to keep the employee in the organization's service (Gillies 1982: 247). According to Gillies, it is estimated that 36% of turnover can be associated with unavoidable causes, while approximately 64% of nursing turnover is of the avoidable type (Gillies 1982: 247). Although nursing service managers often cite pay and family responsibilities as the outstanding factors leading to turnover, research has shown that characteristics of the job itself are usually accountable for turnover.

Regarding pay and family responsibilities, Brief (1976: 57) makes the following observations, among others, concerning turnover among hospital nurses:

1. If money is highly valued, and the work itself does not give the nurse satisfaction, then dissatisfaction with pay occurs. This dissatisfaction leads to turnover.

2. If a nurse experiences strong feelings of responsibility towards her family and derives no satisfaction from her work, she will serve her family instead of staying at the hospital. This leads to turnover.

Reasons for turnover among nurses are not easy to identify; they vary among different individuals and may also depend on the differences in organizational structures and the management of different institutions. After extensive research, Price and Mueller (1981) put forth a causal model which tries to explain the turnover phenomenon among professional nurses. This model argues that job satisfaction is an important variable to take into account when one wants to explain reasons for turnover, but that an 'intent to stay' or a commitment to one's present job is more important in terms of leaving or staying in a particular workplace. It points out that although one might experience a high degree of job satisfaction and a commitment to one's present work, it is the role of outside opportunities which may offer more that which will ultimately determine whether one will stay in one's job or leave (Price and Mueller 1981: 547).

The aspects which underlie job satisfaction according to Price and Mueller (1981: 545) are the following:

- the degree to which a job is repetitive;

- the degree of power or influence one has concerning the speed at which one works, how one perform one's job activities, the sequence of job activities, and the changes one would like to make in one's job;

- the degree to which employees are informed about the priority of work to be done, technical knowledge, and the nature of equipment to be used;

- whether one has close friends among the other employees;
- the total yearly income from the job;
- an employee's feelings regarding the pay received in relation to the effort that is put into the job;
- the employee's perception of the potential for movement from lower positions to higher positions in the organization.

A commitment to one's present job or an 'intent to stay' in one's job usually includes such aspects as the following:

- one's dedication to professional standards — eg membership and active participation in professional associations;
- the degree of one's commitment to family obligations;
- the degree to which one's general training has succeeded in preparing one for positions in different organizations (Price and Mueller 1981: 545–7).

Another viewpoint regarding the causes of turnover focuses not only on the job and its characteristics but on the work environment of the employee. Thus factors such as the following appear to be important for employees at different stages of their work life:

- the overall environment — whether the employee perceives it to be hostile, stressful, and full of conflicts, or calm and rewarding;
- role clarity — ie whether employees know what supervisors expect of them;
- frequent feedback — ie, how often and in how much detail does the employee get feedback on the jobs performed;
- the type of interaction the employee has with her supervisor;
- the number of co-workers an employee has;
- the extent to which co-workers display motivation and positive feelings about their work;
- opportunities to learn new things while doing the job;
- opportunities to use skills and abilities while doing the job;
- opportunities to make independent decisions while doing the job (Seybolt 1986: 27–8).

EFFECTS OF TURNOVER

The higher the turnover rate, the fewer nurses are left to tend patients. Thus when a hospital has a high turnover rate, the quality of care rendered to its patients will suffer. If the nurse administrator is concerned about this lowered quality of care and does not want the patients to suffer, she will have to see that the number of patients is limited so that more-or-less the same patient–nurse ratio is maintained as before.

Although lost employees are usually replaced by new nurses, it is generally assumed that newly appointed employees will take a period of at least six to eight months to become fully efficient in their new workplace.

It is thus easy to see that an institution which suffers from a high turnover rate will also suffer from lower staff morale and less group cohesiveness, which will eventually lead to a decrease in the standard of performance and thus lower levels of care, which will lead to medical and legal risks.

The hospital has to pay for the recruitment of new employees together with their selection and orientation into their new work environment. Furthermore, new employees are generally relatively overpaid for the period in which they are not fully functional because of their orientation phase. The remaining employees usually have to work harder and often have to work overtime as well, which also costs the hospital extra money during the period between resignations and the replacements' achievement of full capacity (Brief 1976: 55).

The lower morale and impairment in the quality of care is also extremely costly when new patients select other institutions for their hospitalization and when costly medico-legal problems occur because of shortages among nursing staff and their decreased level of performance.

ASSESSMENT OF THE COST OF PERSONNEL TURNOVER

The nurse manager who is aware of the actual costs incurred by the rate of turnover in her hospital will be able to make her voice heard when suggesting strategies which might be adopted for the retention of personnel. These retention strategies might involve major policy changes (Jones 1990: 12).

When the costs of nursing turnover are calculated, estimates can be made in terms of direct and indirect costs. Direct costs are incurred by the following activities:

- advertising for, and recruiting, personnel;
- the temporary filling of staff vacancies;
- interviewing and hiring new employees;
- termination of an employee's service.

Indirect costs are incurred by the following:

- the orientation and training of new personnel;
- the lower productivity levels of the newly-appointed nurse.

Advertising and recruiting

The costs for the following activities must all be calculated:

- advertisements in newspapers and journals;
- recruitment personnel doing school visits (time spent and travel expenses);
- the training of personnel for recruitment;
- the salaries of the personnel doing recruitment;
- supplies needed for the compilation of advertisements and for doing recruitment work — posters, transparencies for overhead projectors, films, videos, etc. (Jones 1990: 28–9).

Temporary filling of staff vacancies

Costs to be calculated under this heading include the following:

- the cost of hiring temporary nurses from private agencies, or the cost of paying temporary nurses. The costs of paying these nurses are higher than the normal costs of the nurse in the post;
- if the staff losses result in the hospital having to reduce the number of patients, then the cost of lost income per bed per day must be calculated (Jones 1990: 29).

Interviewing and hiring costs

Interviewing and hiring a new employee involves costs such as the following:

- costs of interviewing — ie time spent by management, supplies needed, processing of applicants;
- costs of hiring a new employee include such aspects as pre-employment physical examinations, payroll processing, and employment processing, eg getting references, filling-in forms, and getting the necessary personal particulars (Jones 1990: 29).

Termination of service costs

When an employee's services are terminated, the following costs are incurred:

- costs of conducting exit interviews;
- the necessary processing;
- payment of unused vacation leave (Jones 1990: 29).

Orientation and training of new employees

This includes the following:

- the costs of the salaries and benefits of the staff who are appointed to do the training;
- supply costs — eg audiovisuals, books (Jones 1990: 29);
- additional costs — eg the hiring of films, payment of outside lecturers, hiring of venues for training, if applicable;
- costs of the decrease in the productivity of newly-appointed personnel.

During the orientation period of newly-appointed employees the overall level of productivity is reduced because they are not functioning at their full capacity. The costs of such reduced productivity could be measured by determining:

1. The average weekly pay for newly-registered nurses.

2. The average number of weeks it takes for a newly-appointed registered nurse to reach 100% productivity.

3. The level of productivity achieved by the typical newly-appointed registered nurse during each third part of the learning period (Jones 1990: 29).

MANAGEMENT OF TURNOVER

When management wants to reduce an excessive rate of turnover there are several paths which can be followed.

Before attempting to lower its turnover rate, each institution should first decide what it considers an acceptable turnover rate for that organization. This will depend on available staff numbers, the number of employees with exceptional skills, the availability of opportunities outside, the level of turnover that is actually desirable in order to avoid stagnation, and the cost of replacing each employee who leaves.

Each institution should also determine why nurses leave the organization. Data should be collected and computerized on such aspects as the length of stay of the average nurse, the reasons for her stay, and the reasons for leaving (elicited through exit interviews carried out by an 'outsider'). The data should be examined carefully to see if any patterns emerge (Marquis 1988: 29). Management must then select measures which will have the greatest effect on lowering the rate, bearing such patterns in mind.

When recruiting, care should be taken not to paint an unrealistically good picture of the organization. The prospective employee should know from the start what it will really be like to work in the organization. A better fit between organizational goals and employee expectations is then possible (Marquis 1988: 29; Wolf 1981: 233).

During the selection and interviewing process, special care must be taken to get an accurate picture of the potential employee (Marquis 1988: 29).

Employees usually do not think of leaving during their first six months. It is nevertheless important to see that their orientation has ensured that they are clear about what is expected from them, that they are able to use a variety of skills, and that positive feedback is given for a job well done (Seybolt 1986: 30; Brief 1976: 56).

During the period after the first six months in their new career and up to the end of the first year, employees get the most satisfaction from their job when they feel that their learning needs are met to the extent that they are able to use their abilities, when they are given sufficient responsibility, and when they are allowed to make some decisions. They want frequent and reliable feedback regarding their growth and their professional activities from their supervisors as well as from their peers. Employees in this stage of their career leave easily when expectations are not sufficiently met (Seybolt 1986: 29).

For the group of nurses who have been employed from one year to three years in an institution there are important factors which will affect whether they intend to stay or leave. The first factor is the amount of autonomy they are allowed in their work, and the second factor is the degree to which they are in agreement with their supervisor regarding the duties which relate to their specific job (Seybolt 1986: 30; Brief 1976: 56).

The nurses who have been working from three to six years in an organization are less likely to leave than the foregoing two groups. However, they are the nurses who may experience burnout symptoms. They are wondering whether the work they are doing bears any real significance and will often need job enrichment so that their jobs will be as exciting as before.

The nurses working in an organization for longer than six years are usually the least likely to leave. The degree to which these nurses agree with each other and with what supervisors expect from them is most important. It is also important to see that this group of employees is kept up-to-date on changes taking place in the organization (Seybolt 1986: 31).

It is clear from the foregoing that nurses want a say in the management of their work and that they must be given the authority to make independent decisions. The more complex the care, and the more uncertain the changes in patients' conditions, the more necessary it is for nurses to act quickly and to intervene appropriately and timeously. It is thus necessary to decentralize management as far as possible so that the nurses in the units will have the biggest possible say regarding matters such as changing methods of recording medications, work schedules, work shifts, patient treatment programmes, applicable nursing care standards, and methods of ensuring that a high quality of care is rendered.

The opportunity to undertake an entire project, or a meaningful part of a project, is important for this group of employees (Brief 1976: 56).

Management may also consider the following recommendations set forth by researchers who studied the turnover phenomenon among nurses:

- Allow nurses to transfer voluntarily between units. This will lessen routinization of the job and permit better utilization of nurses with specialized skills and knowledge (Price 1981: 111). One should aim for the best match between worker and job (Wolf 1981).

- Hold regular weekly meetings, not longer than 45 minutes in duration, during working hours with unit staff to discuss changes in hospital policy and unit administration matters (Price 1981: 112).

- Promote primarily from within the organization. Opportunities for promotion are limited in nursing, so promotions should be reserved for staff who are already employed by the organization (Price 1981: 113).

- Appoint more older married women with children. These nurses tend to have a far lower turnover rate than the younger nurses without families (Price 1981: 114).

- Provide adequate child care facilities.

- Create more part-time positions or, alternatively, make use of the shared or split job principle where part-time nurses are used to fill one full-time post (Wolf 1981: 234).

- Eliminate non-nursing duties as far as possible to lessen the amount of work pressure on permanent full-time staff members (Wolf 1981: 234).

- Make use of a system where new employees who have been out of nursing for a considerable number of years are assisted by working together with a colleague for the first month or two in order to adjust to the realities of the hospital routine.

- Develop career ladders in clinical practice.
- Listen to nurses' suggestions regarding hospital and unit policy and try to put their ideas into practice (Wolf 1981: 236).
- Pay head nurses according to the size and complexity of the units they are managing — the more competent nurses should be assigned to the bigger and more complex units (Wolf 1981: 236).

A variety of approaches may be used to reduce the turnover rate. It must be remembered, however, that not all turnover is bad. In some instances a hospital or organization may be dissatisfied with a large number of its permanent employees. It may not want to reduce the turnover rate because it may want to bring in as many new employees as possible in order to absorb new ideas and to bring about some changes in stagnant routines. Most hospitals do not suffer from this condition and could do well to reduce their turnover rate and stabilize their workforce to a greater extent.

CONCLUSION

Reducing nurse turnover is a challenging task, because it is not caused by any one factor. It is, however, good practice for any nurse manager to try to achieve the following in her organization in order to reduce some of the avoidable resignations:

- maintain a spirit of co-operation and teamwork;
- ensure that supervisors are seen as considerate and responsive;
- try to make the nurses' jobs as challenging and interesting as possible;
- provide ample facilities for staff development and career advancement;
- provide good communication and co-ordination between units/ departments;
- see that nursing administration actively supports the nursing personnel;
- give the nursing personnel as much say as possible in policies, changes, and decisions regarding their own nursing practice and working environment.

References

Brief, A. P. (1976). Turnover among hospital nurses: a suggested model. *JONA*, volume 5, number 10, pp. 55–8.

Gillies, D. A. (1982). *Nursing Management. A Systems Approach*. Saunders: Philadelphia.

Hinshaw, S. A., Smelzer, C. H. and Atwood, J. R. (1987). Innovative retention strategies for nursing staff. *JONA*, volume 17, number 6, pp. 8–16.

Jones, C. B. (1990). Staff nurse turnover costs: part I, a conceptual model. *JONA*, volume 20, number 4, pp 18–22.

Jones, C. B. (1990). Staff nurse turnover costs: part II, measurements and results. *JONA*, volume 20, number 5, pp 27–32.

Landstrom, G. L., Biondi, D. L. and Gillies, D. A. (1989). The emotional and behavioural process of staff nurse turnover. *JONA*, volume 19, number 9, pp. 23–8.

Loveridge, C. E. (1988). Contingency theory: explaining staff nurse retention. *JONA*, volume 18, number 6, pp. 22–5.

Marquis, B. (1988). Attrition: The effectiveness of retention activities. *JONA*, volume 18, number 3, pp. 25–9.

Prestholdt, P. H., Lane, J. M., Mathews, R. C. (1988). Predicting staff nurse turnover. *Nursing Outlook*, volume 36, number 3, May/June 1988, pp. 145–7.

Price, J. L. and Mueller, C. W. (1981). A causal model of turnover for nurses. *Academy of Management Journal*, volume 24, number 1, pp. 543–65.

Price, J. L. and Mueller, C. W. (1981). *Professional Turnover: The Case of Nurses*. SP Medical and Scientific Books: New York.

Seybolt, J. W. (1986). Dealing with premature employee turnover. *JONA*, volume 16, number 2, pp. 26–32.

Wolf, G. A. (1981). Nursing turnover: some causes and solutions. *Nursing Outlook*, volume 29, number 2, pp. 233–6.

CHAPTER 17

STAFF DEVELOPMENT

S. W. Booyens

CONTENTS

INTRODUCTION

The staff members of a health care institution are its most valuable asset and the quality of the patient care rendered by them can be directly related to their knowledge and skills. The nurse manager who invests in the continuous development of her staff gets better patient care results and her personnel become better motivated to perform to the best of their abilities and to stay working in the same institution — especially if such development leads to the fulfilment of higher order needs such as self-actualization and self-expression.

TYPES OF STAFF DEVELOPMENT

Staff development may be seen as a management programme to train and develop staff members. Training and development are aimed at improving the work/job knowledge of staff together with their skills and attitudes towards their jobs. The promotion of personal growth is another important aim. Staff development includes a number of different educational undertakings, namely induction training, orientation, in-service education, continuing education, management training, and organizational development (Gillies 1989: 339).

INDUCTION TRAINING

The new employee has to be orientated towards her new work environment. Induction training is regarded as the first part of the orientation process and it aims to do the following (Gerber, Nel and Van Dyk 1989: 78):

- reduce anxiety and uncertainty;

- save time for supervisors and fellow workers;

- create a positive attitude towards the employer;

- assist the employee to become fully productive as soon as possible;

- assist in creating realistic work expectations.

Induction training is normally the responsibility of the personnel department. All categories of new employees are subjected to the same programme which is conducted during the first few days of an employee's orientation programme.

Aspects which are covered during the induction programme include the following:

- the physical and geographical layout of the institution;

- conditions of service and benefits such as salary scales, overtime payment, leave benefits, night duty, weekend and public holiday duty policies, and recreational activities;

- policies and procedures, such as work schedules, grievance procedures, uniform allowances, leave of absence (sickness, educational, maternity), and SANC registration payments;

- a review of the institution, describing its philosophy, mission, goals, history, culture, structure, norms, and standards, as well as communication procedures. An introduction to the names and offices of the superintendent, hospital secretary, chief professional nurse, and other important authority figures is also recommended;

- safety measures, such as emergency exits, fire extinguishers, and disaster care programmes.

ORIENTATION

Orientation is the personalized training of the individual employee so that she becomes acquainted with the requirements of the job itself. The aim is to achieve effective and productive work performance by the new employee as soon as possible. The newcomer is thus introduced to her supervisor, her fellow workers, to the nursing department where she will work, and to her job responsibilities.

The orientation programme will differ in different departments or units, but the aspects which should be covered when a nurse is orientated to a hospital ward or unit are the following:

1. Physician-related aspects, such as:
    - the allocation of beds to consultants and other doctors;
    - admission days — routine and emergency;
    - theatre days;
    - procedures for referring patients to the outpatient department;
    - days and times of consultants' rounds;
    - calling procedures for consultation with doctors about patients;
    - taking instructions from doctors;
    - conducting rounds with doctors;
    - taking telephonic doctors' instructions.

2. Unit administration aspects, such as:
   - job descriptions of the different categories of personnel;
   - the routine of the unit, eg meal times, medicine administration times, visiting times;
   - routine supply orders;
   - routine maintenance and after-hours emergency maintenance;
   - ordering centrally-stored equipment;
   - porter service;
   - messenger service;
   - routine records, such as daily reports to nursing service managers, census record;
   - rules for off-duty requests;
   - procedures for admission, transfer, and discharge of patients;
   - communication procedures;
   - operation of the patient–nurse call system.

3. Clinical nursing aspects such as:
   - isolation nursing policy;
   - handling of soiled linen;
   - the standard nursing care plans for the most frequently-treated illnesses;
   - patient care records;
   - incident reports;
   - checking of emergency trolley supplies;
   - checking, maintenance and use of resuscitation equipment, eg ventilator, ambubag, defibrillator, oxygen, and suction apparatus (NUA 100-L Study guide 1991: 314).

4. Environmental control, such as:
   - control of noise;
   - maintenance of a comfortable temperature and level of humidity, and control of unpleasant odours;
   - disinfection procedures.

Orientation aspects for a clinic in a comprehensive health service should include, among others, the following aspects (NUA 100-L Study Guide 1991: 314):

- geographical layout;

- working day allocation per type of clinic/service — eg psychiatric service, geriatric service and ante-natal services;

- work rotation within the unit;

- policy regarding immunization procedures;

- methods of ordering and administering medicines;

- different types of patient records;

- days for consultants' visits;

- referral procedures;

- protocols for different diagnostic categories;

- telephonic communication procedures;

- duty rosters and rules for off-duty requests;

- rules and procedures for the use of vehicles and mobile units;

- routine maintenance orders;

- the different types of routine orders;

- checking, maintenance and use of the emergency trolley and resuscitation procedures.

Induction and orientation, if approached systematically, will ease the adaptation process for the new nurse, will lessen errors, and will thus ease the controlling function of the direct supervisor.

IN-SERVICE EDUCATION

In-service education is the education of an employee while she is doing her job or rendering a service to clients in an organization. It thus implies updating, training, educating, and informing the person about the present requirements of the job. Because jobs in the health care services are never static and are subjected to rapid changes, there is a continuous need for the in-service education of health care workers.

In-service education programmes are usually directed towards bringing employees up-to-date about new diagnostic and treatment techniques, the care and operation of new equipment, the optimal use of supplies, and new institutional policy decisions.

According to Mellish and Lock (1992: 174) in-service education is that form of education which:

- is given to people while they are employed;

- is planned deliberately;

- is designed to fill in gaps in learning or to remedy deficiencies in the skills and knowledge of employees;

- aims at more efficient functioning of the employee;

- aims at making the organization function better;

- follows on a period of pre-service education;

- is only a part of continuing education.

Centralized versus decentralized approach

The most cost-effective way to approach the presentation of in-service education programmes is to have a centralized department or section whose main function is the presentation of the in-service education programme to all the nurses from all the different units. This approach, however, does not always achieve the desired results because the in-service educational needs of the nurses working in the different units vary too much due to the specialized nature of nursing at present. A decentralized approach would seem the best, but is often too costly, with the result that a combined approach is recommended. Gillies (1989: 356) advocates an approach where an in-service teacher is assigned to a clinical area and takes an active part in the nursing care of patients in the area, thus detecting care deficiencies which need in-service education. She then does the necessary in-service teaching in her own speciality area for approximately 85% of her time, but spends the rest of her teaching time conducting centralized in-service education sessions.

Assessing in-service education needs

This is usually done by observing employees in the work situation, asking for suggestions from employees by making use of suggestion boxes or making a suggestion form a part of the monthly newsletter from the in-service education department, by the circulation of questionnaires to departments or unit supervisors, and by determining needs which emanate from the perusal of audit reports.

Planning and implementation of programmes

The planning and implementation aspects will include the drawing up of the in-service education budget, the drawing up of the annual and/or monthly programmes, determining time schedules to avoid clashes with service needs, determining the staff members available for conducting sessions, assessing the equipment and material needed, the booking of venues, the different methods of presentation, the notification of in-service sessions, the recording of attendance, the evaluation of the programme, and the carrying-out of long-term follow-up activities in order to assess the effectiveness of the programme over a period of months.

Learning and education principles applicable to in-service education

Readiness to learn

The learner must reach a certain level of maturity in order to learn successfully, but must also have some basic prior knowledge before she can assimilate new knowledge. It is desirable that the employee's basic prior knowledge be known in order to plan and develop learning material which will build onto this pre-existing knowledge base.

Motivation to learn

Children are usually motivated to learn because of their curiosity, but adults are motivated because they want to be able to solve their work-related problems or because they want to increase an area of competence they already have or prepare themselves for an occupation (Gerber Nel and Van Dyk 1987: 195). It is thus essential that in-service education sessions are planned around the employee's expressed learning needs in order to capture their interest. Learners will also be motivated to assimilate the contents of instruction faster if they are told in advance about the benefits that will accrue from learning the presented contents and adopting the required behaviour.

Knowledge of results

The adult learner wants to be given feedback on his performance after he has learned new behaviour. If learned behaviour is heartily applauded or rewarded, this reinforces the behaviour.

Active participation

Adults learn best by actively taking part in their instruction. Recommended methods of instruction are thus projects, exercises, problem-solving sessions, group discussions, and informal discussions. It is also known that better learning will take place if an employee actively performs a particular task according to set guidelines, rather than watching the instructor demonstrate the correct way of performing the task.

Useful knowledge

Adult learners are usually not interested in knowledge which they feel will be of little practical value to them. They want to acquire useful knowledge to integrate into their practical everyday work. The teacher or instructor will thus do well to give everyday practical examples and descriptive case studies which resemble the problems the employee is expected to solve after training (Gillies 1989: 341). Adults should be exposed to training related to actual problems, rather than predetermined theoretical and abstract notions (Gerber, Nel, and Van Dyk 1987: 195).

Individual pace of learning

People differ in their speed of learning and their powers of concentration and comprehension. Teachers often experience the problem that a carefully planned course fits the needs of some students but does not reach the needs of others. The successful teacher of adults must know how to discover the needs and capabilities of individual students and adapt her instructional content appropriately (Hand 1981: 266).

Individual differences

Adult learners are a heterogeneous group with a wide variety of life and work experiences, motivational levels, learning abilities, learning styles, and cultural backgrounds. This means that the subject content and method of instruction must be adapted to suit them. A wide variety of source materials, teaching methods, and audio-visual aids should therefore be employed in staff development activities.

Physical surroundings

Adults are more sensitive to physical surroundings such as adequate lighting, comfortable seating, ventilation, and temperature control than children. They want to receive instruction in comparatively short units, want to cover ground as rapidly as possible, and want to be comfortable (Hand 1981: 264).

Unlearning old habits

Learning involves changes in behaviour. Such changes are difficult to achieve if old ideas, inclinations, and assumptions are not unlearned. These ideas and inclinations must thus be shaken before new thoughts, actions and attitudes can be integrated into the learner's mind. This will make the learner slightly uncomfortable (Gillies 1989: 340).

Training in practical skills that are not for immediate use

When the task to be learned or mastered by the employee is not likely to be practised immediately in the work situation, and when performance of a task must be maintained during periods of stress and emergencies, overlearning should be practised: the trainee must master the skill and then practise it to the point of overlearning in order to retain it for when it is needed. Examples of this type of training are: resuscitation training (for example, normal compression of the heart and mouth-to-mouth-respiration), assembly and use of an ambubag, and the use of respirators and cardiac monitors.

Organization of learning content

The memory span of the adult learner can be increased by grouping the learning content. The adult learner can usually remember three to four orally presented groups and four to six visually presented groups. The more the material to be learned is presented in an organized way, the more likely it is to be assimilated (Sullivan and Decker 1992: 312).

Congenial atmosphere

Adult students appreciate systematic, business-like procedures, but they also welcome a chance to laugh and relax. They want to enjoy the fellowship of their colleagues and want to relate informally to each other. They resent anything bordering on adolescent schoolroom discipline or restraint (Hand 1981: 267). An authoritarian approach will thus be strongly resisted and will accomplish very little learning.

On-the-job instruction

The student nurse is usually taught in the unit or clinical situation by way of on-the-job instruction. The relatively inexperienced nurse is assigned to an experienced nurse, often a preceptor, in order to observe the correct way of performing certain tasks. She is then required to perform them under the watchful eye of the instructor/ preceptor until she is sufficiently skilled to perform them on her own.

This is a cost-effective way of teaching, because necessary nursing services are rendered during the teaching process. The nurse learns by actively practising the new skills or elements of the task until she is proficient, but the instructor/preceptor may not utilize learning theory appropriately, may not evaluate the performance of the trainee nurse correctly, and may neglect to provide the necessary feedback to the student (Sullivan and Decker 1992: 319).

If the professional nurse who serves as instructor or preceptor fully embraces the concept of preceptorship, the training process will be beneficial to both the student and the professional nurse. The role of the preceptor is one of orientator, teacher, resource person, counsellor, role model, and evaluator. The preceptor will benefit in fulfilling this role by having an opportunity to sharpen her clinical skills and by experiencing increased personal and professional satisfaction (Sullivan and Decker 1992: 318).

When an institution considers providing preceptors for nursing students the following aspects must be considered:

- The preceptor's workload will have to be reasonable in order for her to have sufficient time for her preceptor function.

- No 'floating' between units or working double shifts or overtime can be done by a person who must also fulfil the role of a preceptor.

- The correct methods and attitudes regarding the evaluation of clinical skills must be taught to the preceptors.

- A written description that spells out clearly the preceptor's responsibilities with regard to selecting learning experiences and supervising and evaluating the student's progress must be supplied by the training college.

- The role description should explain the required skill level of the preceptor, the amount of time that should be devoted to the student and for meetings, and the degree of commitment required for successful experiences (Limón et al. 1982).

In addition to the above requirements, the preceptors should be adequately prepared for their role by the educational institution; resource persons should be available who are willing to provide guidance and support to the preceptors, and there will be a need for increased communication between the health service and college in planning and implementing the programme (Limón et al. 1982: 19).

The preceptor's role is usually seen as providing a role-model for the inexperienced nurse. Thus the new nurse not only learns actual work-related skills and tasks but also observes the preceptor 'to learn how to set priorities, solve problems and make decisions, manage time, delegate tasks, and interact with others' (Murphy and Hammerstead 1981, as quoted by Sullivan and Decker 1992: 319).

CONTINUING EDUCATION

DiVincenti (1977: 205) views continuing education as that phase of the staff development programme aimed at assisting the employee to keep up to date with current health care trends, increasing her knowledge and competence, and developing her ability to analyse complex health care problems and to maintain sound interpersonal relationships.

Responsibility for continuing education is essentially that of the individual employee, but if management takes the view that employees who are already part of the workforce constitute promising manpower, it can be expected that management will support the individual staff member's continuing education efforts, as well as providing an impetus for continuing education activities at the workplace. There are several methods which may be used to provide and maintain continuing education among staff members:

1. The use of small-group activities in which the staff members of a unit share interesting clinical experiences or other topics of mutual interest with staff members of another unit may inspire some nurses to further their educational training and may encourage others to read relevant nursing literature and so extend their knowledge.

2. The hospital may plan programmes with other health care services in the community with the aim of giving staff members insight into the functioning of different community-based services, of demonstrating and explaining new techniques (such as ultrasound and laser techniques), and of acquainting personnel with the different referral agencies/services in an area.

3. The institution usually supports individual programmes for continuing education, such as degree courses at universities and correspondence or college courses relevant to the nurse's job. In addition, the nurse manager will support attendance at workshops, seminars, conferences, and symposia in order to develop her staff. It is recommended that staff members who are sponsored to attend these educational gatherings, should prepare a written report about the proceedings and share it with the other staff members, so that as many staff members as possible may benefit from one staff member's attendance (DiVincenti 1977: 206).

FURTHER DEVELOPMENT

In recent years the development of managers has become an important aspect of staff development because it was found that, as organizations grew in complexity and the autocratic approach of most managers failed to gain respect from employees, managers no longer motivated them to achieve satisfactory levels of productivity. The development of managers and organizations is described in chapter 18. Together with organizational and managerial development, the management of the careers of staff and training in assertiveness skills are seen as ways of developing staff.

CAREER MANAGEMENT

Career planning is the analysis and specification of an employee's career objectives and the application of various methods to achieve the objectives.

Career development is formal action by an organization to ensure that employees with appropriate qualifications and experience are available when the organization requires their services.

The reasons for career management in organizations are the following, according to Gerber, Nel, and Van Dyk (1987: 298):

- The quality of the employee's work life is improved when she has an opportunity to progress in her career.

- Employees are able to learn new skills with the result that there is always a demand for them.

- Career management of employees decreases an organization's turnover rate.
- The personal job satisfaction of the employee is enhanced when her abilities have been developed and when she is placed in a position which suits her ambitions and abilities.

Career development consists of two main components, namely career planning and career management.

Career planning

1. Self-appraisal. The starting point of career planning is the individual's analysis of her strengths and weaknesses in regard to technical, interpersonal, administrative, and personal skills. The individual must indicate the importance she places on such job characteristics as security, financial rewards, autonomy, influence over others, and socializing with others (Beach 1985: 235).

2. Identify opportunities. A study should be made of trends in the economy, population demography, technology, and public policy. The personnel office in an organization should also publish information regarding the different jobs in an organization.

3. Set goals. After the individual has followed the first two steps, short-term, intermediate, and long-term goals should be set.

4. Prepare plans. The employee should now prepare plans to start to meet these goals, starting off with the short-term ones. It is advisable, here, for the employee to consult her supervisor and a responsible personnel office staff member.

5. Implement plans. In order to implement one's plans, the organizational climate should be supportive. Top level management, and all other levels of management, are responsible for assisting employees to develop their careers by instituting such measures as assignment on special projects, in-service education, and job rotation, for example.

The organization could assist employees in their planning phase by conducting workshops in which participants learn about job and career opportunities in the organization, study the stages of development in adulthood, complete a life projection exercise to envision their lives in ten year's time, and learn how to select a new job and how to be interviewed for it (Beach 1985: 237).

Career management

Beach (1985: 237) describes steps which should be followed in a career management system.

1. Human resource planning

The organization must make an assessment of its current manpower, forecast its manpower needs at various times in the future, and analyse the gap between future demands and projected supply. This should lead to a programme to meet future manpower needs. The analysis of posts will also have to form part of such a programme.

2. Design career paths

Many organizations do not design proper career paths for their employees.

3. Disseminate career information

The personnel department should publish a simple brochure which contains job and career opportunities in the organization. It must be supplied to all employees, and must be up-to-date and reflect the situation realistically.

4. Publication of job openings

All job openings should be publicized by way of bulletin board announcements or newsletters, stating the main duties, the qualifications needed, and the salary scale.

5. Assessment of employees

A well-developed performance appraisal system will assist in assessing the career advancement opportunities of employees. A formal assessment centre in which several evaluation techniques are used to evaluate personnel for managerial positions could also be used for employee development because each employee will receive valuable feedback on her performance on various tests.

Career counselling

Career counselling should take place between an employee and her supervisor during the performance appraisal interview. A resource person from the personnel department could help employees plan their careers and inform them of possibilities regarding training and development. Participants can be assisted in planning their careers during a career workshop (Beach 1985: 240).

Education and training

It is presently the norm to make training and educational opportunities available to all levels and categories of personnel, and not only a selected few.

A career development system works best when employees are adequately informed about careers, jobs, job qualifications, career paths, and job openings, and when selection for promotion is made on merit and not because of favouritism or political connections (Beach 1985: 241).

The nursing literature describes a case where a hospital designed a career development programme to establish a six-step career ladder for registered nurses within four areas, namely management, clinical nursing, research, and education.

The model consists of six phases or levels through which registered nurses may progress. The number of posts at each level is determined by the organization's needs and the available financial resources.

All professional nurses start off at level I and are only in a position to be promoted to the second level after a year's experience. No nurse is promoted automatically from level I to level II. Posts are advertised, applications are made, and the suitable nurses' promotion must be approved by their immediate supervisor and the chief nursing service manager. The same procedure is followed for nurses who want to progress from level II to level III.

The registered nurses are promoted from levels I to VI in the four different areas already mentioned. All the professional nurses in each of the four areas who are on levels I to III are responsible for clinical care. The level III position is designed by the nurse and her manager, and it is required that the occupier of such a post must make a significant contribution to the organization beyond normal patient care activities. These contributions have been found to be particularly valuable to the organization because they include such activities as serving as a unit preceptor and taking an active role in nursing practice or standard committees. The quality of patient care can be increased significantly as a result of the enormous amount of creativity shown by the level III nurses because all the projects which nobody could ever find time for come to fruition.

When level III nurses want to advance to the fourth level, they must first successfully complete a three-month training programme which is conducted by the hospital itself. During this programme, specific projects must be completed by the nurses. The projects must be of benefit to the nurse as well as the organization. They must further be in the area of the nurse's proposed career advancement — eg management, clinical practice, research, or education. Examples of such projects are the compilation of family brochures, orientation guides, and cost-saving programmes.

When nurses advance above level III positions they spend most, but not all, of their time in management, clinical practice, research, or education. The educational level VI nurse, for example, who has a master's degree in nursing education, spends 75% of her time teaching, but must also spend time assisting with research projects, managerial functions, and practical clinical care. The clinical nurse at level VI spends 75% of her time as a clinical nurse specialist, but is also required to spend some time on research, managerial, and teaching functions.

The job descriptions which were developed had to define the expected behaviour for each level, as well as each level's area of specialization from levels IV upwards. Appropriate performance appraisal systems also had to be developed simultaneously (Weeks and Vestal 1983: 29–31).

The career development of employees thus benefits the employee and plays a significant role in an organization's strategy for survival, because successful career development leads to the accomplishment of both the organization's and the employee's objectives.

ASSERTIVENESS AND ASSERTIVENESS TRAINING

Much has been written about nurses' lack of assertiveness. This lack leads to frustration, unmet goals, and mediocre performance (Migut 1982: 13). Lack of assertiveness in nurse managers is evident when they remain subordinate in formulating policies, making decisions, and planning programmes at top level management board meetings (McGillick and Fernandez 1983: 26).

Lack of assertiveness is often conveyed by downcast eyes, a slumped posture, and a whining voice. It is also displayed through the use of a passive–aggressive attitude, avoidance, procrastination, lateness, blatant resistance, manipulation, seduction, and even sabotage (Migut 1982: 14).

The need for assertiveness is widely acknowledged. In order to manage the stress of everyday life, one *has* to become assertive. It is a simple and effective technique to promote and maintain one's personal health and self-esteem. It is especially necessary to become assertive if one is a nurse manager, because the nurse manager must know how to gain power by developing interpersonal and persuasive techniques, building group alliances and coalitions, choosing proper leadership styles, taking risks, and learning confrontation–negotiation techniques (McGillick and Fernandez 1983: 26).

It is thus evident that assertiveness training for nursing personnel and nurse managers will be of tremendous benefit to nursing in general. Migut (1982: 14) maintains that, although changing from traditional passive–dependent habits to assertive behaviour requires patience and courage, everyone benefits from the effort.

According to Morrison and Wirthman (1983), assertiveness training is designed to encourage 'honest, direct, sincere and appropriate expressions of one's thoughts, feelings and beliefs, without infringing upon the rights of others'. It helps nurses allay anxieties which prevent them from functioning effectively as professionals. The impact and value of an assertiveness training programme can be assessed by evaluating the participants' levels of assertiveness before and after training by means of a questionnaire, called the Adult Self-expression Scale (Morrison and Wirthman (1983: 14).

Since assertiveness begins with self-assessment and a decision to change, nursing students should be socialized early in their professional educational programmes to think positively about themselves and their profession. They should be given experience in expressing themselves assertively by verbalizing their convictions, beliefs, and feelings about the health care system and their own nursing care experiences. It is also recommended that nursing management should help nursing personnel to become more assertive through role model behaviour — that is nurse managers acting and expressing themselves in an assertive manner — and through in-service education (Migut 1982: 14).

Assertiveness training may take several forms. Some training may also take place when an individual consciously practises assertiveness principles in order to become more proficient in handling others.

A workshop technique was described by Numerof (1980: 1798–9) in which participants were first asked to complete two inventories, one about people and situations which made them feel non-assertive and the other one to elicit their assertiveness skills regarding speaking up at a meeting, addressing an authority figure, being especially competent, accepting rejection, and discussing another person's criticism with that person openly. The participants also had to list ten strengths that they possessed.

Each participant then had to share his/her strengths, weaknesses, and profile with another person from the group. They thus experienced the sharing of personal experiences within a supportive, structured environment. The entire group then had to meet and share their experiences and what they had learned in the two-person sessions with everyone else in the group.

The participants were afraid to share their experiences, and it was only after the group leader/trainer made a paper ball and suggested to the group that a person may only speak if in possession of the ball that communication started flowing. A person could only get possession of the ball by repeating what the previous speaker had said to his/her satisfaction. In this way the group was pulled together: personal anxiety was lowered and the group members learnt how to communicate and listen carefully to one another. After this exercise, the participants also practised role playing on how to assert themselves with 'nice' supervisors, on how to refuse overwhelming job-responsibilities, and on how to give and receive positive comments about themselves, maintaining confidence in their judgement when challenged and making requests to staff without being aggressive or sounding authoritarian. The participants in the workshop expressed their enthusiasm about the training they received and wanted further training (Numerof 1980: 1796–8).

Another approach to becoming assertive is described by Palmer and Deck (1987: 39–41). The nurse manager consciously practises self-assertive techniques. First and foremost it is considered necessary to change one's outlook from a passive, pessimistic one to an optimistic, positive one in which one expects to succeed. A number of strategies for practice are recommended by Palmer and Deck.

1. Substituting 'you' messages with 'I' messages. Thus instead of saying: 'You made me feel bad about the incident' rather say: 'I felt bad about the incident'. 'I' messages reveal what you stand ready to account for, eg 'I feel...' (moods), 'I understand that ...' (knowledge), 'I think that ...' (opinions), 'I want ...' (desire), 'I decided to ...' (judgements), 'I believe that ...' (commitment).

2. Buying time. When using this strategy the manager expresses her need for time in order to think, plan, or get more information. She would thus say 'I will need more information before I form an opinion', or 'the unit can expect a decision on the matter next week' (Palmer and Deck 1987: 40).

3. Broken record. This is a low-keyed repetition of the same idea, often with slightly different wording in order to deal with attempts to manipulate her; for example 'it is not possible right now', 'no', 'I do not see my way open'.

4. Fogging. To prevent untimely decisions and conclusions and to deal with impertinent questions, or to keep information confidential, the nurse manager should respond by giving partial information, such as: 'the matter is presently under consideration' (Palmer and Deck 1987: 40).

5. Negotiating. When using this strategy the nurse manager first acknowledges the situation — eg 'I need some advice on...'. Secondly, she states what is wanted — eg 'we could benefit from some training'. Thirdly, she asks the other person for assistance in a positive way — eg 'what is your idea on the correct way to solve this problem?' Fourthly, she requests help from someone — eg 'a good idea ... what about sending staff members to that seminar?' (Palmer and Deck 1987: 40).

When the nurse manager has mastered the assertiveness skills she requires for her job, she will be able to present herself more confidently and thus gain credibility as a manager/leader with the result that co-operation from employees for work assignments is more easily achieved.

CONCLUSION

Staff development is one of the essential aspects of the nurse manager's responsibilities. It is, however, a multi-faceted activity/responsibility which comprises a variety of development issues, such as induction training and orientation, in-service education, continuing education, management development, organizational development, career management, and assertiveness training.

References

Beach, D. S. (1985). *Personnel. The Management of People at Work*. Fifth edition. Macmillan Publishing: New York.

Dessler, G. (1984). *Personnel Management*. Reston: Virginia.

Divincenti, M. (1977). *Administrating Nursing Service*. Little Brown: Boston.

Gerber, P. D., Nel, P. S. and Van Dyk, P. S. (1987). *Human Resources Management*. Southern: Johannesburg.

Gillies, D. A. (1989). *Nursing Management: A Systems Approach*. Saunders: Philadelphia.

Hand, L. (1981). *Nursing Supervision*. Reston: Virginia.

Limón, S., Bargagliotti, L. A. and Spencer, J. B. (1982). Providing preceptors for nursing students: what questions should you ask? *JONA*, volume 12, number 6, June 1982, pp. 16–19.

McGillick, K. and Fernandes, R. C. (1983). Reaching for the stars. *Nursing Management*, volume 14, number 1, January 1983, pp. 24–6.

Mellish, J. M. and Lock, M. V.L. H. (1982). *Administrating the Practise of Nursing*. Second edition. Butterworth: Durban.

Migut, P. J. (1982). Self-care for nurses: assertiveness. *Nursing Management*, volume 13, number 2, pp. 13–14.

Morrison, L. M. and Wirthman, M. (1983). Briefs. *Nursing Management*, volume 14, number 9, pp. 12–14.

Nelson, G. M. and Schafer, M. J. (1980). An integrated approach to developing administrators and organizations. *JONA*, volume 10, number 2, pp. 37–42.

Numerof, R. (1980). Assertiveness training. *American Journal of Nursing,* October 1980, pp. 1796–8.

Palmer, M. E. and Deck, E. S. (1987). Assertiveness: phone-calls, memos, and I-messages. *Nursing Management,* volume 18, number 1, pp. 39–42.

Sullivan, E. J. and Decker, P. J. (1992). Effective Management in Nursing. Addison-Wesley: Menlo Park, California.

University of South Africa (1985). *Nursing Administration Study Guide for NUA100-L.* Unisa: Pretoria.

University of South Africa (1991). *Nursing Administration Study Guide for NUA100-L.* Unisa: Pretoria.

Weeks, L. C. and Vestal, K. W. (1983). PACE: A unique career development programme. *JONA,* volume 13, number 12, pp. 29–31.

CHAPTER 18

MANAGEMENT AND ORGANIZATIONAL DEVELOPMENT

Corrie Nel

CONTENTS

INTRODUCTION

The management development programme is a component of staff development that is being increasingly emphasized. The role of the manager is becoming ever more important for the survival of the organization as the competitive milieu and economic constraints oblige health services to function optimally.

The development of managers is aimed at improved managerial efficiency, but unless the organization itself is developed the managers may use their new skills and knowledge to develop and implement plans to do the wrong thing, thus decreasing both the institution's effectiveness and its efficiency (Nelson and Schaefer 1980: 39). Furthermore, the developed manager may not be able to use his newly-developed skills because he may be inhibited by the organization's hierarchical structure, lack of teamwork between departments or sections, and authoritarian inclinations among top level managers.

MANAGEMENT DEVELOPMENT APPROACHES

Early management development activities were mostly programme-centred — ie a programme would be designed and presented to managers regardless of their individual developmental needs. Nowadays management development programmes are more manager-centred because it is realized that managers' personalities, experiences, and abilities differ widely (Stoner and Freeman 1992: 389).

Although the content of the programme must be individualized to meet the needs of particular managers and their organizations, the following topics are commonly included (Gillies 1989: 357):

- political systems;
- economic principles;
- legal constraints;
- types of leadership;
- trade unionism;
- decision-making;
- communication methods;
- statistical analyses;
- interviewing techniques;
- effecting change;
- assertiveness training;

- negotiation with labour unions;
- employment practices;
- performance appraisal;
- management of conflict;
- writing reports;
- performance standards;
- labour contracts;
- information systems;
- risk management.

In general the objectives of management development are (Gerber, Nel and Van Dyk 1987: 267):

1. to improve the present functioning of the manager;

2. to improve the manager's job satisfaction;

3. to develop the latent abilities and potential of managers for the future managerial needs of the organization;

4. to ensure that managers stay updated and stay efficient in their managerial positions.

Understandably, managers at different levels of the organizational hierarchy have different development needs.

The most common needs of managers at the executive level are time management, team building, self analysis, financial management, coping with stress, understanding human behaviour, setting objectives and priorities, holding effective meetings, and decision-making.

The most common needs of mid-level managers are: appraising employees, motivating others, oral and written communication, team building, leadership, holding effective meetings, developing and training subordinates, and selecting employees.

The most common needs of managers at the supervisory level are: motivating others, evaluation, leadership, oral and written communication, discipline, managing time, counselling and coaching, and decision-making (Dignan 1980, as referred to by Dessler 1984: 259).

There are a number of off-the-job and on-the-job approaches to management development.

Off-the-job methods

Off-the-job training methods remove managers from the stresses of the workplace, enabling them to focus on the learning experience.

Off-the-job training is usually conducted in classroom settings where the organization hires consultants or specialist instructors to conduct the development sessions. Some organizations send selected employees to attend management development courses, for example MBA courses at universities, conducted by the department of business leadership or business administration. Classroom instruction is often supplemented with case studies, role-playing, business games, or simulations (Stoner and Freeman 1992: 390). Although most managers prefer on-the-job training by their immediate supervisors, many of the older generation supervisors do not possess the wealth of relevant business knowledge needed by contemporary managers, with the result that the following topics are usually dealt with in a series of short academic courses away from the work setting (Gillies 1989: 358):

- group dynamics;
- economics;
- labour relations;
- accounting;
- cost-benefit analysis;
- techniques for flow-charting;
- job analysis;
- job evaluation;
- programme budgeting;
- grievance arbitration.

On-the-job approaches

The development of managers is an activity which is best undertaken in real-life situations because the individual manager and the particular organization's needs are rather specific.

Designing a management development programme

An external consultant could be appointed to assist in designing the programme. A committee consisting of top managers and the consultant has to take decisions regarding this programme. An atmosphere of trust and support must be ensured in the organization to create a climate of growth.

The educational foundation of management development must be understood. It involves learning for a clearly defined future job, not merely general learning (Nadler and Nadler 1992: 19). The individual and the organization will benefit from education, especially if managers are well educated. Hofmeyr (1990: 108) referred to the fact that 'learning has to be made more active, rather than passive.'

It must also be borne in mind that managers are adults and, in any programme where there are adults in the learning position, managers should actively participate during learning sessions, an informal and friendly atmosphere must be created, and feedback regarding progress should be given regularly (Cherry 1990: 391). In the following discussion, the views of Beach (1991), Gillies (1989) and Gerber (1992) are combined in a plan of action for management development.

1. Objectives should be formulated. The objectives for such a programme could take the following into consideration:

   • improvement of the manager's functioning;

   • improvement of the job satisfaction that a manager experiences;

   • identification of the manager's potential for future leadership;

   • prevention of stagnation among managers due to obsolescence, etc. (Gerber et al. 1989: 267).

   • promotion of the organization's mission and objectives (primary health care, quality nursing).

2. Establish an agreement among top and middle managers.

   • Levels of authority, responsibility, and accountability must be decided upon (Gillies 1989: 357).

   • Analysis of organizational needs is carried out. Specializations and the relationship between positions in the organizational structure should be identified. Defects in present functioning of the structure should be identified.

   • Job descriptions and specification should be studied to decide on future policy regarding appointments/promotions (Beach 1991: 267).

3. Assessment of the organization's assets/talents. Gillies (1989: 357) refers to this stage as an analysis of the effectiveness of managers at each level.

   This analysis includes all the activities related to the functioning of each department or level in the organizational structure. A departmental analysis will indicate the strong and weak links, eg incidents, quality of nursing care identified during nursing audits, and the rates of turnover and absenteeism among employees. The cost-effectiveness of the department will also be reflected in such an assessment. Management talent will be assessed in this analysis (Beach 1991: 267). This is a very positive and motivational step because potential managers and leaders get the opportunity to be identified and noticed.

4. Inventory of management skills (Beach 1991: 267). A profile of each manager is compiled. This profile should include all academic and professional qualifications, biographical information, personal qualities, special competencies, and personal preferences. This profile reflects all experiences and special achievements of the manager and provides information for future planning. All the information mentioned above forms a 'base line of information ... needed to ensure that decisions and interventions are situation-specific' (Gillies 1989: 358).

5. Individual development programmes. The needs of each manager are unique in terms of the profile and the post she holds. Each post has its own needs and demands. It is important to bear in mind that each manager is a human being, and that personal and organizational goals must be congruent in whatever development programme is devised.

6. Development programme for the organization. Gillies (1985: 358) refers specifically to the fact that the development of nurse managers is an educational activity rather than a training activity because it is broader in scope than skill-training and is not task-limited. Courses in leadership, management games, strategic management, financial management courses, and other relevant courses of mutual concern could be offered. Such activities must be recorded for evaluation purposes.

7. Programme evaluation. Large amounts of money and time go into management development (Beach 1991: 268). Top management needs proof of what has been done. Evaluation criteria must be set right at the planning stage of the programme. These criteria must be set by the committee and the consultant in accordance with the objectives of the programme.

8. Avenues to follow to promote management development. The structure and management of the organization should provide opportunities in its daily function to promote management development.

Management committees

The creation of a management committee gives managers the opportunity to be exposed to a wider view of the organization. Planning and policy formulation are carried out at this level. Vision and decision-making skills could be developed at this level too. The management committee is also exposed to the external environment, such as other health organizations, the community, educational departments, and the economic sector. This enables managers to develop a broader body of knowledge and insight.

Participative management

Management committees and ad hoc committees create the opportunity for managers to interact and to put suggestions on the table. Listening and reasoning skills are developed in a management culture where there is mutual concern for an organization. Communication, interpersonal relationships, and knowledge of how to adhere to the protocol procedures of the organization are also developed during participative management sessions.

Job rotation

Job rotation involves shifting managers from position to position so that they can broaden their experience and become familiar with various managerial functions. The nursing service manager, for example, may be assigned to gain experience in the personnel administration section, the general management of patient care section, and the staff development section in a big hospital.

Job rotation can contribute to management development because it exposes the 'new' manager to a new environment. Job rotation involves shifting managers from position to position so that they can broaden their experience and become familiar with various managerial functions. The nurse manager may, for example, be assigned to gain experience in the personnel administration section, the general management of the patient care section, and the staff development section in a big hospital. If a manager spends all her life in the same department she can develop blinkers and this can lead to a very limited approach to organizational matters. A department can stagnate without initiative or new approaches. A new department is also a new challenge for a manager. It is important that job rotation must be part of the management development initiative and should not be applied as a punishment. Reward, acknowledgement, and praise should be part of this strategy.

Coaching/mentoring

Mentoring is the process where an older, wiser, and more experienced person guides and nurtures a younger one, often called the protégé. It has been found that it is especially important for a woman's advancement that she should have a mentor who introduces her to established networks that promote career progress and advancement. The mentor's role encompasses functions such as teacher, guide, patron, advocate, benefactor, and adviser (Vance 1982: 7–8). Both the mentor and the protégé benefit from their association with each other. The benefits for the younger person are found in the fact that the mentor assists the younger person in her intellectual development, eases her entry into powerful work relationships, serves as a role model, provides the necessary insight into the practical realities of the work, and detects and develops the hidden potential of the younger person, with the result that the protégé becomes happier, more competent and self-assured, and her leadership qualities such as risk-taking, sharing, relating to people in an empathetic manner and creativity are enhanced.

The mentor benefits by experiencing personal satisfaction, increased self-confidence, and enhanced self-esteem. The demonstration of her ability to attract a protégé, nurturing her to develop to her fullest potential and become a successful leader herself, enables the mentor to experience her own charisma and success as a leader. The mentor also profits by receiving admiration and affection from the protégé; the protégé later furthers the mentor's ideas and causes, invites her to speak and consult, and introduces her to her own circle of colleagues to share important ideas with them (Vance 1982: 9).

According to Darling (1985: 45), the beneficial effects of mentoring are only possible when there is a proper match between the mentor and the protégé. Characteristics of the protégé which must be taken into account when matching her with a suitable mentor are her experience with authority figures, her pattern of learning, and her stage of professional development.

Training positions

Sometimes manager trainees are given staff posts immediately under a manager — for example the position of assistant to the chief nursing service manager. The trainee is thus placed in a position where she can observe the manager in her leadership role and model herself on such a person.

Understudies

'An understudy is a person who is in training to assume, at a future time, the full duties and responsibilities of the position currently held by his or her superior' (Beach 1991: 269). This approach is directed towards replacing the present manager when he/she is going to leave the organization because of retirement, promotion, transfer, or resignation.

This procedure must be well planned and discussed. More than one understudy may get the chance to gain experience, and they may take turns to act as the 'executive'. These turns give the understudies the required experience in handling daily matters related to the position.

Beach (1991: 270) maintains that the understudy strategy is a practical and quick method of training promising personnel for future positions. Practical learning is emphasized, and the motivation of the understudy tends to be high. There are also disadvantages to this strategy. For example, it does not allow much room for innovation, and not all employees get the advantage of being an understudy.

Planned work activities

The trainee manager may be assigned to important work projects in an organization to develop experience and abilities. Management trainees can be helped to acquire the necessary background information to make sound management decisions by serving on such management committees as the policy and procedure committee, the quality assurance committee, and the disaster committee.

Other activities

Lastly, the fledgling manager will be assisted in developing her communication abilities by making speeches before nursing groups, serving as a hostess for social gatherings, writing formal letters of inquiry, hiring and firing, attending interviews, and gathering experience in the production of software for use in formal presentations or papers (Gillies 1989: 359).

ORGANIZATIONAL DEVELOPMENT

Gerber, Nel, and Van Dyk (1987: 281) describe the following as the objectives of organizational development:

- the improvement of communication between managers at the various managerial levels;

- decision-making by lower level managers who are the nearest to the centre of activity;

- bringing to the surface undercurrents of hostility and conflict in order to make a constructive attempt at removing them;

- improvement of the organization's ability to adapt to change.

Beach (1985: 275) defines organizational development as a

> planned process designed to improve organizational effectiveness and health through modifications in individual and group behaviour, culture and systems of the organization using knowledge and technology of applied behavioural science.

Organizational development is frequently conducted by a consultant (called a *change agent*) who is schooled in the behavioural sciences and who tends to emphasize the 'people' dimensions of organizational effectiveness such as attitudes, norms, values, interpersonal skills, and behaviour patterns.

According to Beach (1985) the values upon which the organizational development movement is built are:

- people are basically good, responsible, helpful, and trustworthy;

- employees need frequent confirmation that they are worthy individuals, and they also need support in their work from their supervisors;

- differences in personality and opposing viewpoints strengthen rather than weaken an organization;

- if employees must be creative and innovative, they must also be allowed to express their feelings of anger, tenderness, and other emotions;

- managers should be authentic, open, and direct in their dealings with employees, because honesty and directness enable people to put their energy into the real problems of the job without spending energy on trying to detect hidden motives and agendas;

- co-operation and teamwork generate a greater volume of production than does destructive interpersonal competition;

- interpersonal conflict should be brought into the open in order to confront it and detect its root causes so that it can be resolved.

The stages in the organizational development process are set out by Gillies (1989) as follows:

1. Problem diagnosis.

2. Gathering of data.

3. Achieving a general understanding of the problem.

4. Achieving group commitment to change.

5. Training of employees.

6. Evaluation of changes achieved through training.

During the diagnosis phase, problems regarding communication patterns, goal setting, planning, decision-making, conflict resolution, and relations between different departments and between superiors and subordinates are investigated.

During the fourth and fifth stages, use is made of workshops, group discussions, written exercises, on-the-job activities, redesign of control systems, problem-solving activities, redesign of jobs, and numerous other methods aimed at changing the attitudes and behaviour of key employees.

Organizational development must not be regarded as a quick cure for an organization's ills. A great deal of effort, and much time, is usually necessary to achieve real and lasting changes (Beach 1985: 281).

Organizational development techniques

Survey feedback

Attitude surveys are conducted among employees to determine their viewpoints regarding salaries, working conditions, and the treatment they get from supervisors, among other things. The survey results are fed back to the employees, and workshops are then held by each manager and/or supervisor with his/her employees where the results of the survey are discussed and solutions to problems are suggested.

Process consultation

A process consultant works with the members of a department in a team and assists them in diagnosing interactional problems that arise between them in their decision-making activities. This consultant counsels individuals and groups to work out more effective behaviour and communication, but does not prescribe to them.

Sensitivity training

This training is developed to help people understand themselves better and to become sensitive to the effects of their behaviour upon others. T-group or sensitivity training is conducted in a laboratory setting where small groups are engaged in uncovering the feelings, emotions, and attitudes expressed by individual group members. The aims are, among others, to sensitize the participants towards the behaviour of others and to improve the ability of participants to analyse their own behaviour continuously in order to establish more effective and satisfactory interpersonal relationships (Dessler 1984: 280).

Transactional analysis

This is a method which was developed by Berne (1972) and his followers to help managers to understand their own ego states and those of others in order to interact with others effectively. The three ego states, namely 'adult', 'parent', and 'child' relate to direct, reality-based interactions; moralizing, judgmental interactionism or emotional, impulsive responses towards others respectively. It also shows the instructional patterns which are commonly found, showing that each individual tends to relate to others from either one of four so-called life-positions, namely (Gillies 1989: 210; Gerber et al. 1987: 224):

- I'm not OK; you're OK;
- I'm not OK; you're not OK;
- I'm OK; you're not OK;
- I'm OK; you're OK.

Managerial grid training

This focuses on individual and team development and was proposed and described by Blake and Mouton (1964). The aim of this method is to change the leadership styles of the organization. Training is conducted in six phases.

1. Phase 1 — the grid seminar. The organization's top management team meets and conducts a seminar during which each manager's position on the managerial grid is determined.

2. Phase 2 — team development. The managers apply the knowledge obtained during the phase 1 seminar to conduct workshops with teams of their own subordinates. The aim of this phase is to implement a problem-solving approach throughout the organization.

3. Phase 3 — intergroup development. In this phase, group-to-group working relationships are examined and ways to move interactions from a typical 'win–lose' pattern to a joint problem-solving orientation are explored.

4. Phase 4 — developing an ideal model. Top managers develop an ideal model for achieving organizational and individual goals. The model could focus on interventions to change structure, technology, and people. The model is evaluated by lower-level managers.

5. Phase 5 — implementing the model. Planning teams are formed for each unit in order to prepare the units for the necessary changes so that they can comply with the ideal model.

6. Phase 6 — monitoring the ideal model. The previous phases are evaluated systematically in order to detect any remaining problems, to assess the progress that has been made, and to see whether there were any further developmental opportunities identified (Szilagyi and Wallace 1990: 826–7).

Team building

This is one of the most frequently used organizational development interventions. A series of off-site problem-solving sessions of two to five days' duration are conducted with a manager and those reporting directly to him/her. Important aims of this exercise are the setting of goals and priorities, the clarification of roles and responsibilities, the identification of problems and conflict, and the improvement of communication between team members. The advantage of this method is the establishment of better communication and problem-solving between and within the different teams (Dessler 1984: 284).

Other interventions

A number of other techniques were developed before the emergence of the organizational development movement.

- Job enrichment. This is the addition of more decision-making, responsibilities, and other challenges to enrich routine jobs.

- Management by objectives. This is collaboration between a manager and a subordinate in order to set work-related objectives, to evaluate the subordinate's progress in achieving them, and to set new ones on completion of the previous objectives.

- Changes in organizational structure. This means the introduction of different organizational designs such as project and matrix organization and decentralization.

- Participative management. This includes participative problem-solving meetings and labour union management and co-operation (Beach 1985: 286).

CONCLUSION

The continuous development of managers is achieved by either off-the-job methods or on-the-job approaches and according to a development programme.

The expansion of any organization into a complex entity over time necessitates a proactive approach in order to address its demands and problems. This requires a programme of organizational development which is often approached through a number of organizational development techniques.

References

Argyris, C. (1992). *On Organizational Learning*. Blackwell: Cambridge Massachusetts.

Beach, D. S. (1985). *The Management of People at Work*. Fifth edition. Macmillan: New York.

Beach, D. S. (1991). *Personnel. The Management of People at Work*. Macmillan: New York.

Cherry, B. S. (1990). Professional development. In Dienemann, J. *Nursing Administration. Strategic Perspectives and Application.* Appleton and Lange: Norwalk.

Cronje, G. J. de J., Newland, E. W., Hugo, W. M. J. and Van Reenen, M. J. (1990). *Inleiding tot die Bedryfsekonomie.* Southern: Johannesburg.

Darling, R. W. (1985). Mentor matching. *JONA,* volume 15, number 1, pp. 45–6.

Dessler, G. (1984). *Personnel Management.* Reston: Virginia.

Douglass, L. M. (1988). *The Effective Nurse Leader-Manager.* Third edition. Mosby: St Louis.

Gerber, P. D., Nel, P. S. and Van Dyk, P. S. (1987). *Human Resources Management.* Southern: Johannesburg.

Gerber, P. D., Nel, P. S. and Van Dyk, P. S. (1992). *Mannekragbestuur.* Second edition. Southern: Johannesburg.

Gillies, D. A. (1989). *Nursing Management: A Systems Approach.* Saunders: Philadelphia.

Hofmeyr, K. B. (1990). *Management education for the nineties. SA Journal for Business Management,* volume 21, number 3, pp. 102–11.

Koopman, A. (1991). *Transcultural Management: How to Unlock Global Resources.* Basil Blackwell: Oxford.

McFarland, G. K., Leonard, H. S., and Morris, M. M. (1984). *Nursing Leadership and Management.* John Wiley: New York.

Nadler, L. and Nadler, Z. (1992). *Every Manager's Guide to Human Resource Development.* Jossey-Bass: San Francisco.

Nelson, G. M. and Schafer, M. J. (1980). An integrated approach to developing administrators and organizations. *JONA,* volume 10, number 2, pp. 37–42.

Stoner, J. A. F. and Freeman, B. E. (1992). *Management.* (Fifth edition). Prentice-Hall: Englewood Cliffs, New Jersey.

Szilagyi, A. D. and Wallace, M. J. (1990). *Organizational Behaviour and Performance.* Scott, Foresman and Co: Illinois.

Vance, C. N. (1982). The mentor connection. *JONA,* volume 2, number 4. pp. 7–13.

PART FOUR:

LEADING

CHAPTER 19

LEADERSHIP

S. W. Booyens

CONTENTS

INTRODUCTION

Numerous definitions of leadership exist. They include the following:

- It is the process which is utilized to direct the behaviour of a group to attain a common goal.

- It is the use of one's skills to influence others to perform to the best of their ability.

- It is an 'interpersonal relationship in which the leader employs specific behaviour and strategies to influence individuals and groups towards setting goals and attaining them in specific situations' (Sullivan and Decker 1992: 181).

- It is a process by which one person attempts to influence others to accomplish some goal or goals.

- 'Leadership results when the appointed head causes the members of his group to accept directives without any apparent exertion of authority or force on his part' (Holloman as referred to by Swansburg 1990: 352).

- It is 'the competencies and processes required to enable and empower ordinary people to do extraordinary things in the face of adversity, and constantly turn in superior performance to the benefit of themselves and the organization' (Charlton 1992: 47).

It is clear from the above definitions that leadership requires a leader and a group of followers who are influenced by the leader, and that the leader's influence is directed at the achievement of work performance or some common goal. Leadership thus requires a *relationship* between people who are to be led (the followers) and the person who is leading them (the leader). The process of leadership is, however, also dependent on the specific setting or milieu in which it takes place. Leadership is thus viewed as a dynamic and interactive process in which three dimensions are involved — the leader, the followers, and the situation — and in which each of these dimensions influences the other two.

Swansburg (1990) quotes McGregor's four variables involved in leadership, namely:

1. The characteristics of the leader.

2. The attitudes, needs, and other personal characteristics of the followers.

3. Characteristics of the organization, such as its purpose and structure and the nature of the task to be performed.

4. The social, political, and economic milieu.

THE DIFFERENCE BETWEEN LEADERSHIP AND MANAGEMENT

It is important to remember that an organization needs both management and leadership. Management and leadership are interdependent, although people at every level in an organization are called upon to exhibit leadership qualities — ie to facilitate productive action.

According to Charlton (1992: 24), Zalesnik distinguished between *traditional management* and *transformational leadership* in terms of a number of dimensions or categories.

Managers tend to rely on systems, while *leaders* tend to rely on people. Managers tend to think of the everyday problems they are faced with in their planning, whereas leaders are more concerned with long-term or strategic planning. Managers thus focus on getting things done and react to everyday pressures and events, while leaders are concerned with the future. Leaders typically develop a vision of the future and a strategy to get there.

In their role interpretations, managers differ from leaders in that they often occupy the implementing role, whereas the leader occupies the guiding, influencing role. The manager usually sees herself as being 'served' by his subordinates, while the leader sees herself as serving others.

Leaders have an active attitude towards goals whereas the manager has an impersonal, if not passive, attitude. For the manager, goals arise out of necessity and are formulated in response to change, in reaction to forces outside the organization. The leader, on the other hand, formulates goals in an effort to influence the organization to bring about change and to create a different future.

In their attitude to work, managers rely on planning, budgeting, and other management tools, and do not want to take too many risks because of their basic survival instincts. In contrast, leaders are prepared to take real risks because they have faith in other people, faith in the judgement of their key executives, and they focus on making the work of their followers purposeful or meaningful in order to motivate them.

Managers are more task-orientated than leaders and are more detached emotionally. Leaders empathize with employees more easily and communicate more freely.

Where power and motivation are concerned, managers use threats and rewards to motivate subordinates, but leaders create a sense of purpose and hope to develop people's intrinsic motivation. Managers use control as a power strategy, whereas leaders give power in order to get power and count on the trust of their employees. From this it is clear that leaders exhibit a strong sense of their own identity and do not rely on others, or their work roles, to achieve a sense of self.

Managers, on the other hand, tend to derive their sense of self from being regulators of an existing order of affairs with which they personally identify.

Regarding change, leaders actively effect second-order or organizational/structural change to create a better future; they change the way people think about the desirability and possibility of innovations and developments. Managers like to maintain order, and sustain the present situation, but are willing to make smaller first-order or functional changes when the need arises.

Managers emphasize the rational assessment and systematic selection of goals, objectives, and processes. Managers are trained in the processes of staffing methods, budgeting, the fundamentals of job description, and performance appraisal techniques (Friss 1989: 248). Leaders use intuitive thinking rather than rational thinking, are prepared to create disorder in order to effect radical changes, and they use power to profoundly change human, economic, and political relationships. They are more innovative than managers because where managers tend to use the left hemispheres of their brains when they think, leaders use both left and right sides of the brain for thinking and are thus more imaginative, flexible, broad thinking, and dynamic individuals.

Lastly, it has been said that managers are there to see that things are done correctly, but leaders are necessary so that the *correct* things may be done correctly (Bennis 1989: 45).

THEORIES OF LEADERSHIP

Research regarding leadership focuses mainly on the elements that result in effective leadership. Thus situations, personal characteristics, and leadership behaviour which would make one form of leadership more effective than another are continually being studied.

Trait theories

During the 1940s and 1950s, research was directed at identifying the individual characteristics or traits of leaders which would serve to differentiate successful leaders from unsuccessful ones.

After many years of research no particular set of traits was found which accurately predicted leadership success.

Some research findings suggest that it is better to view leadership as a relationship between the leader and the situation rather than as a universal pattern of characteristics possessed by certain special people. It may thus be seen that leadership is a human relations function in which different situations will require different leadership styles or behaviours.

Early work on leadership traits maintained that traits were inherited, but later studies suggested that traits could be learned through education and experience.

Despite the fact that trait theory arrived at inconclusive findings regarding leadership effectiveness, it expanded knowledge about leadership. Furthermore, although various researchers arrived at different conclusions regarding the traits needed for effectiveness, some common leadership traits were identified.

In a review of trait research in 1948, Ralph Stogdill identified the following six broad categories:

- physical characteristics;

- social background;

- intelligence;

- personality;

- task-related characteristics; and

- social characteristics.

Physical characteristics

Physical characteristics, such as age, weight, height, and appearance were studied. Although people tend to assign some positive characteristics to a person who is tall, and who has normal weight and a good appearance, there are many other personal and situational factors which will influence the choice and effectiveness of the leader.

Social background

In their investigation of the social background of leaders, factors such as education, social status, and mobility were studied. No consistent links between social background and success in leadership were found, although it was concluded that it is easier for people who have a high socioeconomic status to become leaders, and that leaders today are better educated than they were in the past.

Intelligence

It was generally agreed that leaders should be more intelligent than the group they lead. Numerous studies indicated that leaders have superior judgement, decisiveness, knowledge, and fluency of speech (Szilagyi and Wallace 1990: 387). There is, at present, universal agreement that the effective leader must possess good communication skills. The leader must be able to pick up hidden messages from her followers and must be able to speak and write well. It is through the use of communication that leaders succeed in persuading their followers to pursue a suggested path, to try out new ways of doing their jobs, and to change their thinking about effectiveness and productivity.

Personality

The personality factors which were investigated were alertness, self-confidence, personal integrity, self-assurance, and dominance needs.

A person who wants to motivate others must have emotional maturity and balance, personal control, and integrity. This person will also need a sense of purpose and direction in life and will be dependable, persistent, and objective regarding her own weaknesses and strengths. Mature leaders do what they say they will do and are consistent in their actions. They often work long hours, overcome obstacles, apply themselves intensely to their tasks, and spread enthusiasm among their followers. These people are sure of what they can achieve and do not lack confidence in themselves.

Findings regarding these personality traits were fairly consistent among different research studies, which suggests that some personality traits should be considered in any approach to leadership.

Task-related characteristics

Research into leaders and leadership concludes that leaders are characterized by having drive and initiative, by being achievement-orientated, and by not fearing responsibility, and that they are concerned about both people and results. They often also display creativity and original thinking, which makes them see new solutions to old problems.

Social characteristics

Studies of social characteristics indicate that leaders can socialize with a wide variety of people from all walks of life, that they are approachable, friendly, helpful, and willing to co-operate with others. Their interpersonal skills help them in supervising others and in building loyalty and confidence among their followers.

Research that is directly or indirectly related to leadership traits continues. It is, however, still not clear which traits are the most important ones, which traits are needed to acquire leadership, and which traits are necessary to stay on top. Trait theory does not deal with subordinates, and avoids consideration of environmental influences and situational factors.

Behaviour theories

During the 1950s dissatisfaction with the trait theory approach, which focused on the abilities a leader needed to emerge as a leader, led to a shift of emphasis towards consideration of the behaviour, performance, or actions of the leader. The underlying assumption of this approach was that a specific 'style of leadership' would be more effective for leading a group to attain high productivity and morale than another style.

A number of large research efforts were undertaken after the Second World War to investigate the factors which influenced the behaviour of leaders and to determine the effects of the style of leadership which the leader used on the group's performance and satisfaction.

Two independent leadership dimensions evolved from these studies, namely *consideration* and *initiating structure* (Szilagyi and Wallace 1990: 392).

- Consideration was viewed as behaviour which involved being friendly, trusting followers, showing concern, treating others as equals, taking time to listen, consulting others on important matters, and being willing to accept suggestions. This dimension thus focused on an employee-orientated leadership style.

- Initiating structure is analogous to the task-orientated leadership style and is concerned with such matters as organizing and defining tasks, assigning work to be done, defining procedures, maintaining standards, establishing communication networks, co-ordinating activities, and evaluating the performance of the work group.

Many individual research efforts were conducted in an attempt to determine the effects of initiating structure and consideration on group performance and morale. The underlying assumption of these studies was that the most effective leaders would be both high on consideration and initiating structure. The findings of the studies, however, did not support this assumption.

Another group of research studies into leadership styles differentiated styles according to job- or employee-centredness. The job-centred leadership style focused roughly on the same aspects of leadership as the initiating structure-type, and the employee-centred style on those of the consideration style. Neither increases in task-behaviour nor interpersonal behaviour markedly increased employee performance or satisfaction.

A search for clusters of leadership behaviours was undertaken in an attempt to identify specific patterns or styles of leadership which would be effective in most situations. Several styles were identified.

Autocratic or authoritarian leadership style

This leadership style is characterized by the giving of orders. The leader usually makes decisions alone, and frequently exercises power with coercion. The group usually lacks enthusiasm. This style of leadership is necessary and useful in crisis situations, but in normal day-to-day activities leads to a dependent and aggressive or submissive group of employees who have lost the power of thinking innovatively, are afraid to risk new ventures, are unproductive in the leader's absence, and are apt to be absent from work for the slightest reason.

Autocratic leadership is suitable for crisis situations, for when the entire focus is on getting the job done, or for when it is difficult to share decision-making. It is often referred to as a directive or controlling style of leadership.

Democratic or participative leadership style

This style is concerned with human relations and teamwork. It is particularly appropriate for groups of people who will work together for extended periods of time, when interpersonal relationships can substantially affect the productivity of the group. Decisions are made by the group and the leader. Responsibility for effective work performance or implementation of decisions is shared by everybody.

Group members usually exhibit high morale, are not entirely dependent on their leader, and are thus not afraid to take risks and to think creatively. Their work output is not dependent on the leader's presence or absence, but their general work efficiency is somewhat less than that of a group led by an autocratic leader. Democratic leaders do not issue commands — they offer information, ask stimulating questions, and make suggestions in order to guide the work of the group. They act as facilitators rather than controllers, their criticisms are constructive rather than punitive, and they trust that group members will be committed to accomplish goals that have been set.

Studies show that democratic leadership is not as efficient quantitatively as authoritarian leadership. The work done by a democratically-led group is usually more creative and the group members are more self-motivated, but it takes more time to get the participation of each group member when making decisions and this can be frustrating for people who are impatient and who want a job to be done as fast as possible (Tappen 1989: 37).

Democratic or participative leadership is appropriate when a great deal of co-ordination and co-operation between group members is needed, or when the nature of the work makes close supervision difficult. This is often the case in health care.

Laissez-faire leadership style

Tappen (1989: 37) states that the *laissez-faire* or 'free-reign' leader is generally inactive, passive, and non-directive. This type of leader sets almost no limits, is permissive, has no established goals or policies, and offers very little to a group because few commands, suggestions, or criticisms come forward. These leaders tend to behave inconsistently and will occasionally become directive and issue commands. Group members tend to ignore these attempts at exerting leadership behaviour.

Laissez-faire leadership is often practised by a person who has a great need for approval and is afraid to offend subordinates. She wants to please everyone. This type of manager tends to be preoccupied with her own work (DiVincenti 1977: 59).

In the laissez-faire group, members act independently of each other and often work against each other because there is little co-operation and co-ordination. This often results in apathy and disinterest among group members, or chaotic activity with a rise in frustration levels (Tappen 1989: 37).

When the members of a group are self-directed, highly motivated, and able to co-ordinate activities among themselves, laissez-faire leadership can give them the freedom they need to be creative and productive. In most situations, however, laissez-faire leadership is unproductive, inefficient, and unsatisfactory. This type of leadership is also called 'permissive' or 'non-directive' leadership.

Bureaucratic leadership style

In this type of leadership an insecure leader finds security in following established policies. This leader exercises power by commanding employees to follow relatively inflexible rules. Interpersonal communication is not this leader's strong point. She tends to relate to staff members on an impersonal level. Because of the leader's basic insecurity, she avoids making decisions without having standards or norms which could guide her (Sullivan and Decker 1992: 186).

The behavioural theories suggested the following points:

- Leadership is, in part, a learnt skill. Leaders learn from experience the styles of leadership that work in particular situations.

- Leadership style is flexible and appears to be a function of the situation. The stronger the leader's power base, the greater his or her ability to use a task-orientated style would be. The weaker the power base, the more the leader would depend on a people-orientated style.

- Leadership style is a multidimensional concept because it depends on the nature of tasks to be performed by the employees, the organizational structure, and the characteristics of subordinates (Szilagyi and Wallace 1990: 395).

Situational theories

The work of the trait and behavioural style researchers provided a significant foundation for the study of leadership in organizations because the results strongly pointed to the fact that the situation is the main determinant which affects the leader's style of leadership. In order to determine the leadership style which will fit the situation, the leader must evaluate or analyse the situation. In her evaluation, the leader will assess the following factors in a situation:

- individual differences;
- group structure;
- values;
- attitudes;
- needs and expectations of the leader and of the followers;
- the degree of interpersonal contact which is possible;
- the structure, culture, and climate of the organization;
- the organization's policies and procedures;
- existing communication patterns among group members.

The leadership continuum of Tannenbaum and Schmidt

The way in which leadership needs to vary according to the situation, is illustrated by the leadership continuum of Tannenbaum and Schmidt (Gerber, Nel and van Dyk 1992). This continuum illustrates leadership styles which vary according to the distribution of power or influence from the leader or her followers.

In this model, as illustrated in figure 19.1, the leadership style changes from leader-centredness to a focus on the members of a team, according to the shift of authority/power from the leader to the followers/team members.

From this model, the following comments regarding leadership effectiveness can be made:

1. There is no one single correct leadership style.

2. The successful leader can easily move along the whole continuum of leadership styles and can adapt her style according to the situation.

3. The good leader is sensitive to the environmental, interpersonal, and organizational forces working at a specific moment and adjusts her style accordingly.

4. Team-centred leadership is effective for the achievement of long-term objectives.

5. When a crisis looms, autocratic leadership is necessary.

6. Autocratic action is often needed to achieve short-term objectives.

7. Balance is important. When a balance between team-centredness and leader-centredness is maintained:
   - the brain power of all members is utilized;
   - creativity is enhanced;
   - people feel useful and work is done well;
   - problems are discussed and group involvement is improved;
   - team members become more responsible.

8. It is not advisable for supervisors to use autocratic leadership when they feel that it will be the easiest and quickest way to achieve objectives. They should first try a participative approach. Conversely, team members should not see themselves as co-leaders, refusing to obey any autocratic decisions made.

Figure 19.1 illustrates possible leadership styles and the leader's adjustment of her leadership style to suit the situation. To make this decision, the leader must examine four important areas namely managerial characteristics, subordinate characteristics, group structure, and the nature of the task and organizational factors. According to Milton (1981), as referred to by Gerber, Nel, and van Dyk (1987: 358) and Szilagyi and Wallace (1990: 396–399), these factors can be described as follows:

Figure 19.1: Power base and leadership style according to Tannenbaum and Schmidt

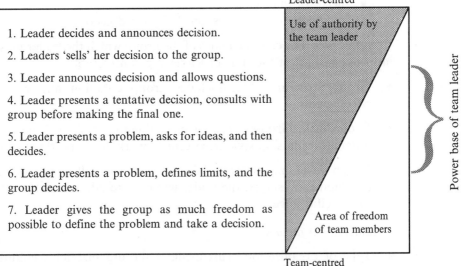

Leader-centred

1. Leader decides and announces decision.

2. Leaders 'sells' her decision to the group.

3. Leader announces decision and allows questions.

4. Leader presents a tentative decision, consults with group before making the final one.

5. Leader presents a problem, asks for ideas, and then decides.

6. Leader presents a problem, defines limits, and the group decides.

7. Leader gives the group as much freedom as possible to define the problem and take a decision.

Use of authority by the team leader

Area of freedom of team members

Power base of team leader

Team-centred

Managerial characteristics. The leader's behaviour in any given situation depends on the following factors:

- Personality — ie how confident the leader is in her ability to lead. Does she possess the necessary background, intelligence, knowledge, insight and experience to be an effective leader?

- Motives, needs, and the value-system of the leader.

- The leader's philosophy of leadership.

- The leader's feelings of security in an unsure situation.

- Past experiences and reinforcement. For example when a leader has become accustomed to an authoritative leadership style during all of her working years she may tend to apply this style herself.

- The trust that the leader places in her followers.

Subordinate factors

- Personality — ie how confident the subordinates are in their abilities. How intelligent are subordinates?

- Expectations and past experiences among subordinates regarding leadership behaviour.

- The leader would determine the measure of involvement allowed in decision-making according to the team members' levels of
  - interest shown in the problem;
  - knowledge and insight regarding problems;
  - identification with organizational objectives;
  - tolerance of ambiguity;
  - need for independence;
  - readiness to accept responsibility for decisions.

Group factors. The characteristics of the group which the leader must influence will affect the style of leadership considerably.

- Group structure. This includes group cohesion and group effectiveness.

- Group task. Groups working on ambiguous tasks will need a different leadership style from groups working on routine tasks.

- Group development stage. When a group is still in one of its developmental stages, the leader will have to adopt a style to fit the specific stage.

Organizational factors

- Type of organization. This includes the organization's culture and structure.

- Rules and procedures. Many organizations dictate the type of leadership required by way of extensive policy and procedural systems.

- Professionalism. Highly trained professionals such as scientists, lecturers, and nurses may depend more on their own educational background and experience to guide them than on the leader's guidance.

- Time. When immediate decisions have to be made, group members cannot be consulted.

- The problem. The simplicity or complexity of the problem will dictate the amount of group consultation needed.

- Power base. The leader's power base will limit or extend his/her influence on group members.

Apart from the above factors, the behaviour of subordinates also has a profound influence on the leader's style of leadership.

Contingency theory

During the 1960s Fiedler introduced his contingency model of leadership to do justice to both the personality of the leader and the complexities of the situation. The theory contends that the effectiveness of a leader in achieving high group performance depends on the need structure of the leader and the degree of a leader's control and influence in a specific situation. The model has four aspects, namely leadership-style assessment, task structure, group atmosphere, and the positional power of the leader. The first aspect identifies what motivates the leader, and the other three describe how favourable the situation is for the leader, ranging from highly favourable to highly unfavourable (Szilagyi and Wallace 1990: 399).

According to Moorhead and Griffin (1989: 330–1) the basic premises of this model can be described as follows:

Leadership-style assessment

The leader's basic personality trait — ie whether she is task- or relationship-motivated — is assessed by a scale called the *least-preferred co-worker scale* (LPC). The leader is asked to mark on a series of sixteen scales (each scale calibrated from positive to negative) the characteristics of the co-worker with whom they have worked who is, in terms of their own preferences, the 'least-preferred' one. An example of the items on the scale is:

$$FRIENDLY\ \overline{8\ 7\ 6\ 5\ 4\ 3\ 2\ 1}\ UNFRIENDLY$$
$$HELPFUL\ \overline{8\ 7\ 6\ 5\ 4\ 3\ 2\ 1}\ FRUSTRATING$$
$$INEFFICIENT\ \overline{8\ 7\ 6\ 5\ 4\ 3\ 2\ 1}\ EFFICIENT$$

(The scale is organized in this manner to force the respondent to read and think carefully.)

When the leader's marks on the scale are assessed and show a fair to high level of esteem for the least-preferred co-worker, she receives a high LCP score. Conversely, if the marks on the scale show that the least-preferred co-worker is held in low esteem by the leader, she receives a low LCP score.

Fiedler believed that the LPC scores do not indicate the value or worth of the co-worker, but reflect how the leader views her least preferred co-worker. Thus he postulated that leaders with high LPC scores are basically more concerned with interpersonal relations than low LPC-score leaders. The behaviour of the high LCP leader is therefore similar to the leadership behaviour which is described as 'employee-centred' or 'consideration' behaviour. Leaders with low LPC scores are viewed as more task-orientated (similar to job-centred and 'initiating structure' leadership).

In motivational terms, the high LPC leader has good interpersonal relationships as her basic goal while the low LPC leader has as her basic goal the accomplishment of tasks, with interpersonal relationships taking second place.

Situational factors

Three factors determining the favourableness of the situation for the leader are, in decreasing order of influence, leader–member relations, task structure, and leader position power.

1. Leader–member relations or group atmosphere. Leader–member relations are classified as either good or poor according to the degree to which subordinates trust, respect, and have confidence in the leader and vice versa.

2. Task structure. Task structure refers to the degree that the structure of the group's task is routine or complex. Task structure has four components:

   - Goal-path multiplicity — this is the number of different ways in which a job can be performed.

   - Decision verifiability — how easily the output can be evaluated.

   - Decision specificity — the degree to which a task has a one correct solution.

- Goal clarity — the degree to which the task has clearly defined goals.

Tasks that are low in multiplicity and high in verifiability, specificity, and clarity are considered to be routine tasks and, in this theory, are considered to be more favourable for the leader, because the leader does not need to be closely involved in defining activities and can thus spend time on more important matters. When, on the other hand, tasks are unstructured, ambiguous, and complex, these will be considered to be unfavourable for the leader because more time will have to be spent by the leader in guiding and in directing the various activities of the team members.

3. Position power. This is the power inherent in the leadership position — in other words the extent to which the leader can influence the behaviour of team members through her legitimate power to reward or coerce. If the leader has the power to assign work, to reward or punish employees, and to recommend them for promotion or fire them, position power is high or favourable.

Fiedler's model assumes that the leader will have most influence and control when she uses a task-orientated leadership style under favourable conditions. Favourable conditions imply that the leader is accepted by followers, the task is structured, and that the leader has strong position power. At the other end of the spectrum it is assumed that the leader's control and influence will be minimal when the leader is not accepted, where the task of the group is relatively complex and unstructured, and when the leader has little position power.

Criticism of this model is mainly directed at its one-dimensional nature. Experience has shown that leadership style is of a multi-dimensional nature in the sense that the style must be adapted according to the variations in the followers' needs which at some times necessitate mainly task-oriented styles, at other times mainly employee-oriented styles, and at other times a fair mixture of both orientations.

Path–goal theory of leadership

This theory is derived from the expectancy theory of motivation and focuses on a particular situation and on the leader behaviours which are appropriate for that situation. This theory assumes that team members are motivated by the leader to the extent that they believe that the leader's actions will help them achieve successful work results. The leader thus affects the performance of her subordinates by clarifying the path, and this leads to desired rewards (goals).

Leader behaviour

There are four kinds of leadership behaviour which are inherent in this theory, as described by Moorhead and Griffin (1989: 334), namely directive, supportive, participative, and achievement-orientated.

- Directive leaders structure the activities of staff in the sense that they schedule the work which must be done, they determine the procedures, and they set standards. This type of leadership can increase motivation because role ambiguity is lessened.

- Supportive leaders create an atmosphere of friendliness, warmth, and support, and consider the personal welfare of their subordinates.

- Participative leaders consult with subordinates before making decisions.

- Achievement-orientated leaders set challenging goals, expect subordinates to perform at their highest level, and trust that employees will not let them down. Strong confidence in the subordinates' innate willingness and motivation to perform at the best of their abilities is displayed.

The path–goal theory of leadership assumes that one leader will display any one of these styles, or combinations of these styles, according to the situation she is confronted with.

Situational factors

The situational factors that the leader will be confronted with will depend on the characteristics of the subordinates, and the characteristics of the environment. The two important personal characteristics of subordinates are locus of control and perceived ability. Locus of control refers to the extent to which individuals believe that what happens to them is the result of their own actions or the result of outside influences which are not under their control. It is believed that subordinates who believe that their own actions are largely responsible for what they achieve prefer a participative leader whereas subordinates who believe that outcomes are controlled by external forces tend to prefer a directive leader. The employee who rates her own ability relatively highly does not like directive leadership.

Environmental factors which influence the situation are the formal system of authority, and the structure of the task and the primary work group (Moorhead and Griffin 1989: 336).

Environmental aspects influence the selection of an appropriate leadership style in the following way. When the structure of the task which needs to be performed is high, directive leadership is not really needed and will be less effective; and when the subordinate receives plenty of social support from the primary work group, the supportive leader will not achieve much.

The path–goal theory of leadership was designed to give a general framework for understanding how the behaviour of leaders and situational factors would influence the behaviour and attitudes of subordinates.

Situational leadership theory

Hersey and Blanchard's approach to leadership behaviour contends that the style of leadership to be used depends on the maturity levels of the followers. Three main concepts are included in the theory, namely: task and relationship behaviour, maturity levels, and leadership styles.

Task behaviour

According to Hersey and Blanchard, this includes specification, organization, and assignment of tasks to team members. The leader also establishes organizational patterns, communication channels, and procedures for performing tasks.

Relationship behaviour

Inherent in the leader's relationship behaviour is the promotion of the behaviour of team members by maintaining open communication channels, provision of socio-emotional support, and psychological stroking.

Maturity levels

Four levels of maturity are described:

- M1 — Low maturity. Low maturity levels refer to subordinates who are unwilling and unsure about how to execute a task. They also do not have the necessary abilities to tackle the task.

- M2 — Low to moderate maturity. This refers to subordinates who do not have the necessary abilities for the execution of the task but are willing to tackle it and possess sufficient self-confidence.

- M3 — Moderate to high maturity. The subordinates have the necessary abilities for the execution of the task, but are unwilling or are unsure about it.

- M4 — High maturity. Subordinates are willing to execute the task and possess the necessary abilities as well as sufficient self-confidence.

Leadership styles

Four leadership styles are described by Hersey and Blanchard.

- S1 — 'Telling' style (directing). In this style, in which only one-way communication takes place, the leader tells her subordinates what they must do, and how and when they must do it, without supplying reasons for her commands. This type of style is seen as mainly task-orientated.

- S2 — 'Selling' style (coaching). The leader, in this style, also directs her subordinates with regard to what must be done, but she tries to 'sell' her ideas and decisions to the subordinates by asking their opinions and by providing socio-emotional support. This type of style is regarded as highly orientated towards both tasks and relationships.

- S3 — 'Participating' (supporting). The leader and the subordinates are engaged in joint decision-making through effective two-way communication. The subordinates have the necessary abilities to partake in decision-making and are encouraged to do so by high relationship behaviour. This type of style is thus regarded as relationship-orientated.

- S4 — 'Delegating'. The leader delegates responsibility for taking the necessary decisions to her subordinates because they are able, confident, and willing to execute the task at hand. This type of style is regarded as low in task and relationship behaviour.

Application

The leader will have to assess the maturity levels of subordinates with regard to the task at hand in order to decide which leadership style would be appropriate.

According to Hersey and Blanchard's model, which depicts the above styles and maturity levels in four quadrants, the appropriate style would be selected as follows:

- The leader who is confronted by M1 or low maturity level subordinates will fare best by applying the S1 or 'telling' style of leadership.

- The leader who has to deal with M2 or low to moderate maturity level subordinates should use the S2 or 'selling' type of leadership where task-behaviour is still high, but should use 'relationship' behaviour to win subordinates over to the leader's viewpoint.

- The leader who has to deal with M3 or moderate to high maturity level subordinates will need the S3 or participative style to encourage and support subordinates to partake in decision-making.

- The leader confronted with M4 or high maturity level subordinates should use the S4 or delegating style, because only a superficial or distant type of supervision is required by these dedicated employees.

This leadership theory is regarded as acceptable because it provides for different styles in different situations. It is similar to Argyris's immaturity–maturity continuum, which suggests that as a person matures she moves from a state of dependence, where structure and directive leadership is needed, through a decreasing need for structure and an increased need for relationship, until a state of independence is reached where there is little need for either structure or relationship in the leader's behaviour style (Marriner-Tomey 1992: 267).

This contingency or situational theory of leadership maintains that the leader does not control the work situation any more than she is controlled by it. Both she and her followers are controlled by the goals which should be achieved. Although there are no particular leadership traits or styles which are effective in all situations, there are guidelines for adapting leadership activities to the needs of the situation. The leader must be regarded by her followers as part of the work group. She must be viewed as superior to her followers in some aspects. It is imperative for the leader to know whether she is more task- or more relationship-orientated, and she should try to adapt these orientations to the situation. Some situations, where the tasks are more ambiguous and the workers are more mature and need to be allowed to work independently, would call for more of a relationship style, and in those situations where the followers are more dependent, not so mature, and prefer more structure in their work, the leadership style should be more task-orientated, with more attention to clear-cut policies and procedures. Where followers are mature and independent and the task is structured, the leader will irritate her followers by a task-orientated approach.

In addition to considering the task at hand and goals to be achieved, the leader must also be influenced to a large extent by the attributes of her followers. When an employee shows a particular attribute by behaving in a certain manner (eg not adhering to set standards of work), the leader interprets this in an effort to understand why the follower acted the way she did and adjusts her behaviour or style accordingly.

TRANSFORMATIONAL LEADERSHIP

The literature makes a distinction between *transactional leadership* and *transformational leadership*. According to Bass, cited by Dunham and Klafehn (1990: 29), transformational leadership is not effective if it stands alone. According to these authors 'the most successful transformational leader must be effective in the day-to-day mundane operations considered to be the purview of the transactional leader' (Dunham and Klafehn 1990: 29).

Transactional leadership tries to effect marginal changes in productivity and attitudes towards the achievement of goals, in a similar way to the situational and behavioural leadership styles. Burns (1978, as referred to by Baker 1990: 43) defines transactional leadership as 'one person taking the initiative in making contact with others for the purpose of exchange of valued things.' In transformational leadership, however, the leader attempts to change the views, attitudes, needs, and values of the followers. The transformational leader uses her influence to lead her followers to higher levels of thinking, or to make them think about old problems in new ways and view the situation in which they find themselves in a new light. The transformational leader typically shares a vision of what can be achieved in the future if people are willing to change certain inhibiting attitudes and certain constricting beliefs about the future, and if they are willing to go along with the leader's enlightened ideas about the path that must be followed to get there.

This type of leadership is viewed by Burns as 'the engagement of one or more persons with others in such a way that the leaders and followers raise one another to higher levels of motivation and morality' (Burns 1978, as referred to by Barker 1990: 42).

Transformational leadership is thus future-orientated and is concerned with change and with the empowerment of others.

According to Barker (1990: 39–40) nurse leaders will need to employ the following strategies in order to achieve transformational changes:

- new visions will have to be created which will make the work of the nurse meaningful and purposeful;

- new, trusting relationships between nurse managers and their staff will have to be created;

- working environments will have to be designed with the purpose of empowering staff members;

- the nurse manager will have to use her own power and her own personality in order to achieve organizational success.

The transformational leader is viewed as a person who is absolutely sure of herself, who can communicate her vision of the future to her followers in clear language, and who can engender trust in the possibility of the achievement of envisioned future goals.

The followers of transformational leadership are developed because they grow intellectually, emotionally, and spiritually. They develop new aspirations, and professional and personal values, and tend to think more creatively.

According to Barker (1990: 43) transformational leadership in nursing is not as rare as one might think and is evident when the following characteristics are apparent in a health care setting:

- a staff retention rate of at least 85%;

- high morale of staff which can easily be discerned;
- staff members display an enthusiastic approach to patient care;

- a team spirit is apparent among staff;

- each staff member can recite the goals and purpose of the unit readily;

- staff members express a sense of achievement and belonging;

- the patients and families who are served are satisfied.

According to Dunham and Klafehn (1990: 29) transformational leaders usually display characteristics such as courtesy, friendliness, belief in the innate worth of people, ability to handle complexity, and ambiguous and uncertain situations, and being lifelong learners. They have a strong belief in themselves and in the success of their organizations; they are aware of their own strengths and weaknesses, and they create excellence in their organizations, which generates trust among employees. In nursing, trust is generated through decentralization and through participation in management.

According to Bennis (1989: 202) the leaders of the future — ie transformational leaders — will all have the following things in common:

- a broad education;

- boundless curiosity and enthusiasm;

- belief in people and teamwork;

- willingness to take risks;

- devotion to long-term growth rather than short-term profits;

- commitment to excellence;

- readiness to take on a challenge;

- vision.

Enabling leadership behaviours

A number of leadership behaviours are distinctively displayed during transformational leadership: the communication of a vision, the establishment of a trusting relationship between leader and followers, empowerment of followers to make decisions and to take risks, the ability to effect change, and self-confidence.

Vision

A vision is a picture of a future state of affairs that is attainable, realistic, credible, and infinitely better than what exists at present. A vision energizes people to act in order to bring about change, and this change leads to the achievement of success and excellence (Barker 1990: 83).

During difficult times, in particular, the creation of a vision gives people energy to go on with their daily toils in order to achieve something better in the future.

A vision has two essential purposes according to Charlton (1992: 50). Firstly, it creates an attractive future, and this motivates people to find their own roles in an organization and to work purposefully towards defined goals. Secondly, it serves to focus people's attention on where the organization is going. This allows the leader and followers to choose those activities which will lead them to the envisioned goal and to avoid wasting time on actions which are not relevant.

According to Barker (1990: 85), a vision provides a frame of reference for decision-making, so that people at lower levels of the organization do not appeal to higher authorities for decisions affecting their daily work but make these decisions themselves because they know the direction in which the organization is going .

A vision, like a mission or philosophy, also provides a framework for the resolution of conflicts. If a vision explicitly communicates the purpose of an organization, an environment is created where commitment to the common purpose is the rule and not the exception. Committed individuals usually muster the emotional resources to be creative and innovative (Barker 1990: 85). Thus by giving the employees of an organization a future vision of how the basic structure/nature of the organization will be changed, hope and commitment are instilled in them. This is cited as essentially the fundamental role of leadership.

Developing a vision statement

The vision statement is different from the philosophy and mission statements of an organization in that it is future-orientated. It describes a desirable future and it is a statement about where energies should be focused (Barker 1990: 89).

When developing a vision statement the leader can seek guidance from the past, by asking questions such as 'what were the past and what are the current strengths of the staff?' and 'what is the present mission of the organization, and what were the past missions?'

Issues presently confronting the organization should be reviewed, along with environmental trends affecting the organization, such as issues and trends in health care. Trends in society as a whole will also have to be reviewed — eg what societal trends will affect health care and nursing (Barker 1990: 86)? The leader will have to review the needs of the customers — in nursing this will be the health needs of patients and society in general.

The leader will also have to question the employees in an organization about their individual dreams and aspirations, both personal and professional (Charlton 1992: 52).

Communicating the vision

The leader can only build employees' commitment to the vision by communicating it to them effectively.

A written statement must not only be published and distributed widely; it must be stressed enthusiastically in meetings, day-to-day encounters with employees, and at gatherings where the leader has to deliver an opening or closing speech.

The language used should be very clear. The vision message is in essence ambiguous because one cannot tell exactly what will happen in future, but it should tell in clear, understandable language, what the organization aims to achieve. In nursing, the vision statement should at least address the future goals regarding the rendering of services to patients, and future aims regarding the management and organization of these services (Barker 1990: 82). Leaders often use metaphors to clarify the vision and to keep employees focused.

The vision statement should be discussed with employees, not simply declared. The values inherent in the statement can be clarified. Employees should be encouraged to give their opinions about the statement. This creates an atmosphere for discussing such aspects as meaningful work, self-esteem, aspirations, and quality patient care.

The leader must be visible, must be available for employees, and must communicate the vision persistently, consistently, and enthusiastically. Getting the nursing staff to commit themselves to a vision is sometimes a long and tedious process, but the leader must exercise patience and persistence (Barker 1990: 91).

According to Charlton (1992: 74–5) excellent leaders communicate a vision which focuses on innovation and creativity among employees, meaningful changes, meaningfulness of work, a purpose in life, and common goals. According to Dunham and Klafehn (1990: 29), referring to Bass, communicating a vision also serves as intellectual stimulation to employees. It makes them aware of problems and, by stimulating thought and imagination and by stressing certain values and beliefs, enables them to solve them. It also encourages risk-taking as a means of problem-solving.

Establishing a trusting relationship

People do not give loyalty to a person whom they cannot trust. Trust is not an inherent part of a leader's position. Trust or credibility must be earned and carefully nurtured over time. It takes patience, consistency, dependability, and unending attention over a relatively long period.

It is not only a case of the leader being trusted by her followers. The leader must also trust the followers to perform to expected standards. The more the leader puts trust in her followers and believes that they will reach high standards, the more they are developed and the better they will perform. The reverse is also true. This notion is called the self-fulfilling prophecy.

The leader who is trusted will find it easier to facilitate change, to motivate employees to follow managerial directions, and to elicit dedication and commitment from staff.

The following aspects are of importance in building credibility:

1. The leader or manager must exhibit knowledge. In nursing, visible clinical expertise serves to instil credibility in a leader.

2. A leader must understand and be able to describe the real world in order to be credible (Davidhizar 1989: 18). The hard and unpopular facts of a situation must not be glossed over. Difficulties must be openly discussed (Hand 1981: 70).

3. Leaders who are willing to admit mistakes and weaknesses and who also show trust in subordinates will generally find that subordinates will confide their own errors and weaknesses to them because they know that the leader will still respect them even if their performance is short of perfection (Davidhizar 1989: 19).

4. The leader will have to spend a good deal of her time with the employees, and must be visible. Involvement with employees is demonstrated by listening to employees, interpreting their body language, and by being sympathetic to and responding to the troubles of subordinates, whether their troubles are of a personal or professional nature.

5. When communicating with employees, the leader engenders trust by being honest and open about organizational problems and the performance of employees. Information which is in the interest of employees is not withheld, but personal secrets and harmful information are not divulged (Barker 1990: 143).

6. When the leader wants to establish credibility, it is essential that actions are planned carefully, that implications of actions are anticipated, that people likely to be affected by plans are consulted in advance and their input utilized, and that plans do not get changed once they are communicated (Davidhizar 1989: 20).

7. The goals which the leader wants her followers to achieve must be achievable. If the goals prove to be unachievable the leader will have difficulty in getting employees to take her seriously when a new set of goals are being put forward. A manager who continuously redefines goals will also not establish credibility (Davidhizar 1989: 20).

8. The trustworthy leader treats people with respect, courtesy, care, and concern (Barker 1990: 152). This type of leader tries to remember people's names and applies tact in dealings with employees (Hand 1981: 78).

9. The leader who can be trusted is consistent in her behaviour and keeps promises. She can be trusted to remember dates. She does not treat a serious situation lightly or with inappropriate humour (Davidhizar 1989: 21). Although consistent in behaviour, the trustworthy leader is flexible and learns from experience.

10. Trustworthy leaders are seen as congruent in vision, word and deed. They are reliable and consistently clarify the values that they wish their followers to follow (Charlton 1992: 80).

11. Lastly, the trustworthy leader is mature, wise, autonomous, competent, goal-directed, emphatic, and has a solid sense of ethics (Bennis 1989).

Empowering followers

According to Barker (1990: 49) 'empowerment is the creation of an environment that ensures that people in the organization get the power they need to innovate and be creative.'

The organizational structure of nursing departments often hinders effective empowerment because of multiple layers of management. Flat organizational structures (eg with only three levels of authority) with wider spans of control (eg one supervisor to 25–75 people) are recommended for effective empowerment of employees (Sullivan and Decker 1992: 9).

Participative management must be practised in order to get all the employees to give their input in problem-solving and decision-making.

Sullivan and Decker (1992: 9) maintain that decentralization of decision-making and the empowerment of employees can only work if staff members are encouraged to take calculated risks. According to them, the organization must develop a culture where risk-taking is rewarded and where failure is acceptable.

The true leader believes in growth, and growth often comes from risk-taking. It is thus essential for the leader to get her followers to make decisions and to make mistakes so that growth can be achieved (Bennis 1989: 97). It is not only the followers that grow by taking risks: the transformational leader, by her very nature, is a person who is not afraid of taking a risk because she knows that 'failure is as vital as it is inevitable' (Bennis 1989: 100).

Empowerment of employees also occurs when leaders take the trouble to enable them to make relevant decisions by supplying them with the information they need. A flow of relevant information must be maintained by making use of meetings, newsletters, memorandums, informal discussions, and formal announcements. Leaders must also have the courage to inform employees forthrightly about what is expected from them and about the results which need to be achieved (Sullivan and Decker 1992: 9).

Empowerment also means decentralizing the budgeting system. Self-control and monitoring costs at the unit level are crucial elements in empowering lower-level employees to take the necessary responsibility for their patient care and unit management activities (Wellington 1986: 38).

Leaders who view people as creative and competent hold a different view from those who operate from the assumption that people are incompetent. A view of people that sees them as essentially incompetent leads to rigid grading systems, status symbols, and hierarchical organizational structures. Leaders who take the other view see the granting of power to employees as a way to get power. They see the empowerment of employees as leading to an expansion of power through the greater involvement of more individuals in decision-making and the implementation of goals. The empowering leader also takes the viewpoint that the leader and follower should be willing to be mutually influenced by one another (Wellington 1986: 38; Charlton 1992: 92).

Effecting change

The transformational leader and the transactional leader view change differently.

The transactional leader usually concerns herself with first-order changes — that is changes within the existing structure or nursing department, such as the institution of a new medication administration system (Barker 1990: 62).

The transformational leader accomplishes second-order change — change that transforms the structure of the organization. For example, a different nurse–patient allocation system, such as the primary nursing method, may be instituted by a transformational leader.

Both types of changes are planned deliberately and thought-out well in advance (Barker 1990: 66).

Creating a sense of urgent dissatisfaction among employees in order to recognize the need for change is not easy. According to Barker (1990: 66), transformational leaders may try the following strategies in order to accomplish this realization among employees:

- Create an environment in which people feel at ease so that they can talk freely, challenge one another, and explore issues.

- Share information about the external and internal environment of the organization widely among employees so that they become aware of challenges facing them.

- Discuss the future with employees in order to create excitement, increase motivation, and stimulate team work.

- Interact with people outside in similar organizations so that key staff members will come to realize that the problems they are facing also appear in other organizations, or that other nursing settings have solved some of the problems successfully.

- The leader can intentionally change management processes — for instance the performance appraisal system — in order to create staff dissatisfaction with the present system and thus create the desire for change.

The leader's management of self

The personality, character, and energy of the leader is a critical factor behind organizational success (Charlton 1992: 85). Bennis and Nanus (1985: 57) as referred to by Barker (1990: 159), consider the most essential personal trait of successful leaders as positive self-regard. The person with a positive self-regard views herself as competent, adequate, capable, useful, independent, and appears confident and assertive (Barker 1990: 159). Positive self-regard is essential because leaders spend about 90% of their time assisting other people in sorting out their problems. It is virtually impossible to manage other people if one cannot manage oneself.

According to Charlton (1992: 88), Bennis and Nanus, in a study of leaders from all spectrums of society, found that positive self-regard was related to emotional wisdom. This emotional wisdom was displayed in the following ways:

- accepting people as they are and using empathy to understand them;

- approaching relationships and problems in present, rather than in past terms;

- treating everybody they come into contact courteously;

- displaying trust in others;

- not requiring constant approval/recognition from others;

- developing self-esteem.

People tend to think about themselves mostly negatively. The foundation of this negative image is usually laid during the first 12 years of a person's life. During this time, the messages that children receive about themselves are mostly negative. This negative image is fixed in the subconscious mind.

Barker (1990: 161) suggests that the subconscious mind can be reprogrammed by using affirmatives and visualization to change the negative self-image to a positive one. Affirmatives are positive messages about oneself. When these messages are repeated over and over again they become entrenched in the subconscious mind. One can thus recite such messages as:

- 'I am an intelligent person';

- 'I am capable of doing my job successfully';

- 'I am a person worthy of the respect of others'.

Visualization is the natural power of the brain to create a mental picture of an event (Barker 1990: 162). The nurse leader can thus visualize pictures of an event that she wishes to accomplish — for example getting her budget-proposal accepted. She should use all five of her senses to visualize the setting — eg the office, its smell, the furniture, her voice as she sets forth her proposal — as well as the successful acceptance of the proposal. Visualization is thus picturing and imagining a future event happening according to one's wishes.

It is also advantageous to develop one's self-esteem by recognizing one's strengths and weaknesses and learning how to compensate for the weaknesses, to set high goals in life for oneself, and to develop one's skills in order to achieve these goals (Barker 1990: 162).

Trying to be perfect in everything one does and trying to avoid making any mistakes is damaging to one's self-esteem. In nursing, rigid enforcement of procedures and expecting perfection in all nursing tasks can damage a nurse's self-esteem (Barker 1990: 163).

Developing self-esteem in others leads to increased morale and productivity. It has also been proven beyond doubt that, where leaders expect followers to achieve high standards, the followers indeed perform better than those following a leader who expects less of them. Superior managers, or successful leaders, have the ability to create high performance expectations of their followers, because they are confident in themselves that they are able to develop their followers to reach high standards.

Developing self-knowledge

Successful leaders are people who know what they are and how to use their strengths and compensate for their weaknesses. They also know what they want, why they want it, and how to communicate their needs to others in order to enlist support and co-operation. According to Bennis (1989: 56) four self-knowledge lessons came forth from his extensive conversations with leaders, namely:

1. You are your own best teacher.

2. Accept responsibility. Blame no one.

3. You can learn anything you want to learn.

4. True understanding comes from reflecting on your experience.

POWER

To lead or to manage requires the use of power. Power is the ability and willingness to influence the behaviour of others. There are multiple sources of power in an organization, and the leader may use a particular source of power depending on the situation. A manager or leader usually possesses all or some of the following six forms of power:

1. *Reward power.* The manager or leader has the power to reward employees for their work in the form of promotions, raises, desired assignments, or formal acknowledgement of accomplishments.

2. *Coercive power.* This is the opposite of reward power: the power the manager has to punish employees who do not conform to expected standards. Punishment may take the form of demotions, termination of services, withholding pay increases, and giving undesirable assignments.

3. *Legitimate power.* This is derived from the individual's position in the organization's hierarchical structure — for example, the chief nursing service manager has more legitimate power than the senior professional nurse or senior nursing service manager. The organization usually sanctions this form of power by giving titles such as 'manager' or 'director' to these sources of power.

4. *Expert power*. This power is derived from an individual's knowledge, skills, and information. The person's expertise gains her respect and power. Useful sources of knowledge are knowledge of the rules, regulations, work flow, and power distribution in an organization as well as expertise in one's own work sphere.

5. *Referent power*. This power is based on a person's attractiveness or appeal. A leader may be admired because of certain characteristics which inspire followers, eg charisma. The extent to which followers are impressed by their leader and are willing to follow her directions is an indication of the extent of this person's referent power.

6. *Information power*. This type of power stems from an individual's opportunity to gain or have access to important information within an organization. Some employees — for example personal assistants or secretaries — sometimes have more informational power than their positions in the organization warrant. Information power is thus not so closely related to an individual's position in a hierarchy as the other sources of power, although it is generally known that the higher one goes in the hierarchy the more informational power one usually possesses.

Apart from the foregoing sources of power, the leader also has personal power — that is, power which is derived from her self-concept and her level of self-esteem.

Her *social power* is derived from the frequency and quality of her interactions with colleagues, superiors, and subordinates. Social power is increased when she succeeds in exerting her will on others and is decreased when she is allowed to be influenced by others.

According to Gillies (1989: 410–11) the nurse manager should seek power for selfish as well as altruistic reasons. The nurse manager needs power to survive in the tough world of internal institutional politics, to be able to compete for scarce funds for her nursing department, and to bring about transformational changes in nursing practices.

CONCLUSION

In this chapter the difference between leadership and management was outlined, together with the theories of leadership and the different leadership styles found among managers such as the autocratic, democratic/participative, bureaucratic, and laissez-faire leadership styles. Situational leadership was discussed, and the variables to be taken into account when assessing which leadership style to follow — the organization, the leader and the followers — were described. The sources of the leader's power were outlined briefly, and the leadership style of today, namely transformational leadership, was discussed at length.

References

Barker, A. M. (1990). *Transformational Nursing Leadership*. Williams and Wilkins: Baltimore.

Bennis, W. (1989). *On Becoming a Leader*. Hutchinson Business Books: Kent.

Charlton, G. D. (1992). *Leadership: The Human-Race*. Juta: Cape Town.

Davidhizar, R. (1989). Managerial credibility. *Nursing Administration Quarterly*, volume 13, number 3, pp. 17–21.

DiVincenti, M. (1977) *Administering Nurse Service*. Little Brown: Boston.

Durham, J. and Klafehn, K. A. (1990). Transformational leadership and the nurse executive. *JONA*, volume 20, number 4, pp. 28–33.

Friss, L. (1989). *Strategic Management of Nurses*. National Health Publishing: USA.

Gerber, P. D., Nel, P. S. and Van Dyk, P. S. (1992). *Mannekragbestuur*. Southern: Johannesburg.

Gillies, D.A. (1989). *Nursing Management: A Systems Approach*. Saunders: Philadelphia.

Hand, L. (1981). *Nursing supervision*. Reston: Virginia.

Hersey, P. and Blanchard, K. (1982). *Management of Organizational Behaviour: Utilizing Human Resources*. Prentice-Hall: Englewood Cliffs, New Jersey.

Marriner-Tomey, A. (1992). *Guide to Nursing Management*. Fourth edition. Mosby: St Louis.

Moorhead, G. and Griffin, R. W. (1989). *Organizational Behaviour*. Houghton Mifflin: Boston.

Sullivan, E. J. and Decker, P. J. (1992). *Effective Management in Nursing*. Addison-Wesley: California.

Swansburg, R. C. (1990). *Management and Leadership for Nurse Managers*. Jones and Bartlett: Boston.

Szilagyi, A. D. and Wallace, M. J. (1990). *Organizational Behaviour and Performance*. Scott Foresman/Little Brown: Illinois.

Tappen, R. M. (1989). *Nursing Leadership and Management*. F. A. Davis: Philadelphia.

Wellington, M. (1986) Decentralization: how it affects nurses. *Nursing Outlook,* volume 34, number 1, pp. 36–9.

CHAPTER 20

WORK MOTIVATION

Karien Jooste

CONTENTS

INTRODUCTION

Why are some nurses dedicated to improving the quality of nursing care whereas others put minimal effort into their job? The answer to this question is that they have different levels of motivation.

It is not easy to motivate employees since individuals differ in what motivates them. Motivation is influenced by the personal characteristics of an individual and by the various conditions that exist in the organization (Chung 1977: 17).

MANAGEMENT APPROACHES TO IMPROVE MOTIVATION

Frederick W. Taylor (1856–1915) is generally recognized as the father of the scientific management approach. This approach emphasized that the best way to increase an individual's working capacity/output was to improve the work methods used by the workers. This approach proposed that an organization should be planned and run on a rational basis in order to create more efficient administration and higher production. Management should focus on the structuring and instrumentalization of tasks, separating themselves from human affairs and emotions. The use of monetary incentives, such as merit increases, profit sharing, and bonus systems was recommended to enhance or maintain the productivity levels of the more productive employee.

The bureaucratic approach focuses on how an organization can be protected against internal and external disturbances. A hierarchical structure and a system of rules are characteristic of the control and co-ordination of such an organization. This approach suggests close supervision and tight control of employees, which may undermine their motivation. Max Weber (1864–1920) was called the father of the bureaucratic system. He saw rules, rather than people, as forming the basis of an organization.

The scientific administration approach consists primarily of a pragmatic development of the bureaucratic idea and gives directions regarding how to manage an organization efficiently. As in the bureaucratic approach, the emphasis is upon internal efficiency (Robertson and Smith 1985: 4). Lyndall Urwick (1891–1983) described the managerial process as involving planning, co-ordinating, and controlling. The following managerial concepts became known as a result of his managerial views:

- balance of authority with control;

- departmentalization;

- proper utilization of personnel;

- span of control;

- unity of command; and

- use of general and special staff.

The human relations approach started in the 1940s and focused on the effect that people had on the success or failure of an organization. This approach stressed a concern for interpersonal relationships and focused on how the needs of an individual could be harmonized with the goals of the organization. The main focus was on individual needs and the improvement of workers' morale and co-operation rather than on the needs and structure of the organization. Other concerns of the human relations approach were group dynamics, leadership, and communication. Individuals were encouraged to develop their potential and managers were supposed to assist them in fulfilling their needs for accomplishment, recognition, and a sense of belonging.

The above traditional approaches demonstrate that an organization must explore different options to motivate its employees. It must control the behaviour of its employees, and guide it in the direction most favourable for the organization as a whole. At the same time the organization must ensure that these individuals remain sufficiently motivated (Robertson and Smith 1985: 4).

As a result of the evolution of these approaches, nurses are asking much more from their organizations; instead of nurses simply serving their organization, they want to know how the nursing organization can contribute to the quality of their work life and to their personal and professional development. All these approaches have resulted in a shift of emphasis from the extrinsic rewards of work to the intrinsic rewards. These changes force us to look at jobs from the viewpoint of nurses as employees as well as from the viewpoint of the organization.

While earlier approaches to job design implied a technologically-determined view of human behaviour at work, current views hold that behaviour is a product of both technological factors and human factors (Robertson and Smith 1985: 5).

Current views of work are more inclusive. There is a developing body of theoretical knowledge about people at work, produced by behavioural scientists, as well as a more informed approach to the general problem of managing organizations. In addition, wider social changes are significantly modifying the ways in which we view work and organizations (Robertson and Smith 1985: 3).

Three key managerial approaches towards motivation in the work situation will be discussed and are set out in table 20.1: the traditional model, the human relations model, and the human resources model. Every nurse manager has her own theory about motivation. Most of these theories fit in with one of these models.

The traditional model

The traditional theory is based on views that have been held by managers over the years concerning their subordinates. The underlying assumption in the traditional model is that people act to maximize their self-interest (Petri 1986: 340). This model is based on the following assumptions:

- the key task of management is to solve problems of inefficient production;

- it is the responsibility of management to find the right employees for the job and then train them in the most efficient methods;

- tasks should be simple and repetitive;

- management should put in place a wage incentive system so that workers can maximize their income;

- production problems can be solved by either changing the methods for performing the job or by modifying the wage incentive programme;

The greatest danger for an organization operating with these assumptions is that such assumptions tend to be self-fulfilling. If employees are expected to be indifferent, hostile, and motivated only by economic incentives, the managerial strategies that are utilized to deal with them are very likely to train them to behave in precisely this fashion (Petri 1986: 341).

The human relations model

The human relations model is based on the assumption that employees are motivated by satisfactory treatment. The social context of work life has become increasingly relevant to the motivation of workers. More attention has been given to group dynamics and interpersonal relations in the workplace. The concept of simulation training was developed to help leaders develop sensitivity and skill in managing people in groups. Simulation training methods focus on here-and-now experiences and:

- make it possible for individuals to obtain personal insight into their own and others' reactions and feelings about commonly-shared group events;

- improve both the interpersonal skills of the manager and the overall functioning of the group (Petri 1986: 341).

Table 20.1: Three models of managerial motivation

Traditional model	Human relations model	Human resources model
Assumptions	*Assumptions*	*Assumptions*
1. Work is inherently distasteful to most nurses.	1. Nurses want to feel useful and important.	1. Work is not inherently distasteful.
2. What nurses do is less important than what they earn for doing it.	2. Nurses desire to belong and to be recognized as unique individuals.	2. Nurses want to contribute to meaningful goals which they have helped establish.
3. Few nurses want or can handle work which requires creativity, self-direction, or control.	3. These needs are more important than money in motivating nurses to work,	3. Most nurses can exercise far more creativity, responsibility, self-direction, self-control, and intelligence than their present job demands of them.
4. Most nurses choose not to take responsibility for decisions.	4. Most nurses want to feel important for the nursing service.	4. Most nurses are eager to show their abilities.
5. Most nurses are not able to solve their work problems.	5. Most nurses want to be informed about events that will influence them in future.	*Policies*
Policies	*Policies*	1. The nurse manager's basic task is to make use of 'untapped' human resources.
1. The nurse manager's basic task is to closely supervise and control nurses.	1. The nurse manager's basic task is to make each nurse feel useful and important.	2. She must create an environment in which all members may contribute to the limits of their ability.
2. She must break tasks down into simple repetitive, easily learned operations.	2. She should keep subordinates informed and listen to their objections to her plans.	3. She must encourage full participation on important matters, continually broadening subordinates' self-direction and control.
3. She must establish detailed work routines and procedures, and enforce these firmly but fairly.	3. The nurse manager should allow subordinates to exercise some self-direction and self-control on routine matters.	4. The nurse manager should help nurses to set meaningful objectives.
	4. The nurse manager should have an open-door policy and keep herself updated on cultural differences.	5. The manager should give nurses opportunities to prove themselves, to think for themselves, and to solve their problems, to do their own work-planning and to set their own priorities.
	5. The manager should encourage social activities.	

Traditional model	Human relations model	Human resources model
Expectations	*Expectations*	*Expectations*
1. Nurses can tolerate work if the pay is decent and the boss is fair.	1. Sharing information with nurses and involving them in routine decisions will satisfy their basic needs to belong and to feel important.	1. Expanding nurses' influence, self-direction, and self-control will lead to direct improvements in operating efficiency.
2. If tasks are simple enough and nurses are closely controlled they will produce up to standard.	2. Satisfying these needs will improve morale and reduce resistance to formal authority — nurses will 'willingly co-operate'.	(Mol 1990: 15–20; Petri 1986: 343)

The human resources model

The human resources model is a comprehensive approach that emphasizes the employee's participation in important and relevant matters. The expectation is that, when an employee's influence and authority are expanded, the employee will be self-directed and motivated to perform well. In this way the needs of both the worker and the organization can be integrated (Petri 1986: 342).

ORGANIZATIONAL FACTORS INFLUENCING MOTIVATION

The important aspects of organizations influencing motivation (individual or group) are organizational structure, technology, and organizational climate.

Organizational structure

To function effectively many organizations need to divide the tasks to be performed between individuals, units, divisions, and departments. This division of tasks brings with it a need to co-ordinate the work of separate sections and people. Organizations need different structures — eg a hierarchical structure or a matrix structure — to deal successfully with these needs. The structural dimensions of organizations determine, for example, the extent to which specialized tasks are allocated to employees and the degree to which rules and procedures are written down. These dimensions may effect the motivation of employees in the work situation.

Technology

Different structural factors — eg span of control and unity of command — can be connected to the technology used in an organization. Complex interrelationships exist between structural factors, technology, and the employee's motivation, attitude, and behaviour in an organization.

Organizational climate

It is generally accepted that the organizational climate is a function of both the individual person and the organization and depends on the interaction between the two (Robertson and Smith 1985: 13–14). Different employees can develop different views of the same organization and may experience the climate of the organization in different ways.

THEORIES OF WORK MOTIVATION

Motivation theories can be divided into content theories and process theories.

Content theories focus explicitly on the content of motivation, such as those factors or needs within an individual that energize, direct, sustain, or stop behaviour. They are the factors that motivate nurses in the nursing environment.

Process theories emphasize how the motivation process works. They attempt to identify how motivation occurs in the workplace (eg in the nursing environment) and are concerned with the processes by which motivational factors interact to produce motivation.

Table 20.2 indicates some of the differences between these two types of motivation theories. Theories of motivation can be divided into the following three broad categories:

1. Need theories
   - Maslow's need-hierarchy theory
   - ERG theory
   - Herzberg's motivator-hygiene theory

2. Cognition theories
   - Expectancy valence theory
   - Equity theory
   - Goal-setting theories

3. Reinforcement theories
   - Organizational behaviour modification approach

Table 20.2: Types of motivation theories

Content theories	Process theories
1. Attempt to develop an understanding of fundamental human needs (physiological, safety, security, and self-esteem needs).	1. Direct an individual's effort into performance.
2. Emphasize the specific factors that motivate an individual.	2. Attempt to develop understanding of the psychological process involved in motivation.
3. Imply that motivational factors may reside within the individual (eg human needs) or within the environment of the individual (eg job characteristics)	3. Focus on the dynamics of motivation, from the initial energization of behaviour, through the selection of behavioural alternatives, to actual effort.
4. Emphasize individual needs or the rewards that may satisfy those needs.	
	4. Include expectancy theory, equity theory, goal-setting theory, and behaviour modification (cognition and reinforcement theories).
5. Include need hierarchy, existence related growth theory and two-factor theory (need theories).	
6. Include the following examples: satisfying people's needs for pay, promotion, and recognition.	5. Include the following examples: clarifying the individual's perception of work inputs, performance requirements, and rewards.

Need theories

Need theories assume that individuals possess internal needs that motivate them to exert effort. Different people have different needs at different times, so they require different motivators. Important motivators of behaviour include a need to feel competent, to be self-determining, in control, fully functioning, advanced, to grow, and to be self-actualizing. The basic thrust of need theories is that individuals need to believe that they have an effect on their environments. From the perspective of the nurse manager, if her intent is to motivate a nurse, need theory argues that she should find out what needs the nurse as an individual, is trying to satisfy. Need theories of motivation are closely related to the human relations and behaviour science approaches to employee motivation.

Maslow's need-hierarchy theory

One of the most influential content theories is the need hierarchy model, developed by Abraham Maslow, which claims that human motives develop sequentially according to a hierarchy of five levels of need (see figure 20.1). Maslow's theory is also called a dynamic theory of human motivation (Halloran 1986: 227).

Needs lower on the hierarchy (physiological, security, and love needs) are more powerful and must be satisfied before needs higher on the hierarchy (esteem and actualization needs) will be triggered.

Figure 20.1: Maslow's need hierarchy

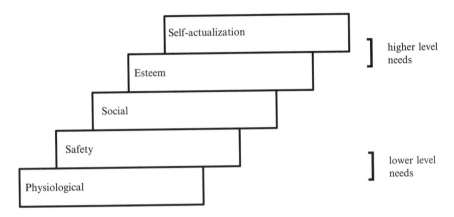

From: Bernhard and Walsh (1990: 87); Flude (1991: 111); Halloran (1986: 229–30); Longnecker and Pringle (1984: 417); Lunenburg and Ornstein (1991: 91); Petri (1986: 289); Robertson and Smith (1985: 20).

The theory states that higher level needs partially emerge when lower level needs have been partially met or satisfied. It also advances the hypothesis that lower level needs decline in strength on satisfaction while higher level needs grow in strength the more effort is exerted in an attempt to satisfy them. As lower level needs are satisfied, the higher needs become increasingly prominent in controlling behaviour.

Maslow asserted that a satisfied need is no longer a motivator. This applies only to the lower needs, however. Satisfaction of the higher needs leads to an immediate desire for more 'higher level' experiences (Robertson and Smith 1985: 21) For example, if a nurse has reached the stage where she has completed her studies for a basic degree, she is often motivated to strive for the attainment of higher qualifications — eg a master's degree.

Maslow considered the first four levels of needs to be needs that result from deficiencies in the person's life — ie behaviours related to the first four categories are motivated by a deprivation of those things necessary for full development (Petri 1986: 291).

Self-actualization needs can never be fully met. As people become more self-actualized, their need for self-actualization increases (Siegel and Lane 1987: 376).

At the level of the need for self-actualization, an individual's behaviour is motivated by what Maslow termed the being needs. These are values such as truth, honesty, beauty, and goodness, and they provide meaning to the life of the individual. At this level, individuals are no longer motivated by deficiencies but are motivated to grow and become all that they are capable of becoming.

Table 20.3: Fulfilment of Maslow's needs in the working environment

Need level	Satisfaction/general factors	Organizational factors
Physiological:	Highest priority needs (necessary for survival) that have little practical importance as motivators. Needs for food, water, warmth, activity, shelter, sleep, sex, oxygen, etc.	Working conditions: heat and air conditioning, basic salary.
Security:	Basic requirements for safety and security that dominate behaviour in times of emergency. Needs such as protection against danger, threat, deprivation, safety from physical, social, and financial attack, shelter, clothing, growth and stability.	Wages, salaries, medical and life insurance benefits, safety regulations, safe working conditions, job security, job regulations, fringe benefits, retirement plans.
Social:	Involve personal relationships and being part of a group. The need for belonging, association, acceptance by one's fellows, giving and receiving friendship and love, a sense of communal involvement, being loved by someone and having someone to love, giving as well as receiving affection.	Provide employees with social activities (exercise groups, hospital committees, etc.). Recent studies show that teamwork and teamspirit are often more important than individual achievement, Quality of supervision, compatible work group, professional friendships.
Esteem:	Needs for positive, high evaluation of oneself. 1. Self-esteem (self-confidence, independence and freedom, achievement and strength, self-respect, feeling worthwhile). 2. Esteem from others (the need for status, recognition as an individual, the need to win praise and approval, appreciation, respect from one's fellows, feeling of importance).	Titles, promotion, certificates of achievement, private office and secretary. Status symbols, challenging work, advancement in organization, achievement in one's work.

Need level	Satisfaction/general factors	Organizational factors
Self-actualization	Doing what one is best suited for. The need to realize one's potential. Continued self-development, self-expression, self-fulfilment, utilizing one's human capabilities to the full. The need to be creative, to be totally committed to achieve so that one develops to the limit of one's potential.	The content of work: challenging work, advancement in the organization, achievement in work.

Maslow barely touches on the role of environmental factors in the development of his hierarchy, despite wide recognition among psychologists that behaviour can only be fully understood as a result of the interaction between the individual and his environment (Robertson and Smith 1985: 21–2). Maslow's theory holds some obvious implications for work behaviour, but there are also difficulties in trying to relate the theory to work processes. One such problem lies in the fact that people do not necessarily satisfy their higher-order needs through their jobs or occupation (Robertson and Smith 1985: 22).

Maslow's need-hierarchy theory has two major implications. Firstly, it is clear that different individuals are at different places in the hierarchy and that the same person may be at different places at different times (Siegel and Lane 1987: 376). All individuals cannot be motivated in the same way. Secondly, the theory implies that since employees are motivated by higher level needs, their jobs should be designed to allow these higher level needs to be satisfied at work (Siegel and Lane 1987: 377).

Existence, relatedness, and growth theory (ERG theory)

Alderfer's existence, relatedness, and growth theory (Alderfer 1969, 1972) is a modification and reformulation of Maslow's need-hierarchy approach. Alderfer attempted to empirically generate and test an alternative to Maslow's theory. Need hierarchy theory suggests that an individual must satisfy the lowest level of need before moving on to the next level. It is assumed that movement along the hierarchy occurs in one direction — ie upwards. Alderfer, however, proposed that individuals can also move down the hierarchy under certain conditions. According to Sullivan and Decker (1988: 182) the frustration of higher-level needs lead to an individual focusing upon the next lower level need in the hierarchy. For example, a nurse manager whose ideas for new staff development programmes are continually rejected becomes frustrated with her job. Alderfer's theory predicts that this manager will eventually adapt to the frustration by moving down the hierarchy and consequently directing her energies to lower-order need fulfilment. This nurse manager might focus on pay and job security instead of creating new ideas for staff development (Petri 1986: 344).

Figure 20.2: Alderfer's modified need hierarchy

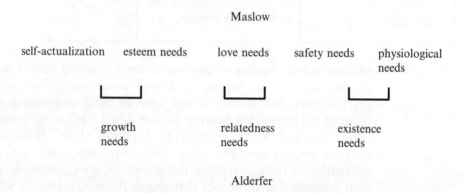

Alderfer suggested that this process of frustration and regression allows some employees to channel their energies constructively, even though the fulfilment of higher-order needs is blocked (Petri 1986: 344).

The idea that people do adapt and try to cope with their frustration as best they can is an important one, making ERG a useful and innovative contribution to work motivation theory (Petri 1986: 345).

Instead of five levels of need, as suggested by Maslow, Alderfer proposed three basic sets of needs. They are the following:

1. *Existence needs* relate to Maslow's lower-order needs and can be satisfied by pay, fringe benefits, and safe working conditions (Petri 1986: 345). These are material needs such as the desire to have food, water, housing, money, and furniture (Siegel and Lane 1987: 377).

2. *Relatedness needs* correspond to Maslow's belonging and esteem needs and can be satisfied by social attachments and group membership involving co-workers, supervisors, family, and friends (Petri 1986: 344). They involve the need to share one's thoughts and feelings with other people and to have those people share theirs in return (Siegel and Lane 1987: 377).

3. *Growth needs* correspond to Maslow's self-actualization needs and can be satisfied through the search for personal and career development and through creative work and home activities (Petri 1986: 344).

Alderfer's theory is concerned about how people move from one level of need to another and suggests that more than one need may be operative at a time.

Herzberg's motivator-hygiene theory/two-factor theory of motivation

Herzberg's two-factor theory relates to both work motivation and job satisfaction since it assumes that conditions which enhance job satisfaction act to heighten work motivation (Siegel and Lane 1987: 379; Sullivan and Decker 1988: 182). The two-factor theory proposes that human beings have two basic sets of needs regarding work motivation — ie extrinsic needs and intrinsic needs. Different elements of the work experience can serve to meet these two sets of needs.

Herzberg proposed that two major categories of job factors, hygiene factors and motivators, affect the attitudes and behaviour of employees (Longenecker and Pringle 1984: 417).

The hygiene or extrinsic factors of a job relate to such aspects as satisfactory pay, adequate supervision, enlightened policies and administration, good working conditions, and job security. The intrinsic or motivating factors relate to such aspects as recognition and praise, autonomy in one's work, opportunities for promotion, and the sense of achievement an individual experiences for a job well done.

Herzberg found that the factors that make a job satisfying are different from the factors that make it dissatisfying. Offering nurses more pay (hygiene factor) does not replace the nurse's need for doing fulfilling work (motivator).

According to Herzberg's theory, job dissatisfaction is not the opposite of job satisfaction: it is an element of satisfaction which lies on a different level. Employees who experience job dissatisfaction are dissatisfied with the hygiene or extrinsic job factors. This feeling of job dissatisfaction will most likely lead to behaviours such as absenteeism, voicing of grievances, or quitting one's job. When employees are satisfied with the presence of hygiene factors — ie satisfactory pay and good working conditions —— they will come to work and do their jobs, but they may not experience positive motivation or job satisfaction because the intrinsic or motivating factors may not be present. In other words, the employees will not experience sufficient autonomy in their job, promotional opportunities, and a sense of achievement in performing their work. The motivating factors, if present, make individuals satisfied with their jobs, produce positive attitudes, and help them increase their productivity.

Intrinsic needs are expressed in attempts by nurses to become all that they are capable of becoming, by exploring and conquering challenges posed by their nursing environments (Longenecker and Pringle 1984: 418). Nurses need challenges, a sense of achievement, and a feeling of accomplishment in nursing practice in order to feel fulfilled. The nurse manager should thus not be too inhibited by nurses who complain about their workload when she wants to set a quality assurance programme in motion.

According to the two-factor theory the absence of all motivators induces neutral feelings and nurses will be neither satisfied nor dissatisfied (Siegel and Lane 1987: 380).

Some individuals are more motivated than others in general. They are more inclined to set goals for themselves and to set things in motion to achieve these goals.

Three characteristics of the self-motivated achiever

1. Self-motivated achievers like to set their own goals.

2. Achievers set moderate goals, and select goals that are tough but practical.

3. Self-motivated achievers prefer tasks that tell them how well they are doing at all times by providing measurable feedback (McClelland, as quoted by Halloran 1986: 233).

Implications of need theories for nurse managers

1. Making the nurse's job more interesting.

   - Determine the boundaries of the job by developing job descriptions and promoting staff development programmes so that problems fall within the competence level of the nurse.

   - Promote appreciation of the nursing service as a whole and encourage involvement of nurses in all aspects of the nursing service related to their jobs.

   - Set targets that 'stretch' the nurse's capabilities but are attainable within the limits of the authority delegated to her.

2. Giving the nurse scope for achievement.

   - Recognize achievement by nurses and so promote feelings of active involvement.

   - Promote constructive feedback on all levels of performance (Flude 1991: 113).

3. Promote two-way communication in the nursing service:

   - Ensure that all nurses are aware of the factors influencing their nursing practice and those affecting the nursing service in general by informing them at regular meetings or through a regular attractive internal newsletter.

- Ensure that an adequate and effective feedback system exists for communication with the nurse manager. This can be achieved by being available: by doing rounds on a regular basis — eg bi-weekly or monthly — or having a business lunch with representatives from various nurse committees.

4. Give nurses responsibility.

- Allow nurses the freedom to institute and implement courses of nursing action within the policies of the nursing service — eg to institute changes regarding work methods which will improve the quality of care rendered to the patients and the productivity of the care givers.

5. Prospects for advancement.

- Regularly review nurses' performance and consult with them so that you can develop career paths which are sensitive to their performance and ability.

- Create a nursing environment whereby nurses are trained and developed to enable them to take advantage of opportunities which arise (Flude 1991: 112–14).

The main management objective should be to create conditions where nurses can achieve their own goals by pursuing the objectives of the organization.

Table 20.4: Similarities in need theories of motivation

View of motivation	Lower level needs	Higher level needs
Maslow	Physiological, safety, social	Esteem, self-actualization
Herzberg	Need to avoid unpleasant-ness	Need for achievement and growth
Alderfer	Existence and relatedness needs	Growth needs

Cognition theories

These assume that learners interact with their environments (Bernhard and Walsh 1990: 107). They tend to focus on the information processing capabilities of individuals rather than their needs and assume that individuals rationally assesses their working environment and gather information to make decisions. These theories explain motivation in terms of rational, thinking human beings.

Cognition theories help us to understand how nurses make choices in their workplace, based on their beliefs, perceptions, and values. Such theories assume that the performance of organizational activities is seen by an employee as an instrument for obtaining organizational rewards (Chung 1977: 36).

Expectancy valence theory (valence–instrumentality–expectancy theory)

Victor Vroom developed the expectancy theory during the 1960s. It is based on Kurt Lewin's field theory and has been expanded by other theorists. According to Marriner-Tomey (1988: 234) this theory states that people are motivated by how much they want something (valence) and by their estimation of the probability of getting it (expectancy) (Sullivan and Decker 1988: 188).

$$motivation = valence \times expectancy$$
$$M = V \times E$$

$$
\begin{aligned}
M &= E \times I \times V \\
M &= motivation \\
E &= \text{belief that effort will lead to desired performance} \\
I &= \text{belief that performance will give desired outcome} \\
V &= \text{value of reward}
\end{aligned}
$$

Figure 20.3: Expectancy theory

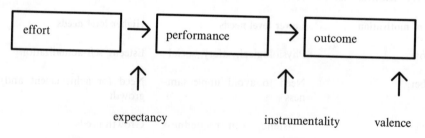

The expectancy theory has been further developed. It states that human motivation is affected by the value of outcomes (rewards). The employee will be motivated to work towards the organizational goal if she:

- believes that her performance will lead to a desired outcome — eg that her efforts will lead to the satisfaction of a personal goal;

- believes that the outcome is worth the effort (Halloran 1986: 236; Marriner-Tomey 1988: 235).

Motivation and performance are influenced by the individual's view of the links between effort and performance (E), and between performance and outcome (I), and the value (V) that the outcome has (Robertson and Smith 1985: 28).

The basic idea underlying expectancy theory is that motivated behaviour results from a combination of individual needs, the value of goals available for the individual to achieve, and the individual's expectance of achieving the goal (Petri 1986: 218).

What is important in the notion of expectancy is not the actual relationship between effort and performance but, rather, what the person involved believes the relationship to be. Many nurse managers, for example, stress that a nurse's belief in her ability to reach certain performance targets is an essential ingredient for achievement (Robertson and Smith 1985: 27).

The nurse manager should be sensitive to a nurse's feeling of self-worth and should strive continuously to improve it. This can be achieved, for example, by listening intently to an employee when discussing what the employee is satisfied or dissatisfied with in regard to her career or when discussing her career goals. It can also be achieved by recognizing the employee who does exceptional work (not only by praise but also by enhancing her work through job enrichment), by identifying employees with low self-esteem, and by bringing each one in for a private conversation in order to assess their specific personal and career needs. Expectancies are generally regarded as being built up through past experiences (Petri 1986: 218).

The theory recognizes that there are significant differences between people in terms of the outcomes that they find attractive. A student nurse who does not relish the idea of winning a certificate for outstanding examination results will be unlikely to put in the amount of learning that would lead to this outcome, for example. Each nurse is motivated by different outcomes.

Implications of expectancy valence theory for nurse managers

Nurse managers should motivate staff by discussing the relationships between work and outcome and should reward desirable behaviour appropriately. Outcomes may be external rewards (pay, promotion etc) or internal rewards (feelings of increased self-esteem or self-actualization etc) (Longenecker and Pringle 1984: 418).

The manager should do the following:

1. Find out what particular outcomes or rewards are valued by each nurse. This could be assessed through questionnaires or interviews.

2. Be specific about the precise behaviours that constitute good levels of performance (eg good interpersonal relationships).

3. Ensure that the desired levels of performance are reachable.

4. Ensure that there is a direct, clear, and explicit link between performance at the desired level and outcomes/rewards. Nurses must be able to observe and experience the connection between performance and outcome. If this is not clear, and if it is not seen to work, motivating expectancies will not be created in the nurses' minds.

5. Check that there are no conflicting expectancies.

6. Ensure that changes in outcome are significant enough to serve as motivators.

7. Check that the system is treating everyone fairly (Robertson and Smith 1985: 29).

8. Ensure that nurses perceive that job performance will lead to the outcomes they desire. This requires managers to be alert and consistent in providing such extrinsic rewards as recognition and salary increases.

9. Increase nurse's expectancies that effort will result in better performance. This could be accomplished through staff training and development programmes or job descriptions which help nurses to channel their efforts in the proper direction (Longenecker and Pringle 1984: 420).

Implications of expectancy valence theory for nursing organizations

1. Design pay and reward systems so that:
   - desirable performance is rewarded (ie merit rating);
   - the relationship between performance and reward is clear to the nurses. It could, for example, be explained during group discussions and during in-service training sessions.

2. Design tasks, jobs, and roles so that nurses have an opportunity to satisfy their own needs through their work — but do not assume that everyone wants the same things. Every nurse is a unique being.

3. Individualize the nursing organization. It is important to allow nurses opportunities to influence the scope of work they do and also other aspects of organizational life such as the reward systems or the fringe benefits offered (Robertson and Smith 1985: 30). It is important to involve nurses when policies are formulated regarding aspects of the ward which directly affect them — eg the programme of daily washes for patients.

Equity theory

Equity theory (Adams 1965) is concerned with defining what individuals in our society consider to be fair and studying their reactions to being in situations that they perceive as unfair (Siegel and Lane 1987: 397).

Equity theory suggests that effort and job satisfaction depend upon the degree of equity that an individual perceives in the work situation (Sullivan and Decker 1988: 189).

Individuals need to feel that they are getting fair treatment at work in terms of their contributions to the job (eg skills, ability, education, experience, their effort) and the rewards they receive for working (eg pay, fringe benefits, recognition, praise, promotion, prestige).

People need to feel that they are being treated fairly when they compare themselves with others (Robertson and Smith 1985: 42). Employees working long hours on a difficult, demanding, and highly-skilled job will, in most cases, feel that they should benefit more than those working shorter hours on an easier job (Robertson and Smith 1985: 42–3). Equity does not motivate a change in behaviour; rather, inequity motivates a change in behaviour that may increase or decrease actual effort and job performance (Sullivan and Decker 1988: 190).

The theory has four basic postulates:

1. Individuals strive to create and maintain a state of equity.

2. When a state of inequity is perceived, it creates tension which the individual is motivated to reduce or eliminate.

3. The greater the magnitude of the perceived inequity, the greater is the motivation to act to reduce the state of tension.

4. Individuals will perceive an unfavourable inequity (eg too little pay) more readily than a favourable one (eg receiving too much pay) (Siegel and Lane 1987: 398).

A state of equity is depicted by the following equation:

$$\frac{Person's\ outcomes}{Person's\ inputs} = \frac{Other's\ outcomes}{Other's\ inputs}$$

An example will help to explain these basic concepts. Imagine that you provide nursing care in a unit with another nurse. Both of you are paid exactly the same salary at the end of the month. As you perceive it, you have greater inputs. You have worked for the nursing service longer, you perform nursing care duties faster, and you have attended in-service training programmes more often. This situation makes you feel you are treated unfairly since you perceive your inputs as not being rewarded to the same degree as are those of the other nurse. The theory predicts that you will attempt to eliminate the tension you feel as a result of the perceived inequity (adopted from Siegel and Lane 1987: 398).

It is also interesting to note that research on why nurses in provincial hospitals are leaving the service and/or feel dissatisfied with their jobs has pointed out that one of the important reasons for dissatisfaction was the fact that all professional nurses and senior professional nurses were on the same salary scale as their peers irrespective of the amount of work they had to do. Senior professional nurses in charge of busy surgical or medical wards in an academic hospital, or in charge of a highly complex intensive care unit, felt demotivated because they were on the same salary scale as a senior professional nurse in charge of a quieter ward in a rural hospital. These nurses felt that, because they had to function in the complex, stressful, and ever-changing environment of the academic hospital, and because of their added responsibilities regarding the teaching of student nurses, they should be on a higher salary scale than their colleagues who practise in rural clinic or hospital settings.

Equity theory suggests several alternative strategies that individuals use in order to reduce inequity or restore equity. These include behavioural changes such as reducing the quantity or quality of work, or perhaps convincing the manager to give one a raise, or quitting the job. Cognitive changes to restore equity could involve selecting a different reference person with whom you compare your own inputs, or deciding that you are going to change your own inputs in the work situation in the future (Siegel and Lane 1987: 399).

Implications for nursing of equity theory

Despite the importance of reducing inequity, it is difficult to apply equity theory in organization settings — especially in a nursing setting. A relatively large measure of inequity is found regarding the work input between different nurses in the same unit, even if they work together as a team. This is not easily resolved, because of the varying nature of a number of factors in the nursing setting — eg daily variation in patient numbers, in nursing personnel numbers, and in the acuity levels of the patients. The nursing profession tends to treat too many nurses as equals. The nurse manager should conscientiously identify those nurses who are performing exceptionally and should try to acknowledge their higher quality work. This acknowledgement need not always be in the form of promotions or pay increases; it could be in the form of appointment as the chairman of a committee or it could involve giving the nurse more challenging work.

Goal-setting theories

Path–goal theory attempts to identify the situational aspects affecting the leader's leadership behaviour by examining the effect of the leader's behaviour on group members. The theory examines conditions where the leader's behaviour affects the group member's satisfaction. The degree to which the leader exhibits consideration determines the individual's perception of available rewards. On the other hand, the degree to which the leader initiates structure — ie the degree to which concern with the work or organizational goals are emphasized — determines the individual's perception of paths, or behaviours, which will lead her to her goal (Bernhard and Walsh 1990: 64). Goal-setting theory is based on three basic propositions:

1. Specific goals lead to higher performance than do general goals such as 'try your best'.

2. Specific difficult goals lead to higher performance than specific, easy goals — provided the goals are accepted.

3. Incentives such as money, knowledge of results, praise, participation, reproof, competition, and time limits affect behaviour only if they cause individuals to change their goals or to accept goals that have been assigned to them (Sullivan and Decker 1988: 193).

According to the path–goal theory, the leader initiates structure to show members how their actions will lead to goal attainment and reward. Leaders use consideration to make the path to the goal easier by helping the individuals remove barriers. Consideration and the initiation of structure increase motivation and satisfaction to the extent that they clarify the path to the goal (Bernhard and Walsh 1990: 64).

The presence of supervision helps to ensure the acceptance of goals. Supervisors who are frequently with their nurses are likely to have nurses with higher productivity than supervisors who are frequently absent (Sullivan and Decker 1988: 193–4). Supportiveness, and encouragement for those nurses who are facing difficult tasks, contribute to nurses accepting high performance goals and obtaining high levels of performance. The more participation the nurses have in setting these goals, the more they will be motivated to achieve them.

The motivational functions of a nurse leader include:

1. Increasing the number and types of incentives available to nurses to motivate them to attain work goals.

2. Making paths to incentives easier to travel by:

- reduction of roadblocks and pitfalls such as demands and pressures in the workplace;
- increasing opportunities for personal satisfaction (Longenecker and Pringle 1984: 444).

Reinforcement theories

Reinforcement theory emphasizes the environmental control of behaviour. Research supports the importance of both response–reward relationships and of rewarding desired behaviour.

The organizational behaviour modification approach

Organizational behaviour modification uses the principles of operant conditioning to influence the behaviour of people at work. Organization behaviour management is concerned primarily with the acquisition and maintenance of correct responses and with the extinction (or reduction in frequency) of incorrect ones.

Several terms must be understood before these areas can be covered: these include *stimulus, response,* and *reinforcer.*

- Relevant stimuli in the organization can be one's co-workers and the work setting.
- Responses — for example the achievement of productivity levels or absenteeism — usually have consequences.
- When the consequence of a particular behaviour increase the probability that a similar behaviour will be repeated under similar stimulus conditions, that consequence is a reinforcer. Examples of relevant potential reinforcers in an organization are salary, fringe benefits, and personal recognition and praise (Siegel and Lane 1987: 384).

The amount of money (a reinforcer) earned by salesmen on commission clearly depends on their job performance. The more they sell, the more they get paid. Other employees — eg nurses — are paid on a non-contingent basis. Their monthly pay cheque arrives in a fixed amount irrespective of the quality of job performance during the preceding pay period. It is clear that a reinforcer which is directly contingent upon one's work performance will be more powerful than one which is not so directly tied to it (Siegel and Lane 1987: 385).

Organization behaviour modification theorists state that a behaviour cannot be acquired or learned until after it has been reinforced. The employee must make the connection between her actions and their consequences. Learning tends to occur most rapidly when reinforcement is continuous — ie when the correct response, or some portion of the correct response, is rewarded after each occurrence (Siegel and Lane 1987: 386). Responses that are either punished or not reinforced will be eliminated.

Using the principles of operant conditioning to influence the behaviour of nurses at work, involves five steps:

1. Identifying the critical behaviours that need to be changed. The manager must thus pinpoint what nurses actually have to do, what they are failing to do, and what is worth changing. Focus on observable behaviour only. Specific examples of behaviour such as 'arriving late for meetings' must be identified. The individual will probably not be motivated to change behaviour by statements like: 'Your behaviour is unsatisfactory,' but rather by a statement such as the following: 'You have arrived late for our staff meetings on the past three occasions. This is unexcusable. Please try to be punctual for staff meetings in future.'

2. Measure the frequency of the critical behaviours. Is there really a problem? Before intervening make sure that you are not assuming that a once-off example of undesirable behaviour necessarily means that the behaviour will recur.

3. Carry out functional analysis of the behaviours. This step involves identifying:

    *   the stimuli that precede the behaviour — for example a nurse who is consistently sick when the manager is going to undertake ward inspections. In this case the manager's inspections consistently precede and produce sickness;

    *   the contingent consequences — ie the consequences in terms of reward or punishment that influence the behaviour concerned. This step involves understanding the behaviour involved and providing a starting point for ideas on how to improve matters.

4. Develop and implement an intervention strategy. Develop a strategy that could be used to influence performance. Various strategies may be used but the use of positive reinforcement encourages good performance. Punishment for various reasons is much less useful. The closer the reinforcement is to the behaviour that one wants to influence, the greater will be the likelihood that future behaviour will be affected.

5. Evaluate the effects of the intervention. Evaluation can be conducted in several rigorous ways, but busy managers will probably simply examine whether things have improved or not (Robertson and Smith 1985: 35).

Organizational implications of organization behaviour management

The manager should make sure that:

1. the employee knows what is expected — performance standards should be realistic and clearly communicated;

2. the employee is able to fulfil the expectations that are required of her;

3. the consequences of effective job performance are weighted positively for the employee in the form of a promotion, bonus, or salary increase;

4. immediate, specific, and positive feedback about the consequences of effective and ineffective job performance is provided to the employee;

5. improvements in employee job performance are reinforced (Siegel and Lane 1987: 389).

Behaviour modification approaches do have drawbacks and limitations and some question the ethics of such deliberate and controlled modification of people's behaviour (Robertson and Smith 1985: 35).

GENERAL CONSIDERATIONS FOR PROMOTING MOTIVATION AMONG NURSES

1. Recognize small gains as well as large ones.

2. Give feedback during performance as well as at the conclusion of the delegated assignment.

3. Communicate vision and a sense of purpose.

4. Include nurses in policy formulation as far as is possible.

5. Boost self-confidence.

6. Provide rewards and punishments according to success or failure in achieving goals.

7. Promote management by objectives.

8. Proper job analysis in an organization promotes motivation because it forms a basis for career planning.

9. Reward success due to effort and ability.

10. Punish failure resulting from lack of effort.

11. Nurse managers must be taught about motivational strategies for personnel during their formal preparation phase.

12. Personnel development programmes must address the learning needs of staff in order for them to be able to advance in their career paths.

13. Provide a clinical promotional ladder in the service.

14. Effective career path counselling promotes motivation.

15. Institute quality circles in the service.

16. Provide opportunities for work enrichment.

17. Maintain an open, informal, friendly atmosphere in the organization where people feel free to speak their minds without fear of retribution.

18. Develop effective listening skills.

19. Remove any organizational barriers to success, if possible — eg too much red tape.

20. Maintain flexibility regarding the scheduling of work rosters.

21. Trust your subordinates so that they are able to trust you.

22. Delegate according to the abilities of your personnel and delegate authority in order to develop staff.

23. Merit rating of nurses should be done according to criteria agreed upon by nurses themselves.

24. Periodic re-evaluation of nursing procedures and tasks should be undertaken by the manager in direct consultation with her subordinates.

25. Evaluation of the work performance of personnel must take place on a regular basis, must follow a continuous pattern, and must be undertaken according to objective criteria which are known to everyone in the service.

26. The work of the nurse should be made as challenging as possible and should contain enough responsibility and authority to ensure that a sense of accomplishment and achievement can be derived when the work is carried out well.

27. Be as flexible regarding the hours of shift work as is possible.

28. The nurse manager who is perceived as trustful and supportive, and who evaluates fairly and gives adequate feedback, promotes motivation (Marriner-Tomey 1992: 335).

29. The nurse manager who readily shares information about the organization, consulting nurses on organizational problems and decisions and sharing information about the results, is also seen as promoting productivity (Swansburg 1990: 377).

30. Sources of dissatisfaction frequently quoted by nurses in research studies are: poor planning, an excessive workload which leads to poor quality of work, unco-operative physicians, unclear rules and regulations, unreasonable pressure, understaffing, non-nursing duties, and unqualified managers (Marriner-Tomey 1992: 335).

CONCLUSION

Motivating nurses to provide quality nursing care is a difficult problem for most nurse managers. They often want simple, practical ideas for motivating personnel but there is no easy solution to personnel problems. Tight controls, close supervision, excessive rules and regulations, and threats of dismissal do not achieve the objective. The opposite approach — ie excessive permissiveness, trying to satisfy every demand of employees, and achieving harmony at all costs — also does not motivate personnel. Many managers try to apply an approach which is somewhat in the middle of these two extremes (Swansburg 1990: 377). It is advisable for nurse managers to apply a number of different motivational approaches which will fit the particular work setting.

References

Barnum, B. S. and Mallard, C. O. (1989). *Essentials of nursing management, Concepts and context of practice.* Aspen: Rockville.

Bernhard, L. A. and Walsh, M. (1990). *Leadership. The key to the professionalization of nursing.* Second edition. Mosby: St Louis.

Chung, K. H. (1977). *Motivational Theories and Practices.* Grid: Columbus, Ohio.

Flude, R. (1991). *People for Business. The Key to Success.* Graham and Trotman: London.

Garner, J. F., Howard, L. S. and Piland, N. F. (1990). *Strategic Nursing Management. Power and Responsibility in a New Era.* Aspen: Rockville.

Gerber, P. D., Nel, P. S. and Van Dyk, P. S. (1991). *Management Resources.* Second edition. Southern: Johannesburg.

Halloran, J. (1986). *Personnel and Human Resource Management.* Prentice-Hall: Englewood Cliffs.

Hersey, P. and Blanchard, K. (1982). *Management of Organizational Behaviour: Utilizing Human Resources.* Prentice-Hall: Englewood Cliffs.

Longenecker, J. G. and Pringle, C. D. (1984). *Management.* Sixth edition. Merrill: Columbus.

Lunenberg, F. C. and Ornstein, A. C. (1991). *Educational Administration. Concepts and Practices.* Wadsworth: Belmont, California.

Marriner-Tomey, A. (1992). *Guide to Nursing Management.* Mosby: St Louis.

Mol, A. (1990). *Help! Ek is 'n Bestuurder.* Tafelberg: Cape Town.

Petri, H. L. (1986). *Motivation Theory and Research.* Second edition. Wadsworth: Belmont, California.

Pinder, C. C. (1984). *Work Motivation. Theory, Issues, and Applications.* Scott, Foresman: London.

Robertson, I. T. and Smith, M. (1985). *Motivation and Job Design. Theory, Research and Practice.* Institute of Personnel Management: London.

Siegel, L. and Lane, I. (1987). *Personnel and Organizational Psychology.* Second edition. Irwin: Homewood, Illinois.

Sullivan, E. J. and Decker, P. J. (1988). *Effective Management in Nursing.* Second edition. Addison-Wesley: Menlo Park.

CHAPTER 21

MANAGEMENT OF CHANGE

S. W. Booyens

CONTENTS

INTRODUCTION

Nowadays it is expected that nurse managers should have the vision to plan and implement change. In the fast-changing world in which the nurse manager operates, she must develop skills that will enable her to accomplish change effectively. The ability to manage change successfully and to be resilient and flexible, has become the hallmark of an efficient and happy leader.

Change occurs continuously in nursing because of the dynamic health care scene. Traditional methods of managing change are no longer always appropriate.

COMMON CHARACTERISTICS OF CHANGE

Managers who are aware of the common characteristics of change will not easily be overwhelmed by changes; they will be prepared to analyse change systematically. They should be aware of the following.

1. Plan. A plan may be drawn up in advance to outline the process of change, or a plan can be allowed to emerge as the issues in the change process become clearer. A planned change is *structured* when timetables for various activities are drawn up, and it is *unstructured* when the solution is open-ended (Szilagyi and Wallace 1990: 765).

2. Power. Power concerns the issue of who is making the decisions about change and on what basis. When subordinates are skillful enough and sufficiently informed, it is better to delegate some power to them. This aids decision-making. When subordinates do not possess sufficient skills and information to participate, top level managers tend to make the decisions, although the view of top level managers that subordinates are not skilled enough to participate may be questioned by the subordinates and may thus dilute the enforcement of top-level decisions.

3. Relationships. An approach to change can be *personal* or *impersonal*. When the leadership style or characteristics of a manager or supervisor are analysed with a view to training a person to change her style or characteristics, a personal approach is used. An impersonal approach, on the other hand, would view certain styles of leadership and their effects on subordinates and the necessary changes to be effected in them from a general point of view. The way that people in the manager's sphere of authority feel about a personal or impersonal approach would dictate how the manager would go about effecting necessary changes among supervisors.

4. Tempo. The speed and the depth of the process of change are reflected in its tempo. A change can be effected by starting out with minor changes which will build up to a major change over time, or it may be done by initiating a number of major changes right from the start.

The manager must consider these four elements when contemplating change. It is also essential to remember that the critical variables in change are the organizational structure (rules, regulations, policies), the work ethic and procedures (work methods, work standards), technological approaches, the people (attitudes, motivation), and the environment (external and internal) which all interact with one another. A change in one area will influence the other areas. The manager should therefore not settle on an approach to change before first examining the problem, the personnel, the environment, time constraints, resources, and the goals to be achieved (Szilagyi and Wallace 1990: 766).

MODELS OF CHANGE

There are numerous models of change; some describe change on a macro-level (ie organizational level), and some on a micro-level (ie functional level). It must, however, be remembered that no perfect model has yet been developed which can be applied in every type of organizational setting or in all circumstances. An eclectic view of organizational change and development which incorporates a number of techniques or strategies, taking into account the situation at hand, is recommended.

Macro-level model

When change is viewed on the macro or organizational level, the following model as depicted by Moorhead and Griffin (1989) and Szilagyi and Wallace (1990) is relevant.

The first step is an examination of *external forces,* such as political, social, and economic factors, and *internal forces,* such as the morale of employees, leadership effectiveness, and whether there are delays in communication. Next, the specific problem areas must be recognized and diagnosed. In other words, the problem must be defined. The third step would involve the identification of the goals or objectives which must be achieved by the process of change.

In order to implement the change process, it is necessary to select a change agent or agents who will facilitate the process. This is the fourth step. The fifth step in the cycle involves the identification of constraints, resources, structures, technology, people, and resistance to change. Once the constraints have been identified, the identification and selection of an appropriate approach is considered in step six.

The seventh step involves the implementation of the change taking into consideration the timing, depth and the location of the process. Step eight is concerned with measurement, evaluation, and control aspects. In this step the change agent and the top management group evaluate the degree to which change is having the desired effect. Progress towards the goals or objectives to be achieved is measured, and adjustments in the change process are made if necessary.

Micro-level model

On the micro-level, Lewin (1951) described three steps in his theory of change.

The first step is called the process of *unfreezing*. This process involves unfreezing or loosening old attitudes, ideas, and beliefs, and the development of a feeling of a need to change. The induction of guilt and anxiety, removing a person to a new environment, and punishment for undesirable attitudes are techniques that are sometimes used for unfreezing. If an individual experiences stress in a given situation, she may also be motivated to change. It is, however, recommended that the manager should be careful in using the above methods to unfreeze old habits because it is essential that trust be developed between the people suggesting change and the people who are asked to implement the change.

The second step is termed *moving to a new level*. During this step, plans are made for the implementation of change and information about the envisaged change is collected and discussed. Potential problems are debated, and solutions are sought. The plan for change is then implemented and the transition period to a new working level is started (Haynes 1992: 635).

The third step is the *refreezing of new patterns*. During refreezing, the new patterns are integrated into one's personality and working methods. This process needs to be reinforced, because personnel tend to return to their old habits once the initial effort that effected the change is no longer applied. This process of refreezing or stabilization needs to be reinforced by positive feedback, constructive criticism, and encouragement. Other stabilizing factors are changes in organizational structure and procedures that support the overall change.

According to Lewin (1951), an organization which is not engaged in an active process of change is in a state of *equilibrium*. This state of equilibrium is brought about by the fact that the driving forces — which are forces for change — are balanced by the restraining forces — the forces which are acting against change. Change can only be brought about if the driving forces are in a stronger position than the restraining forces, with the result that the previous state of affairs is uprooted or toppled over. In order to achieve this, the manager should identify the restraining forces and selectively remove them. Once this is achieved, an imbalance is created and the preponderance of driving forces will cause change to occur. The greater the number of driving forces, and the more potent they are, the greater the degree of change will be (Wilson 1992: 30).

STRATEGIES TO EFFECT CHANGE

Change theorists have proposed three major categories of change strategies — empirical–rational, power–coercive, and normative–re-educative. Each strategy is based on different assumptions about what will effect a change in a person's behaviour. Each strategy will create change, but the consequences and ease of change will vary. Each strategy has a different focus. The appropriateness of each of these strategies will depend on the situation in which the change must occur, as well as on the people whose knowledge, beliefs, and behaviour patterns need to change (Haffer 1986: 19).

Empirical–rational strategy

The basic assumption underlying this strategy is that people are rational beings who will readily adopt change if it can be justified rationally and if they can perceive some gain from the change. The focus of this strategy is thus the provision of knowledge so that a person or group makes a rational decision to change. An example of this strategy would be the education of a group of nurses about the results of research findings, such as audit findings, in order to get them to change their documenting behaviours or attitudes.

This strategy frequently does not bring about lasting change because people do not always act rationally. Although knowledge does affect our behaviour, there are also a number of other factors affecting our motivation to change. Among these factors are our hierarchy of needs, our perception of potential gain, our value systems, past experiences with change, the length of time spent practising the old behaviour, and tolerance for risk and ambiguity (Haffer 1986: 18).

This strategy is, unfortunately, the one most frequently used by nurse managers, since they tend to believe that providing knowledge will effect the necessary changes among their rational employees.

Power–coercive strategy

The basic underlying assumption of this strategy is that people with less power will follow the plans, direction, and leadership of those who possess greater power. The idea behind this strategy is that power, in some form, should be applied to bring about change. People are thus pressurized, manipulated, coerced, or forced to comply with the authority's wishes. This strategy does not deny the rationality or values of people, but acknowledges the need to use some form of power to effect change.

Examples of the use of this strategy are strikes, peer pressure, economic coercive power, authoritative power which creates policies and legal rulings, and moral power which induces guilt or shame.

The use of this strategy often leads to strong resistance. It is, however, frequently used when there is already high resistance to change or when high resistance is expected. The changes which are made as a result of this strategy often do not last. As soon as the person demanding the change is absent, the changed behaviour tends to disappear. This strategy will bring about change quicker than other strategies, and is sometimes necessary if an immediate change needs to be instituted. If a lasting change is desired, it should be combined with other strategies.

Normative–re-educative strategy

The underlying assumption of this strategy is that the people who need to change should participate in the identification of the problem, the selection of solutions, and the choice of methods to bring about the change. People are viewed as having habits, values, and norms. Change will only occur once commitment to old norms and values decreases to a point where new norms are accepted.

This strategy involves clarification and modification of habits, values, and attitudes, and re-education to accept new or changed habits, values, and attitudes. This changing of beliefs and attitudes needs to take place in a setting where there is trust, support, and assistance regarding the clarification of values and the solving of problems. The change agent must thus be accepted, and she needs to be sensitive to people's perceptions and values (Haffer 1986: 20).

Examples of the use of this strategy are seen in small group counselling and in organizational development programmes, where it is usual to collect data about the organization, to give feedback about the data and its analysis to appropriate people, to plan ways to improve the system, and to train internal change agents. When the internal change agents can create a trusting and open relationship with the other employees, the appropriate setting is established for their re-education.

The normative–re-educative strategy takes the longest period of time to effect change, but if beliefs, values and attitudes need to be changed, then this strategy will bring about better results than the other two.

Adapted situational leadership change model

Haffer (1986) proposes a model for effecting change, adapted from Hersey and Blanchard's situational leadership model. This model outlines the strategy of change in accordance with the willingness and ability of the group or individual subjected to change.

According to this model, there are four positions which the individual or group could take in terms of their willingness and ability to change. There are also four kinds of facilitating strategies which the change agent would choose from, according to the position taken by the individual or group.

The first position is where the group or individual is unable and unwilling to change, and incompetent, unsure, and insecure about change. The appropriate strategy is a power–coercive one where the group or individual is told what must be done. Specific directions are given, close supervision is provided, the 'how', 'when' and 'what' of the task is spelt out, and support given until change starts.

The second position is where the group or individual is frequently willing to undertake the change, but is unable, and lacks the skills, to bring about what is needed. The appropriate facilitating strategy is an empirical–rational one, where selling is used. They are thus provided with the necessary knowledge and a demonstration of what is required. Direction and supervision are decreased, and support is given for change efforts.

The third position demonstrates an ability to effect the change but an unwillingness to act because the group or individual lacks the confidence or motivation. The appropriate facilitating effort is a participative one which involves both the empirical–rational and the normative–re-educative strategies. The group or individual is thus involved in decision-making about what should be changed and how it should be done, increasing self-direction is encouraged, and a decreased need for support is evident.

The fourth position of the group or individual shows a willingness and ability to effect change, as well as competence and self-directed behaviour. The appropriate strategy is the normative–re-educative one, where the client decides how, when, and where the change should be brought about. The facilitator delegates authority for implementing the change to the individual or group, providing little direction and little support because they are self-directed.

RESISTANCE TO CHANGE

Resistance to change is a natural human characteristic, rooted in basic human needs and perceptions. Lancaster identified two types of resistance associated with change:

1. Resistance due to the nature of the change, and

2. Resistance due to misconceptions and inaccurate beliefs concerning the change process (Haynes 1992: 637).

Other researchers identified the following reasons why individuals tend to resist change:

- *Habit*. To do a job in the usual way is easier than learning an entirely new way of doing it.

- *Security*. Some employees like the security of doing things in the same old way. While ever-increasing changes are going on around them, the sameness of the job and the organization provide a measure of security in their lives.

- *Economic considerations*. Employees often fear that changes will mean that they will no longer have a job. Many nurses tend to reason that the incorporation of computers in the hospital setting would mean fewer nursing jobs.

- *Fear of the unknown*. Some people fear anything which is unfamiliar to them. However, most employees resist change not because they fear anything unfamiliar but because they fear that certain contemplated changes will make it more difficult for them to get something worthwhile accomplished in their jobs in the available time-span.

- *Lack of awareness*. People may not resist change actively, but may fail to recognize a small change in a rule or a procedure and thus may carry on according to the familiar pattern due to lack of awareness. People tend to pay attention only to those things which are of real interest to them.

- *Misunderstanding*. If the goals of the change process are not made clear to employees, the employees may resist the process because they may tend to think that the top managers want to bring change about just for the sake of change.

- *Belief that the proposed change is not sensible for the organization*. It is natural to expect resistance if the employees have the view that nothing of value can be gained by the proposed change.

Resistance to change may also come from the following organizational factors:

- *Sunk costs*. Organizations may not be willing to implement a change for the simple reason that no money is available for such a change. It is often the case that all of the available resources are being used in order to maintain the status quo, and this can have the result that there are no additional resources available to spend on a process of change.

- *Threats to powerful coalitions.* Power relationships and the status of people in the organization often shift when changes occur. When the change process is geared to the empowerment of more individuals in an organization, power and status become dispersed, with the result that the middle managers often lose some power and status.

- *Indictment of leadership.* When leaders complain about the problems facing their organizations they recognize that the need for change shows up the limitations of their past decisions and actions (Barber 1990: 70).

In the health care field, barriers to change may emanate from the following:

- *Expectations of autonomy among health care personnel.* Doctors, nurses, radiographers, physiotherapists, and other health care professionals are accustomed to a relatively high degree of autonomy. When proposed changes impose formal methods for increasing productivity and quality of care, professionals often tend to view these as an imposition on their independence and autonomy, with the result that they tend to resist them.

- *Loss of prevailing advantage.* When changes will directly affect the perceived power of nurses and doctors, strong resistance can be expected.

- *Programmed behaviour.* Rules, regulations, procedural manuals all serve to create a programmed way of doing the work in a hospital. While this behaviour is necessary in order for the health institution to function effectively, it also tends to stifle innovation and change. Official constraints on behaviour thus often significantly suppress the implementation of change (Johnson and Boss 1991: 9).

- *Resistance from informal key staff members.* Although it is recognized that the support of the formal key staff members, such as supervisors and managers, is essential in effecting any lasting change, powerful informal groups, such as physicians, are also regarded as key personnel as far as support for change is concerned. If they do not support a change, it will be extremely difficult to get it accepted and implemented — if it can be done at all.

- *Inter-organizational agreements.* When agreements between organizations or health care institutions are made, these agreements may inhibit change more effectively than any internal obstacle. For example, when medical staff hold posts in more than one hospital, or are shared between a hospital and a university, staffing agreements limit the hospital when making changes which may affect these agreements. Similarly, if a number of private hospitals are owned by one company, certain changes in one hospital may affect the other hospitals in the group.

MANAGING RESISTANCE

Managers should view resistance to the proposed change as a cue to re-examine the merits of the envisioned change. Resistance can be seen as a constructive force if it gets managers to rethink their decision to make a change, if they are prompted to search for new ways to reach their goals, and if it leads to more communication with employees.

The following approaches are recommended in order to overcome resistance to change:

1. Education and communication. Accurate information that allows people to understand the reasons for the proposed change will help them to accept that change. Communication will help to dispel fears of the unknown. It should clearly indicate the plan for the change and the goals of the change, and must be a two-way process. The use of training programmes to increase employees' awareness of the problems that must be overcome by the change process will aid in overcoming resistance. Education and communication are time-consuming activities.

2. Participation and involvement. When the people who are affected by change are called upon to help design the change process, their resistance may be reduced. Involvement in the planning process is especially important when people's commitment is essential for the successful implementation of the change. This approach is, however, time-consuming, and should be managed properly. It is a useful strategy when resistance is caused by a focus on restricted or limited change and a lack of awareness of the types of problems which must be overcome (Moorhead and Griffin 1989: 714).

3. Facilitation and support. When problems arise among employees from a fear of the unknown, stemming from the employees' desire for security, facilitation and support are needed. The manager may also need to arrange additional training sessions if employees are having difficulties in adjusting to new methods. Emotional support must be given until the new ways of doing things are entrenched, otherwise people may fall back on the working

methods used before the change. Facilitation and support also take up a lot of time.

4. Negotiation and agreement. When the implications of the change process are such that some employees may lose their jobs or their expected benefits, negotiation should be used in order to reach an agreement about how the change will be implemented. Negotiation is useful when resistance is encountered due to power relationships being threatened, and particularly where a group has considerable power to resist (Moorhead and Griffin 1989: 714).

5. Manipulation and co-opting. When the above strategies are not successful in managing resistance, some managers resort to covert methods to influence employees, such as imparting only selected parts of the available information, or including key members of resistance groups in the designing process. By the inclusion of members of groups who will probably not offer resistance in the planning phase of the change process, it is hoped that their support for the implementation of change can be won. Manipulation and co-optation, however, can lead to problems later on when people feel that they have been manipulated to accept change.

6. Explicit and implicit coercion. Managers may use coercion explicitly or implicitly when all other methods of overcoming resistance have failed or where speed is essential, and when the people who are initiating the change are in a powerful enough position to enforce it. Employees may be threatened that they will lose their jobs, be demoted, or transferred if they do not comply with the change. This is a speedy method which may overcome any kind of resistance, but may seriously affect the attitude of employees towards authority figures in the organization in general (Szilagyi and Wallace 1990: 786).

7. Establishing trust. When a trust relationship is established between managers and employees it is far easier to implement changes than when one party does not trust the other.

8. Plan the change in stages. When the initial planning is done and the change process is designed in a way which involves the accomplishment of various stages it is easier to implement change than when the process is not planned beforehand. When the plans outline the stages involved, the people who must bring about the change in each stage, the time in which the implementation must be completed, as well as the results which are expected at the end of each stage, the employees stay informed about the progress and results of implementation (Beyers 1984: 37).

COST OF CHANGE

The cost of change is not always considered by managers because they only tend to think in terms of the advantages which will emanate from the change. According to Beyers (1984), however, the following costs should be taken into account when change is designed and implemented:

1. The time of the people who are doing the planning and implementation of the change.

2. Payment for consultants or experts from sources outside the organization.

3. Materials to be printed. Examples are: letters, memos, questionnaires, surveys, and written plans.

4. Other resources which are needed, such as equipment and supplies.

5. The time, materials, and space which are needed for instruction.

6. The time, materials, and people needed to evaluate the results of the change.

These costs are usually of more concern when change is introduced as an 'extra' project, over and above the usual routine work. When change is part of the normal work routine the costs may be less pronounced because time and materials would be utilized for routine activities in any case. Even minor changes involve an extra input of time, energy, and printed materials, however.

STEPS IN THE CHANGE PROCESS

When change is contemplated in an organization, the wise manager will understand that, in order to effect change, communication must take place and participation must be achieved between all departments of the organization right from the start. In order to bring about change effectively, the following steps, which are adapted from those recommended by Bolton, Aydin, Popolow, and Ramseyer (1992), may be used.

Step 1: Define the goals of the project

The project team members inform the entire staff of each department of the manager's wishes to bring about a change to improve service. Each staff member in a department must give an input by stating how he/she sees the future of the organization and the measures which need to be taken to achieve this vision of the future. The common threads or ideas are extracted from the employees' visions, and are moulded into a common vision for the future. The goals which need to be achieved can then be defined.

The project team leaders will also have to ensure that the defined goals are compatible with broad organizational planning for the future — ie the organizational strategic plans.

Step 2: Decide who will lead the project

It is necessary for change agents or change facilitators to keep on communicating their vision for the future to individuals at all levels in the organization. They must also devote large amounts of time to daily coaching and encouragement of the change process. It is thus necessary to select people who are devoted to bringing about change to act as leaders of the project.

Step 3: Obtaining commitment from managers

It is necessary for the employees in the organization to feel that everybody in it is actively supporting and working towards the change goals. The commitment of key managers must be felt and seen.

Step 4: Build the change process incrementally by setting specific objectives to be attained

If incremental objectives are set, the change process achieves the easier objectives first before attempting the more complicated ones. This encourages the participation of employees. They become more committed because they build on successful ventures. The goals of a large project are thus broken up into achievable smaller chunks or objectives.

Step 5: Emphasize the main goal to be achieved

The major goal of the change process, ie to improve patient care services, needs to be emphasized continuously because individuals and departments may fall into the trap of setting narrow objectives which may well promote productivity or effectiveness in their departments but which might jeopardize the efforts of other departments or the efforts of the whole change process.

Step 6: Provide continuous support

The different interdepartmental working groups must be supported continuously. If they started to change some aspects of their work before the new change project was initiated, the change process must build on these past changes, and the facilitators should not try to alter these efforts because employees might become discouraged. It is necessary to emphasize realism by focusing on what works.

Step 7: Teach employees new ways to define and solve problems

The facilitators need to train departmental supervisors and leaders of smaller work groups to think more globally in their approach to problems — ie to think from the perspective of the total organization when they are seeking solutions to problems. In this way, new and more effective ways of problem-solving are developed, which are often more satisfying in the long-run.

Step 8: Communicate the change-process

An ongoing plan for communication about the progress of the change process is developed. Informal weekly and monthly one-page bulletins about the progress of the project in the organization will assist in keeping employees informed and committed until all the goals have been achieved (Bolton et al. 1992: 15–19).

REASONS FOR CHANGE

The nurse manager is functioning in an ever-changing environment. In society at large we all face the following changes and must adapt to them:

- A growing world-wide population.

- Limited resources.

- Grave ecological problems.

- Faster acquisition of knowledge and communication.

- Increasing interdependence among organizations.

- Different political and religious ideologies.

- Constant or frequent replacement of leading figures, or frequent transition of power from one head of state to another (Conner 1992: 11).

The following factors, among others, threaten the stability of health care organizations:

1. Increased demands from patients. People nowadays have been made more aware of health and health issues, and of the benefits of staying healthy, with the result that consumers of health care have become more assertive in their demands. They want up-to-date technology to be used if they are sick, and want services to be cost-effective and convenient.

2. Advances in medical technology. These produce entirely new approaches to the treatment of diseases. Apart from the demands that this places on staff who must constantly adapt to new

technological changes, hospitals are often saddled with continuous requests for the latest technology to replace earlier machines and devices. The result is that most of the hospital's capital is consumed by investment in the state-of-the-art technology which leaves them with no extra money to implement other necessary changes (Johnson and Boss 1991: 6).

3. The short duration of the hospitalization of patients. Because it is so expensive to hospitalize a patient, the continuity of patient care is complicated by shorter stays in hospitals and increased specialization, as well as the increased use of outpatient facilities and home-care.

In the nursing profession, the nurse executive or nurse manager is expected to focus more on what will be required in future than on what is required at present. The nurse manager is expected to sustain an environment for nurses that provides high staff morale and quality patient care in a climate of revolutionary change and ever-shrinking resources (Collotan 1986: 6).

She will have to bring staffing ratios into balance with new payment systems, be extremely flexible regarding scheduling patterns, will have to develop highly sophisticated norms for staffing, patient classification systems, and indices of workload measurement. The nurse manager will also have to work in closer collaboration with doctors and administrative managers to help sustain quality of patient care. She will also have to become committed and take an active part in the strategic planning of the institution in which she is functioning (Collotan 1986: 6).

She will have to study projections of future demographic changes, evolving technology, and changing societal values about health and health care in order to make predictions and to arrive at a number of possible future scenarios, so that strategies may be developed for meeting health care requirements in future (Beyers 1984: 38).

FORCES WHICH PROMOTE OR INHIBIT CHANGES IN NURSING

Research has identified the following forces, both inside and outside institutions, which would either facilitate or hinder changes in health care settings.

Factors from outside which would promote change were identified as:

● Adequate and flexible facilities.

● Support from a school of nursing which could provide well-educated nurses.

● A positive image of the hospital/institution.

- Recognition of the need to improve.

- An organizational commitment to quality and patient care.

- Recognition of the key position of nurses regarding the institution's accomplishments (Taft and Stearns 1991: 16).

- New technology.

Factors from within an institution which would promote change include the following:

- Appointment of new personnel.

- Satisfying organizational structures or recognition for the need for change in the working patterns.

- Clear role descriptions.

- Recognition of the work of nurses from patients, families, and the hospital.

- Use of innovative nursing care models.

- Recognized standards of practice for each nurse category.

- Commitment from nurses to patients, the profession, and change.

- A strong and visible leadership from especially the chief nurse manager, but also the other nurse managers, with good relationships between staff and leaders.

- The involvement of nurse managers in all the strategic planning processes in the institution.

- A recognition by medical and administrative leaders of the essential role played by nurses in a hospital.

- The participation of all nursing levels in decision-making.

- Improvement in the salary structure for nursing

- Well-managed implementation of change.

- Appropriate financial and informational support for change.

- A balance between centralization and decentralization.

- Commitment to change from hospital leadership.

- Good interdisciplinary relationships.

- Willingness to let go of tradition.

Factors from outside which would inhibit change were identified as:

- Unpredictability in the environment.

- Threatening legal regulations.

- Insufficient resources to maintain the status quo.

- A negative image of the hospital.

- A long-standing paternalistic health care culture.

- Short-term planning.

- Absence of shared care values in the organization.

- A history of poor relationships among the different members of the multidisciplinary team (Taft and Stearns 1991: 16).

Factors from within the institution which would hinder change were, among others, the following:

- increasing demand for productivity together with inadequate resources (time, money, staff development) for innovation;

- low morale, poor performance, and high staff turnover;

- an insufficient number of well-trained personnel;

- a lack of nursing practice standards;

- not recognizing the contribution of nursing;

- bureaucratic red tape and rigidity;

- lack of support and commitment from leaders in the institution;

- insecurity, fear of risk-taking, and lack of self-confidence among staff members;

- a tightly controlled nursing structure;

- overcommitted leaders and staff members: the 'too busy' syndrome;

- inadequate leadership with lack of consensus for change among nursing staff members;

- sunk costs.

THE TEN STAGES OF CHANGE

Change has personal and emotional effects on the employees who are affected by it. The nurse manager who is aware of these issues and who knows how to deal with them should experience more positive results from the change than those managers who are not. According to Perlman and Takacs (1990), the following ten stages or phases of change should be taken into account:

The first phase — equilibrium

In this phase the employees are functioning productively because their personal and professional goals are congruent with those of the organization. They are contented and comfortable with the status quo. When external changes put pressure on the organization to change, the status quo becomes endangered with the result that employees become uneasy. Managers should make employees aware of the environmental factors which will necessitate change, but should not lecture them about productivity and competition (Perlman and Takacs 1990: 33–4).

The second phase — denial

In this phase the employees try to maintain the status quo and actively resist the changes that are taking place. The energy they previously used to maintain normal functioning is now increasingly used by their resistance efforts with the result that they are left depleted of energy and depleted of emotional strength, which leaves them somewhat unbalanced, thinking illogically. They do not always attend the training sessions which are meant to promote the change process. The manager should not threaten these dissident employees that they must 'attend or else'; managers should rather use active listening skills to accommodate the feelings expressed by employees. Managers should also learn what parts of the change dissident employees are accepting, and then build on this. Workshops in which the management of stress is addressed are recommended during this phase.

The third phase — anger

During phase three the employees realize that the status quo cannot be maintained because they do not have enough energy to maintain it in the face of the challenges which confront them. They become angry and vent their anger on the managers. Managers need support and reinforcement in order to deal with their own frustrations and to deal with their employees. They should use active listening skills and assertiveness skills to talk openly with their employees, to listen empathetically, to teach new problem-solving skills, and to get employees to do some introspection to detect the real reason for their anger.

The fourth phase — bargaining

During this phase the employees try to bargain the change out of existence. They want to negotiate and bargain with the manager, as if to say 'we will go this far in assisting you to institute the change, if you will do the following for us'. Although this phase may appear to be rational or logical, when a type of compromise is reached it often leads to no change at all taking place. During this phase the manager will need conflict management skills and win–win negotiation skills.

The fifth phase — chaos

This phase is characterized by a diffusion of energy. Employees feel powerless and at a loss because nothing seems to work any more. Managers and employees begin to wonder if any of their previous efforts were worthwhile. Managers should accept this state of flux, and spend time discussing pessimistic views that have been expressed, emotions, and the direction that change should take.

The sixth phase — depression

Self-pity, emptiness, and longing for the good old days are felt. Managers can alleviate this by informing the employees as thoroughly and as quickly as possible about change. Expressions of sorrow must only be *accepted* by managers, not answered or denied.

The seventh phase — resignation

People accept the reality of change at last and no longer resist it. They accept it, however, with no enthusiasm. Managers should not prod too much or criticize lack of enthusiasm; they should let employees function at their own pace.

Phase eight — openness

The employees are open to the change process. Managers will now have to repeat the procedures, policies, and objectives of the change again, although it may seem unnecessary.

Phase nine — readiness

Employees are finally willing to use energy to explore the new structure. Managers should direct them by assigning tasks, monitoring results and providing guidelines.

Phase ten — re-emergence

In this phase the change becomes operational. Employees re-invest their energy in the organization and in themselves, become proactive and initiate projects and ideas. Managers should help redefine career paths and the organizational mission and culture, and clarify roles and functions.

THE NURSE MANAGER AS A CHANGE AGENT

The change agent provides the environment for change to occur and actively spurs it on by doing the following:

- clarifying and identifying the problem;
- getting the available resources together;

- getting different people to work together in order to reduce resistance;
- giving support and encouragement until refreezing has occurred (Haynes 1992: 636).

The nurse has not traditionally been trained to fulfil a leadership role, or to be ready to act as a change agent or facilitator of change. Nurses often find themselves unable to resist negative changes being thrust upon them. The change agent should be able to distinguish between necessary and unnecessary change and should resist unnecessary changes. If nurses are not ready to act as change facilitators, they risk change being imposed on them by people from outside the profession. Nurses, and especially nurse managers, should thus develop themselves to become facilitators of change. Lancaster and Lancaster (1982), as referred to by Haynes (1992), suggest that nurse leaders develop the following characteristics in order to become successful change facilitators:

- sufficient self-confidence to lead;
- the ability to communicate clearly and to listen effectively;
- the ability to make decisions;
- trusting and respecting other people;
- planning and organizing abilities, which include effective delegation, guidance, directing, and co-ordinating skills;
- patience and consideration for other people's needs;
- perseverance;
- considerable energy;
- adequate knowledge of the field in which they lead;
- the ability to control their feelings in various difficult situations.

Health style changes for nurse managers

The nurse manager who is fatigued, who works extremely hard to meet constant deadlines, who believes that honest hard work will solve most problems, and who is in an organization where most of the executives are inflexible and threatened by new ideas and change, will probably not have the vision or the willpower to initiate and motivate the necessary changes. Such a nurse manager needs to consider the following lifestyle changes:

1. Self-assessment and professional and personal goal-setting. The manager assesses her strengths and weaknesses herself by listing them on a personal record and indicating areas where

improvements are necessary. After a period of five years a follow-up assessment is done in order to evaluate if improvements were, in fact, carried out. This assessment of strengths and weaknesses usually leads to a new view of the job, which leads to renewed commitment. It may, however, lead to a change of job or career.

2. Set aside some personal time for which no activities are planned in order to do some introspection and to recharge batteries. An early morning walk or jog is a good start to the day if it allows time for reflection on past events and future plans.

3. Networking. It is wise to build up a network of colleagues who are nurse managers and health executives. These networks stimulate the nurse manager to think about old problems in new ways, they are important support structures in times of stress, and they provide camaraderie, useful advice, information regarding job opportunities, and opportunities for leadership roles for young managers (Burk and Bice 1991: 18).

4. Lifelong learning should be seen as an enriching experience and should not be perceived as an added burden. Attendance at seminars, workshops, and conferences on a regular basis assists in this process of continuous informal education.

5. The manager should surround herself with staff members who view change as a positive force and who are always willing to accept and implement changes where needed. Their enthusiasm usually rubs off on the manager, who then displays an enthusiastic and visionary attitude to change, which will spur subordinates on to take risks instead of 'playing it safe' all the time.

6. Maintaining a healthy interest in outside activities helps to keep a proper perspective on life and work. Whether the chosen activity is gardening, reading, sport, or community involvement, it makes the manager a well-rounded individual who is more resilient to the stress of daily work problems.

7. Mentoring. The manager who can periodically turn to a mentor for a realistic perspective, or who serves as a mentor, is fortunate and experiences continuous growth and renewal.

8. The manager must learn to view past mistakes as opportunities for learning and should not always see them in a negative light.

9. A sense of humour is necessary to maintain perspective in a very serious occupation. Religious faith and spiritual values serve as an anchor in times of trouble, and personal relationships with family and friends serve to stabilize life (Burke and Bice 1991: 21).

CONCLUSION

The changing world environment, and especially the rapidly changing health care environment, compels the nurse manager to plan and implement changes in nursing care settings. Models of change and strategies and steps to change in an organizational setting are all geared to overcome the natural phenomenon of resistance to the change process. Forces both inside and outside the organization that inhibit or promote changes were listed, along with the characteristics which the change agent or facilitator of change needs in order to get the change process going.

References

Barber, A. M. (1990). *Transformational Nursing Leadership*. Williams and Wilkins: Baltimore.

Beyers, M. (1984). Getting on top of organizational change. Part I. *JONA*, volume 14, number 10, pp. 32–9.

Bolton, L. B., Aydin, C., Popolow, G. and Ramseyer, J. (1992). Ten steps for managing organizational change. *JONA*, volume 22, number 6, pp. 14–20.

Burke, G. C. and Bice, M. O. (1991). Renewal and change for health care executives. *Hospital and Health Services Administration*, volume 36, number 1, pp. 15–23.

Collotan, J. W. (1986). The changing environment: guest editorial. *JONA*, volume 16, number 4, p. 6.

Conner, D. (1992). The management of change: welcome day 29. *JONA*, volume 22, number 8, pp. 10–12.

Haffer, A. (1986). Facilitating change: choosing the appropriate strategy. *JONA*, volume 16, number 4, pp. 18–22.

Haynes, S. (1992). Let the change come from within. *Professional Nurse*, July 1992, pp. 635–8.

Johnson, J. A. and Boss, R. W. (1991). Management development and change in a demanding health care environment. *Journal of Management Development*, volume 10, number 4, pp. 5–10.

McGovern, W. N. and Rodgers, J. A. (1986). Change theory. *American Journal of Nursing*, May 1986, pp. 566–7.

Moorhead, G. and Griffin, R. W. (1989). *Organizational Behaviour*. Houghton Mifflin: Boston.

Perlman, D. and Takacs, G. T. (1990). The 10 stages of change. *Nursing Management,* volume 21, number 4, pp. 33–8.

Szilagyi, A. D. and Wallace, M.J. (1990). *Organizational Behaviour and Performance.* Scott, Foresman: Illinois.

Taft, S. W. and Stearns, J. E. (1991). Organizational change towards a nursing agenda. *JONA,* volume 21, number 2, pp. 12–21.

Wilson, D.C. (1992). *A Strategy of Change.* Routledge: London.

CHAPTER 22

DECISION-MAKING AND PROBLEM-SOLVING

S. W. Booyens

CONTENTS

INTRODUCTION

Decision-making forms an integral part of problem-solving. Both are integral parts of nursing management. The effectiveness of a nurse manager is measured by the quality of her decisions.

Decision-making forms the core of the management process since a decision is a prerequisite for any significant action by either the manager herself or by her subordinates (Gillies 1989: 439). To function successfully, the nurse manager must consistently demonstrate problem-solving skills in situations which change both frequently and rapidly. She is also in a position where she has to make decisions despite the fact that she does not always have the full picture of the situation or all the relevant facts at hand. Good decision-making by the manager, however, creates a climate for sound interpersonal functioning and may foster good decision-making by subordinates.

The nurse manager must be able to make sound decisions and make them in a relatively short timeframe. Her decisions must be appropriate and rational, must move her organization in the right direction, and must enable it to meet its objectives. Rules, regulations, resources and circumstances change constantly and the nurse manager needs to be poised to react appropriately. This will become evident from the decisions she is making.

THE ELEMENTS OF DECISION-MAKING

The nurse manager never makes decisions in a vacuum. A number of elements are always present in any decision that is made. These elements include the problem at hand, the abilities and personality of the decision-maker, the process that is to be followed in making the decision, and the environment in which the decision has to be made. Factors in the environment which would influence the decision would typically include the following: the mission of the organization, the type of organization concerned (eg hierarchical or horizontal), the cultural and social sphere in which the organization operates, the economic climate both inside and outside the organization, the resources available, and the main characteristics of the consumers of health care and of the employees of the health care organization.

DECISION-MAKING MODELS

Decision-making models include the normative model, the descriptive model, and the branch approach.

The normative model

This model was proposed by Adam Smith 200 years ago. It rests on the assumption that in any given situation where a decision has to be made, all the possible choices, consequences, and political outcomes of each are known, and that the decision will involve choosing the alternative which will ensure the greatest measure of satisfaction (Lancaster and Lancaster 1982: 23). The normative model characterizes the decision-maker as a completely rational, all-knowing, hedonistic calculator who approaches any problem in a chronological series of steps to find the desired answer.

The steps are as follows (Lancaster and Lancaster 1982: 24):

1. The definition and analysis of the problem.

2. The identification of all available alternatives.

3. Evaluation of advantages and disadvantages of each alternative.

4. The ranking of all the alternatives in the order in which they are likely to meet the desired objective.

5. Selecting the alternative which will achieve the greatest measure of satisfaction.

6. Implementation of the decision.

7. Following up the decision.

The normative model is analytically precise, but it is frequently criticized because the assumption that there are clear-cut choices among the identified alternatives is often not correct in nursing management. A nurse manager might, for example, be faced with the problem of an urgent request to open a new four-bed unit. Examine the following aspects which she will have to consider:

- Aspect 1: the hospital superintendent and important doctors will be satisfied.

- Aspect 2: a whole contingent of staff has to be found for the unit. The staff must be drawn from a number of already poorly-staffed units.

- Aspect 3: the hospital will gain community acceptance by opening up this new added facility.

- Aspect 4: the quality of patient care in the units that staff will have to be drawn from is not satisfactory, mainly because of staff-patient ratios.

- Aspect 5: the nurse manager will be seen as effective and efficient and will gain esteem in the eyes of the hospital administrator if she opens this unit.

- Aspect 6: the costs of the orientation and in-service education programmes which will be essential for the staff members to work in this unit have to be borne by the nursing department, although they were not budgeted for.

The descriptive model

It is usually found that the nurse manager must base her decisions on incomplete information about a problem. The nurse manager is often faced with problems which are not clearly and correctly defined, and it is not always possible or feasible to try to obtain full information about the problem because of limitations of time, money, or people (Lancaster and Lancaster 1982: 24).

In the descriptive model, the decision-maker is viewed as a person who solves a problem logically on the basis of known or easily obtainable information. Instead of seeking an optimal solution, managers tend to establish a set of minimal objectives that they will seek to accomplish and which they can comfortably consider as acceptable alternatives (Lancaster and Lancaster 1982: 24).

In the descriptive model, the manager thus first establishes an acceptable or satisfactory goal. Thereafter, subjective perceptions of the problem are defined. Acceptable alternatives which might solve the problem are then identified and evaluated. A satisfactory alternative is selected, and the decision is implemented and followed-up (Lancaster and Lancaster 1982: 24).

The branch approach

When using this approach, the manager perceives the problem or managerial challenge at hand and develops her decision or final goal by making small changes which build and follow-on, one after the other, until the final goal is reached. Thus basic policy decisions are not made in a final once-and-for-all fashion, but small-scale decisions are made, one at a time (Gillies 1989: 450–1). In this type of decisional approach, the nurse manager is using the outcomes of each of the earlier small decisions to guide her in her approach regarding the next decision that must be made. This type of method decreases the nurse manager's need for facts since, at each decision point, she only needs to consider those facts that relate to the present small intended change that she is considering (Gillies 1989: 451). This type of decision strategy could be followed by a nurse manager who is serious about improving the quality of nursing care in her institution considerably but is cautious about making unacceptable big changes on a once-and-for-all basis. She thus makes a series of small changes over an extended period of time until she reaches her goal of a substantial increase in the quality of patient care.

THE STEPS IN THE DECISION-MAKING PROCESS

Step 1: Recognizing the problem

Problems are not always what they appear to be. Although identifying a problem is an essential prerequisite for decision-making, it is the most complex step in decision-making because failure to correctly identify a problem leads to wrong decisions and solutions, or no solutions at all. It is easy to get caught up in the symptoms and never identify the real underlying problem (Lancaster and Lancaster 1982: 25; Bandman and Bandman 1988: 139).

It is thus helpful to state specifically what is wrong and what improvements appear to be feasible so that the nurse manager is in a position to gather facts, investigate possible causes, and determine the real problem (Lancaster and Lancaster 1982: 25)

The definition of the problem should not be too general (eg 'a nursing shortage') because a globally-defined problem is too difficult for a nurse manager to investigate and to solve. On the other hand, when a problem is defined in terms that are too specific it effectively restricts the number of alternative solutions that can be applied to solve it (Bandman and Bandman 1988: 139).

When evaluating a problem, the nurse manager must look at both the problem's importance as well as its potential for being solved. Nurse managers are sometimes faced with high priority problems which cannot be solved by their efforts alone (such as a problem of a high absenteeism rate because of occupational illness and injuries resulting from the fact that the institution does not have an occupational health service).

Nurse managers must usually establish priorities for dealing with problems. Three ways of choosing priorities are:

- The first problem encountered is the first problem solved.

- Problems which can be solved immediately are given preference over time-consuming ones.

- Crisis or emergency problems take precedence over all the others (Lancaster and Lancaster 1982: 25).

Step 2: Gathering relevant information

The urgency and type of problem to be solved will determine whether information-gathering will be instantaneous or whether it will involve an extensive search over a prolonged period of time. A search for information usually consists of an internal and an external search. With the internal search the nurse manager searches her memory for similar problems in the past and their solutions, her prior experiences with that particular type of problem, and ideas regarding the education and training of her employees and the organizational policies which might hinder or assist in the search for solutions.

During the external data gathering process the nurse manager consults external sources. The external sources of information may be specific knowledgeable individuals, records of meetings where similar or related problems were discussed, or policy manuals and regulations. Another source of information is the database information system of the institution. This provides a timely flow of up-to-date information (Lancaster and Lancaster 1982: 26).

The amount of information sought, or the intensity with which this is undertaken, is influenced by several factors, eg:

- The urgency and type of problem — eg 'is the problem of a routine administrative type or is it a strategic one?'

- The availability of information.

- The ability of the decision-maker to endure the tediousness of the data-gathering effort.

- The degree of risk that the decision involves. (The risk may be financial, psychological, social, or physical in nature. In general, the higher the risk, the more information is gathered.)

- The type, quality, and amount of information stored in the decision-maker's memory, and the ability to recall it.

- The decision-maker's personal confidence in her decision-making abilities. Less experienced managers, who are not so confident of their decision-making abilities, generally gather a considerable amount of information to support their decisions. Experienced managers, by contrast, may have made many similar decisions and thus feel more comfortable about the outcome of their decisions. They therefore need minimal supporting information (Lancaster and Lancaster 1982: 26).

A common problem that follows the gathering of information is that of deciding what to do with it and how to use it most effectively. Several tests may be useful:

- The *test of adequacy* asks if there are sufficient data collected to generate possible conclusions.

- The *test of accuracy* asks whether the information gathered is accurate. Inaccurate, vague, or ambiguous information is worse than useless because it can lead to an inaccurate conclusion and a wrong decision.

- The *test of relevance* asks whether the collected information is relevant for the problem at hand, because irrelevant information may obscure the clarity and directness of the decision-making process (Bandman and Bandman 1988: 141–2).

Step 3: Evaluating alternatives

The alternatives may be evaluated in sequential steps — eg the advantages and disadvantages of the first alternative are evaluated, then those of the second alternative, and so forth. Another approach would be to evaluate them in a comparative fashion. In this approach, all the available alternatives are evaluated simultaneously. When evaluating the disadvantages of each alternative, the amount of risk involved in each possible outcome is determined (Lancaster and Lancaster 1982: 27).

Step 4: Selecting an alternative

The selection of the best alternative is often complicated by the fact that the constantly changing environment in health matters causes uncertainty regarding the possible success or failure of a prospective solution. A further complicating factor is the interaction of activities with each other. One activity usually does not achieve a goal without having some positive or negative influence on another goal. This is illustrated by the case of the hospital superintendent who makes decisions to control the hospital's expenses at the cost of inconveniencing the nursing staff to the extent that the nursing turnover rate is increased considerably. The argument followed when selecting a possible conclusion must be as valid and sound as possible. One must critically scrutinize the effects that each conclusion/alternative might have in order to arrive at the best decisions (Bandman and Bandman 1988: 143).

Step 5: Post-decision activities

This step is usually called *implementing the decision,* but the necessary follow-up which must be carried out is more than just the implementation of a decision. Good decisions lose their effectiveness if they are improperly implemented. The nurse administrator should therefore ask the following questions before implementing the decision (Lancaster and Lancaster 1982: 28):

1. What must be done?

2. In what sequence must it be done?

3. Who should do it?

4. How can the necessary steps be most effectively accomplished?

The importance of communicating the reasons for the decision and the logic of the decision to everyone who will be directly or indirectly participating in its implementation cannot be overemphasized. The nurse manager who is able to tell her subordinates in clear and concise language what must be done and why is in a position to enhance the subordinates' willingness to implement the decision. Even the best decision will not achieve the desired goal if the people who are to implement it are not motivated to do it, or if they are willing but do not understand fully what must be done and why it must be done.

Because the nurse manager cannot be sure that the implementation of her decision will automatically meet the desired objective, she must monitor the actual results against the planned results. If deviations occur she should reassess the original objective to be achieved, the method of achieving it, and the actions formulated to achieve it and, if necessary, she must make the required modifications (Lancaster and Lancaster 1992: 28).

TYPES OF NURSING MANAGEMENT DECISIONS

The nurse manager's decisions originate from three distinctive fields, ie:

- from authoritative communications from her superiors;

- from cases referred for decisions by her subordinates;

- from cases originating from the initiative of the nurse manager herself (Barnard and Beyers 1982: 27).

Decisions emanating from instructions from superiors

The nurse manager is faced with these type of decisions when she must decide on the nursing staffing mix she is going to use in her institution, or the number of beds she is willing to staff with nursing personnel in order to stay within the allocated budget for the salaries of nursing personnel in a specific budget year.

Decisions emanating from cases referred by subordinates

These cases arise from the subordinates' incapacity to decide for themselves, because the situation is new or unfamiliar to them, because there are conflicting orders confronting them, or because the necessary authority to decide has not been delegated to them.

The effective nurse manager minimizes this type of decision as far as possible by deciding only about cases which are important or cannot reasonably be delegated (Barnard and Beyers 1982: 27).

Examples of this type of decision are when the nurse manager has to resolve personnel conflicts, or when she has to resolve a relationship problem between the nursing staff and the supporting services, or when the nursing staff are confronted by unreasonable or unfamiliar patient care requests from the medical staff.

Decisions arising from the initiative of the nurse manager

There is much incentive to avoid raising, and taking decisions on, those issues which nobody else is in a position to raise effectively. One's failure to raise the issues will usually not be attacked (Barnard and Beyers 1982: 27).

The nurse manager could easily tell others, as well as herself, that the pressure of her daily workload is too heavy to raise any additional issues. However, it is often an implied condition of service that the occupant of such a senior post should have the will and the energy to make decisions on such matters as the change from functional nursing to team or primary nursing in her institution, or the decision to allocate unit budgetary responsibilities and accountability to unit sisters, or the decision to change the in-service education system from a centrally-organized one to a decentralized departmental one in her institution.

The decision not to decide

According to Barnard, the fine art of executive decision-making involves refraining from making decisions on questions which are not pertinent at the time, not making decisions prematurely, not making a decision which cannot be made effectively, and not making decisions that others should make (Barnard and Beyers 1982: 28).

Not making decisions regarding questions which are not pertinent at the time is good sense. Not deciding questions prematurely means that one does not allow oneself to become prejudiced. Not making decisions that cannot be made effectively is to refrain from destroying authority. Not making decisions that others should make preserves morale, develops competence, fixes responsibility, and preserves authority (Barnard and Beyers 1982: 28).

TOOLS AND TECHNIQUES FOR DECISION-MAKING

The work of the nurse manager has become increasingly demanding and complicated. The environment in which she functions is complex, with intense demands and competition for scarce resources. Most of the decisions which must be made involve varying degrees of uncertainty. The probability of reaching effective and appropriate decisions depends largely on the appropriateness, quality, and amount of information available on which to base a decision. A number of decision support tools and techniques are available to aid the nurse manager in making managerial decisions.

Simulation, models, and games

Simulation is a way of using models and games to simplify a problem by identifying the basic components of the problem and then arriving at a solution by trial-and-error. Through simulation the manager may compare alternatives and their consequences. This is a useful tool when trying to arrive at decisions regarding a contemplated organizational change (Marriner-Tomey 1988: 10).

Models are used to aid decision-making because they represent the real situation, but provide a simplified version of it. The more variables are added to a model, the more realistic but cumbersome it becomes. The more simplified a model becomes, the more useful it is for quantitative analysis and prediction (Marriner-Tomey 1988: 11).

Since the environment in which nursing management decisions must be made is a highly complex one, however, a comprehensive model will usually be called for.

Management games are used to train personnel in decision-making by simulating real-life problem situations in a laboratory setting (Marriner-Tomey 1988: 11).

Decision trees

A decision tree is a graphic display of the available alternatives, the outcomes, risks, and information needs for a specific problem over a period of time (Marriner-Tomey 1988: 11). The process begins when two or more alternative decisions are taken for a specific problem at hand. The problem, and each alternative decision, is displayed graphically on a piece of paper. The probable consequences of each alternative decision are then displayed opposite each decision. The decision tree does not depict an obviously correct decision, but it allows the manager to base her decision on a consideration of various alternatives and the probable consequences of each one (Marriner-Tomey 1988: 11).

Linear programming

Linear programming is a sophisticated short-cut technique in which a computer can be used to determine solutions. Linear programming is dependent on linear relationships — ie relationships where a constant ratio exists between the change in one variable and the change in another variable. Many decisions do not involve linear relationships, but when these relationships exist and the problem is complex and involves thousands of possible choices, this technique is extremely useful (Marriner-Tomey 1988: 15).

For example, a school of nursing might use this technique to determine the size of classes, the number of students, and the numbers of tutors by feeding into the computer equations containing such variables as the students' need to enrol in particular classes, the number of students, the number of tutors qualified to teach the course, and the hours available to conduct the course (Marriner-Tomey 1988: 15).

The pay-off table

This method aims to provide decisions based on statistics. A methodical approach is followed whereby probabilities are assigned to various possible outcomes (Kerrigan 1991: 3). The pay-off is the key component in the selection of an option. Table 22.1 depicts data from a theatre complex of a large hospital where paper gowns are used. It has been determined that, on a weekly basis, there is a 60% probability that 300 gowns will be used and a 40% probability that 350 gowns will be used. The cost of 300 gowns is R30.00 and the cost of 350 gowns is R35.00. If there were a shortage of gowns, a special order would entail an extra cost of R10.00. Thus, if 300 gowns are available and the amount used during the week is 300, the cost is R30.00. If 300 gowns are available but 350 gowns are needed, the cost will be R40.00 (R30.00 for the available ones plus R10.00 for the special order). If 350 gowns are available and 300 used, the cost is R35.00. If 350 gowns are available and 350 are used, the cost is R35.00 (adapted from Kerrigan 1991: 3–4).

Table 22.1: A pay-off table

Alternatives	Results 300 (0.6)	Results 350 (0.4)
300	1. R30.00	2. R40.00
350	3. R35.00	4. R35.00

Although there is only a 0.4 probability that 350 gowns will be used, it is obvious from the above that alternative no. 4 will be the best in relation to the pay-off it provides.

Computers

Computers, when used correctly, can obtain information faster and more efficiently than paper-based record systems. Their applications in management information systems include, among others, patient classification systems, management of supplies, the scheduling of staff, information and management of budgets, and statistical and administrative reports (Marriner-Tomey 1988: 16).

A number of computer programs are available for use in hospital management to support the decisions that are taken by nurse managers. The databases of most of these *decision support systems* (DSS) programs include:

- internal files — eg payroll, patient days, patient accounts;

- external files — eg public health reports, governmental statistics;

- managerial files. Included in these files are the manager's ideas, insights, logic, experience, and style — these might, for example, be in the form of estimates of the need for a certain hospital service.

The database is organized in a special manner to enable the manager to retrieve data on request. The database in a DSS is managed by software called a database management system (Turban 1982: 36).

The applications of the DSS are varied and include statistical analysis, building mathematical models for analysis, or forecasting, and are especially useful for answering 'what-if' questions — eg 'what changes in hospital rates are necessary to achieve a 10% increase in net profit?'

Advantages and limitations of quantitative tools

Quantitative tools encourage a rational, systematic approach to problem solving. In other words, they encourage disciplined thinking. While the human mind can only consider six to seven variables at a time, these tools may evaluate thousands of interrelationships simultaneously (Marriner-Tomey 1988: 15). Decisions which are made with the use of quantitative tools are likely to be superior to decisions that rely heavily on judgement. Unfortunately, many managerial decisions have to be based on intangible, unmeasurable factors and these situations will reduce the effectiveness of the tools. Another aspect which must be considered is that mathematical expressions are based on certain assumptions. If these assumptions are not true for any given situation, the tool in question will become entirely worthless (Marriner-Tomey 1988: 16).

PROBLEM-SOLVING STYLES

There are several styles which can be applied when solving problems. We now discuss several ways in which the issue of problem-solving styles can be approached.

The Vroom and Yetton model

When this model is used for decision-making, a manager makes a choice between five methods of decision-making. She makes this choice according to her own perception of the problem, her personal characteristics, and the assessment that she makes of her own and her subordinates' capabilities. The five methods are as follows:

- Autocratic 1: the manager solves the problem herself by making use of whatever information is available to her at the time.

- Autocratic 2: the manager recognizes that she lacks the necessary information to solve a particular problem. She then approaches her subordinates to get the necessary information from them, informing or not informing them about the nature of the problem. The subordinates are only required to give information, not opinions or tentative solutions.

- Consultative 1: the manager discusses the problem with subordinates on an individual basis. She does not bring them together as a group. She then makes a decision which may or may not represent the opinions and suggestions of the individuals consulted.

- Consultative 2: the manager shares the problem with a number of her subordinates in a group session in order to get their opinions and suggestions. Her subsequent decision may or may not reflect her subordinates' influence.

- Group: the manager, acting as a chairman or discussion leader, shares the problem with the group. Ideas are generated, alternative solutions evaluated, and a final agreement is reached by consensus. She adopts and implements the solution which has the support of the total group (Gillies 1989: 454; Marriner-Tomey 1988: 19).

Experimental use of this model demonstrated that the two autocratic types of decision-making result in more rapid decisions, that subordinates support decisions reached by the consultative methods more than the autocratic methods, and that decisions resulting from the group style elicit the strongest commitment from subordinates (Gillies 1989: 454).

A number of rules regarding the selection of the appropriate method when faced with a problem emanate from this model:

1. If the quality of the decision is important and the manager does not have enough information or the necessary expertise to solve the problem by herself, the autocratic 1 method should be eliminated automatically.

2. If the decision's quality is important for achieving the goals of the institution, and if the subordinates in general lack commitment to the institutional goals, the group method should be eliminated.

3. If the quality of the decision is important for achieving institutional goals, the manager lacks the necessary information, and the problem is unstructured, do not choose the autocratic 1, autocratic 2 or consultative 1 methods. Subordinates will have to be consulted after giving them full knowledge of the problem.

4. If acceptance of the final decision is of decisive importance in terms of its effective implementation, and if it is not certain whether the subordinates will accept an autocratic decision, do not choose the autocratic 1 or autocratic 2 methods.

5. If acceptance of the solution is decisively importance for its effective implementation, if it is not certain that the subordinates will accept an autocratic decision, and if there is a likelihood of conflict over the final solution, shy away from the autocratic 1, autocratic 2 and consultative 1 methods. Face-to-face interchange among subordinates will be needed to resolve the conflicts.

6. If decision's quality is of little importance, if its acceptance is critical for successful implementation, and if subordinates are unlikely to accept an autocratic decision, do not use either the autocratic or consultative methods. Only the group method will ensure acceptance of the decision — and this is the only relevant consideration (Gillies 1989: 455; Marriner-Tomey 1988: 20–1).

Psychological types

The ideas of the Swiss psychologist, Carl Jung, regarding the different personality elements found among people have been refined by Briggs and Myers in the Myers–Briggs Type Indicator (MBTI) which measure one's problem-solving style. The MBTI is currently extremely widely used as an aid in management development. The instrument is used to measure the overriding tendency of an individual to use one of four problem-solving styles. The individual's style will depend on how a problem is perceived and how a conclusion regarding the problem is reached. The four decision-making problem-solving style categories are (Mosley, O'Brien and Pietri 1991: 7):

- sensing and feeling;

- sensing and thinking;

- intuitive feeling;

- intuitive thinking.

Sensing and feeling

Managers who use this decision-making/problem-solving style approach decisions from a factual standpoint. Their feeling orientation make them sympathetic, tactful, and highly receptive to the approval of others. They are also open and trusting in their relations with others. They usually have favourable expectations of others and tend to develop an effective team spirit among their subordinates. Their strength is their human relations, but they tend to tolerate inadequate performance longer than warranted and find it difficult to discipline others (Mosley et al. 1991: 7).

Sensing and thinking

Managers using this type of decision-making style tend to be more comfortable working on problems related to numbers or things, rather than people. People in careers such as engineering, applied science, and construction are often of the sensing-thinking type. They are usually exceptionally conscientious in carrying out duties and responsibilities. Their major strengths lie in carrying out short-term planning, implementation, organizing, and controlling managerial functions. Their areas of weakness are usually long-term or strategic planning and delegating effectively (Mosley et al. 1991: 7).

Intuitive thinking

Managers falling into this category focus on changes and possibilities in an objective, impersonal manner. These managers enjoy complex, unstructured problems, and running organizations. Many entrepreneurs and top managers have this problem-solving style. They are often dynamic leaders with vision who approach new challenges with enthusiasm. One weakness of these managers is that they become so involved with the overall mission that they may lose sight of important details and facts. A further weakness is that they expect excellence from others, but might fail to give praise when this excellence is achieved. They tend to be quick to criticise when things go wrong (Mosley et al. 1991: 8).

Intuitive feeling

This type of manager tends to focus on changes and possibilities but views these from a personal standpoint of serving other's needs. These managers have good conceptual skills and know-how and practise participative management. They usually possess good communication skills and are enthusiastic. The two major weaknesses of these managers are the fact that they tend to over-delegate without implementing controls to see that the delegated assignments are carried out properly, and their reluctance to discipline subordinates (Mosley et al. 1991: 8).

Implications for management

Individuals with different problem-solving strategies invariably tend to clash, making working together difficult. For example, a manager who is strongly intuitive might want to move a group that is trying to solve the problem with him to other issues seemingly unrelated to the issue to be addressed, while most of the members of the group are of the sensing type and feel that a more realistic approach to the problem at hand is necessary (Mosley et al. 1991: 9).

Rowe decision style inventory

According to the Rowe decision style inventory, a person is usually categorized according to his/her decision-making style by one of the following four descriptions:

- directive;

- analytical;

- conceptual;

- behavioural.

The description of each category of style is depicted in figure 22.1. According to research conducted by Ala and Jones, nurses in administration tend to have slight left-hemisphere dominance in their brains but the difference is not a marked one (Ala and Jones 1989: 52). It is important for managers to identify their own decision-making/problem-solving preferences and to become conscious of subjective preferences regarding certain problems.

BASIC DECISION-MAKING STYLES

The astute manager usually has a good understanding of her subordinates' abilities and knowledge, and of the situation which calls for decision-making. She will thus choose the appropriate decision-making style by following the undermentioned guidelines:

- If none of the subordinates have experience or information on a specific area, they cannot contribute to the decision. The manager thus makes an authoritative decision by herself and tells them what to do.

- If the subordinates have some knowledge of a subject, they may be capable of contributing to (but not making) the final decision. The manager should thus seek their help in a consultative manner and make the final decision herself, after considering their input.

- If the subordinates have quite a bit of experience, they can take some of the responsibility for making the decision. The manager should thus use a facilitative strategy to share the decision-making process with them.

- If the subordinates have a thorough understanding of the subject and are willing to deal with it, the manager should delegate. The subordinates are given both the problem and the authority to make a decision (Hersey and Blanchard 1988).

Figure 22.1: Rowe decision style inventory

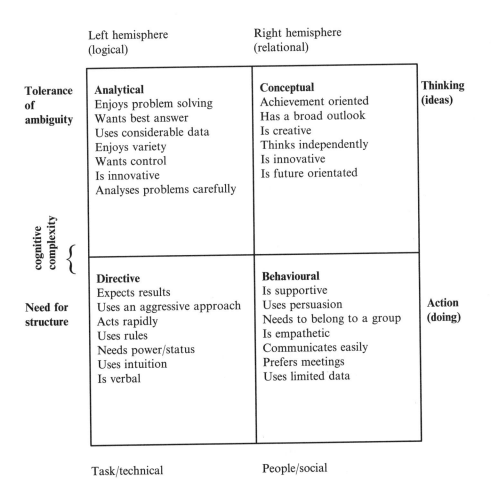

(Adapted from Ala and Jones (1989: 53)

Another approach to some basic decision-making styles is governed by the abilities and knowledge which the subordinates possess as well as the type of decisions which must be made. This approach incorporates the following four styles: directing, guiding, supporting and delegating (Hersey and Blanchard 1988: 418–9).

The directing style should be used when non-negotiable types of decisions are made, such as rules, regulations and clearly defined procedures. The subordinates lack the ability or understanding to make decisions regarding these matters and so the manager gives specific direction where it is needed, makes the rules clearly understood, and maintains tight controls when necessary (Hersey and Blanchard 1988: 418–9).

The guiding style is appropriate when the subordinates want to be involved but lack the ability and understanding to make a decision. The manager involves the subordinates in the decision-making process, but the decisions come primarily from the manager. This type of strategy is used when decisions are made on how to implement managerial strategic decisions. By utilizing this strategy, the manager orientates her people to new assignments, builds their understanding and their abilities, explains decisions, answers questions, and provides coaching and guidance when these are needed (Hersey and Blanchard 1988: 418–9).

The supporting style is appropriate when the manager must be involved in the decision-making process since feedback must be given to a higher authority about the decisions made. This style is used when subordinates possess both the abilities and the understanding to make the decisions. The manager's role, with this style, is to keep the group in setting objectives, to encourage participation of all group members when necessary, to provide support, and to build and maintain confidence among the subordinates responsible for the decision. (Hersey and Blanchard 1988: 418–9).

The delegating style is used when the subordinates are willing, knowledgeable, and able to make the decision themselves. Examples of such decisions usually occur when subordinates must decide what their defined job responsibilities should be. The manager's role in this situation implies that she gives the necessary authority to the subordinates to make decisions and subordinates are given as much responsibility as they can handle. This approach gives people freedom to do their job well (Hershey and Blanchard 1988: 418–9).

Group decision-making

Although group decision-making seems to be increasing nowadays, there is a debate regarding its effectiveness. The advantages of a decision made by a group are the following:

- A group can provide more information regarding a specific problem to be solved, and more variables are thus considered before the final decision is made.

- Non-programmed or novel decisions are made more effectively by using the efforts of a group, because a group is more effective in establishing objectives and identifying and evaluating alternatives as wider knowledge and a broad range of viewpoints are available. A group is also more likely to accept a solution which carries a risk (and to try it out) because responsibility for the decision is carried by the group as a whole and not by one individual (Lancaster and Lancaster 1982: 166).

- If an important change has to be made, it is better to get a group to decide to make this change because management will need the commitment of at least a substantial group of personnel to effectively implement the change — eg a change from functional nursing to team nursing.

The disadvantages of group decision-making are the following:

- It usually takes longer for a group to reach a decision than when an individual is responsible for it.

- In some groups there are strong social pressures for conformity of thought and action, reducing the likelihood of innovative decisions (Gillies 1989: 453).

- All too often, open and honest group discussions are hampered by a feeling of pressure to conform, fear of reprisal, and the influence of a dominant personality who is perceived to have greater status than the others (Lancaster and Lancaster 1982: 166).

- In a group it is possible for an exceptionally strong individual to dominate group discussions to the extent that give-and-take among group members becomes impossible. The decisions reached in such a climate may be of a lesser quality than those reached by an individual, because the most acceptable solution is apt to be a compromise between the best and the worst alternatives (Gillies 1989: 453).

Group decision-making methods

Brainstorming is a method in which the members of a small group, preferably with 10 to 12 members, rapidly generate as many solutions to a problem as possible. The emphasis is on the quantity of the solutions proposed, not so much the quality. As many alternatives as possible should be generated, so judgement regarding the quality of the proposed solutions is deferred until enough alternatives have been put forward to ensure the inclusion of several potentially useful ideas (Gillies 1989: 432).

This method of problem-solving is most effective when group members have similar organizational status, but have a variety of different experiences between them. The group should be told 24 to 48 hours in advance what the problem is that they will have to deal with. The brainstorming session should begin by informing the group members that a large number of ideas are needed in rapid succession, that wild and crazy ideas are not only acceptable but desirable, and that criticism of ideas is forbidden (Gillies 1989: 432). Towards the end of the session the group members should take each new idea generated and evaluate it for originality and flexibility. The more promising ideas are then set aside for extension or refinement later on. Two days after the brainstorming session the facilitator should contact group members to collect any ideas which they have been generating after the session, because some people produce their most creative ideas only after a period of incubation (Gillies 1989: 432).

The *nominal group technique* is a method where members of a group can identify and prioritize goals or solutions to a problem under non-threatening conditions (Gillies 1989: 451).

The technique stimulates creative thought and the prioritizing of problems, solutions, or goals. It is designed to minimize the effect of inhibitions in group members where there is a mix of high and low status members. The group should ideally consist of not more than five to eight people. If a group is large, it is advisable to divide it into smaller groups. The sum total of the different groups' decisions is then established at the end of a session.

While seated together in a group setting, each member lists a number of solutions to the problem during a period of silent formation of ideas. The period could be five or ten minutes, or even up to half an hour if the problem warrants it. The problem or concept must be clearly formulated and presented in writing to the group beforehand. The group leader then asks for one solution to the problem from each member and writes it down on a blackboard or transparency sheet. The group leader then asks for another solution from each member, and this process is continued until all the recommendations or solutions are listed. A solution is only listed once. If another member presents a similar one, the second solution is not listed. The entire group then discusses the solutions in turn, clarifying and elaborating each one.

Each group member is then asked to write down on a separate piece of paper the five best solutions to the problem, according to her own view, and to prioritize these by numbering them from one to five accordingly.

The group leader then collects the pieces of paper and makes a list of the solutions which were numbered first or second, or even third. The results are then communicated to the group. When there is more than one group involved, all the number one solutions are totalled. A final group decision is taken from the pool of solutions (Gillies 1989: 452; Swansburg 1990: 304; Muller 1988: 23).

Another method which eliminates the inhibitory effects of differences in status and personality incompatibilities on group decision-making is the *Delphi method* (Gillies 1989: 452). With this method, the decision-makers never come face-to-face with each other. They remain anonymous throughout the decision process (Gillies 1989: 452). The group leader selects a number of key employees who possess the necessary experience and expertise to make worthwhile contributions.

A questionnaire is sent to each member, asking for opinions and suggestions on an important issue to be resolved. The aim is to elicit a large number of responses in order to be able to compile a list of goals or research priorities at the end of the exercise. The completed questionnaires are returned anonymously to the group leader, whereafter a summary of the subjects' responses is made.

A second round of questionnaires is mailed to the subjects. Included in this second questionnaire is a summary of the responses in the first round, together with direct quotations from respondents as needed in order to clarify their different viewpoints and concerns (Gillies 1989: 452).

The second questionnaire asked the respondents to react to the list of goals, solutions, or research ideas compiled from the first response. The respondents vote for or against each idea/goal/ solution, and they must also indicate their agreement or disagreement with the prioritizing of these ideas/goals/solutions. They must give their reasons if they do not agree with the prioritizing. When the second round of questionnaires is returned, the leader summarizes the responses and reports the refined and perhaps reprioritized goals/solutions to the respondents, asking for their response. Repeated cycles of questionnaires and summaries of responses are generated until consensus is reached concerning a handful of goals/solutions that have been modified and re-ordered to the point where they are all acceptable to the group members who took part in the exercise (Gillies 1989: 452).

Fishbowling is a method designed to improve the quality of a group decision by ensuring a fair and full hearing for each member's opinions and suggestions. The members of the group sit in a circle surrounding a single empty chair. The leader explains that no member of the group may start a discussion without occupying the single middle chair. The speaker occupying the chair will then introduce his viewpoint on the matter to be discussed and explain his opinion in detail. The other members of the group may not interrupt the speaker while he represents his ideas. When he is ready, he will indicate this and the members of the group may then address questions to the speaker. The person in the chair may not relinquish his central position until he is satisfied that his viewpoint has been adequately understood by all group members (Gillies 1989: 452). When all members of the group have had an opportunity to state their opinions as occupants of the middle chair, any member of the group may then propose a recommendation for acceptance by a higher authority or for implementation as a group activity by again occupying the central chair. The session is ended when a majority vote is reached for a recommendation coming from the central chair occupant. The fishbowling technique provides for an orderly group discussion by eliminating irrelevant discussions and distracting cross-talk (Gillies 1989: 453).

PITFALLS IN DECISION-MAKING

The nurse manager can succumb to a number of pitfalls which will affect the quality and effectiveness of her decisions.

When the nurse manager remains an authoritarian controller of the behaviour of others at heart, she will fall into the trap of not consulting her subordinates adequately before a decision is made. By controlling decision-making and preventing those affected by the decisions from participating in the process, she will alienate them. The subordinates may then lack the necessary commitment to put the decisions into practice (Swansburg 1990: 230).

A common pitfall is inadequate fact-finding. Before a decision is made, wide and varied sources of information from authorities on the subject should be consulted. It is not necessary to consult with these authorities personally; their publications can be reviewed (Swansburg 1990: 230).

The pressure of time, resources, and priorities renders the decision-making process in nursing management complex. It is not always possible to obtain all the necessary facts. This produces a measure of uncertainty in the decision-maker, especially when a choice has to be made from multiple alternatives (Swansburg 1990: 230).

When the decision, the reason for it, and the manner in which it should be implemented are poorly communicated to the individuals who are responsible for its implementation, the expected results are often not realized.

If the steps of the decision-making process are not followed, the results of the decision-making process will probably not be as anticipated (Swansburg 1990: 230).

IMPROVING DECISION-MAKING

Apart from the strategies which have already been mentioned for improving decision-making, it is necessary to add the following recommendations.

A successful manager is one who stays informed about decisions being made at various levels in the organization, deals with those decisions requiring her level of expertise, supports the implementation of decisions made by responsible employees, and credits the decision-maker (Swansburg 1990: 230). Managers who make all the decisions themselves convey a lack of trust in the abilities of subordinates and do not contribute to the development of loyalty and self-esteem among those subordinates. According to Wrapp, good managers do not make policy decisions; they concentrate on a limited number of significant issues, identify areas where they can make a difference, judge how hard to force an issue, give a sense of direction to the organization through open-ended objectives, and spot opportunities that will permit others to make decisions and plans for implementation (Wrapp 1967, as quoted in Swansburg 1990: 230).

Managers must also realize that there is a place in the decision-making process for intuitive reasoning abilities. Intuition is a powerful tool guiding executive decision-making.

According to Leo, productive, structured, efficient thinking eliminates irrelevant facts, moves one towards achieving one's goals, enables one to largely ignore the uncertainties inherent in any situation, and get quick management approval for one's decisions because one's thought processes seem logically impeccable (Leo 1984). He stresses, though, that it is necessary to plunge periodically into the outside world of uncertainty and ambiguity; that quantitative analysis makes a contribution to, but is not a substitute for, intelligence, scepticism, and common sense (Leo 1984). He proposes that managers employ lateral thinking periodically when faced with problems in order to think innovatively and creatively. This involves forcing oneself to forget all one knows about a subject, and letting new data, concepts, thinking patterns, and possibilities get into one's mind and receive a fair trial (Leo 1984).

Top managers usually utilize intuitive thinking as one of their tools in guiding their decisions. In an extensive research study by Agar in the 1980s it was found that there are eight conditions in which top-level managers usually make use of intuitive thinking when faced with problematic situations:

- when a high level of uncertainty exists;

- when little previous precedent exists;

- when variables are not easily predicted by scientific measures;

- when 'facts' are limited;

- when the available facts do not clearly point the way to go;

- when analytical data are of little use;

- when several plausible alternative solutions exist to choose from, with good arguments for each;

- when time is limited and there is pressure to come up with the right decision (Agar as quoted by Swansburg 1990: 230–1).

CONCLUSION

There are several strategies and models which the nurse manager can use to arrive at effective decisions. There are also a number of tools and techniques which can assist in decision-making. Decisions can be made by following a rational way of thinking as well as by using an intuitive thinking method. The nurse manager is confronted by a wide range of issues that require her to make decisions, but she should take care not to decide on issues that employees lower down the hierarchical structure could decide on for themselves.

References

Ala, M. and Jones, C. (1989). Decision-making styles of nurses. *Nursing Management,* volume 20, pp. 52–4.

Bardman, E. L. and Bardman, B. (1988). *Critical Thinking in Nursing.* Appleton and Lange: Connecticut.

Barnard, C. and Beyers, M. (1982). The environment of decision. *JONA,* March 1982, pp. 25–9.

Frolic, M. F. (1989). Decision support systems: essential for quality administrative decisions. *Nursing Administration Quarterly,* volume 14, number 1, pp. 1–8.

Gillies, D. A. (1989). *Nursing Management — A Systems Approach.* Saunders: Philadelphia.

Hersey, P. and Blanchard, K. H. (1988). *Management of Organizational Behaviour.* Fifth edition. Prentice-Hall: Englewood Cliffs, New Jersey.

Kerrigan, K. (1991). Decision-making in today's complex environment. *Nursing Administration Quarterly,* volume 15, pp. 1–5.

Lancaster J. and Lancaster, W. (1982). *The Nurse as a Change Agent.* Mosby: St Louis.

Lancaster, W. and Lancaster, J. (1982). Rational decision-making: managing uncertainty. *JONA,* September 1982, pp. 23–7.

Leo, M. (1984). Avoiding the pitfalls of managementthink. *Business Horizons,* May/June 1984, pp. 39–42.

Marriner-Tomey, A. (1988). *Guide to Nursing Management*. Mosby: St Louis.

Mosley, D. C., O'Brien, F. P. and Pietri, P. H. (1991). Problem solving styles determine managers' approach to making decisions. *IM*, September/October 1991, pp. 6–9.

Muller, M. E. (1988). Probleemoplossing nominale groeptegniek. *Nursing RSA*, volume 3, number 9, September 1988, pp. 5 and 23.

Swansburg, R. C. (1990). *Management and Leadership for Nurse Managers*. Jones and Bartlett: Boston.

Turban, E. (1982). Decision support systems in hospitals. *HCM Review* Summer 1982, pp. 35–41.

CHAPTER 23

MANAGEMENT OF CONFLICT

S. W. Booyens

CONTENTS

INTRODUCTION

Conflict may be defined as a situation in which two or more parties become aware of the fact that what each party wants is incompatible with the wishes of the other (Hein and Nicholson 1990: 328).

A degree conflict is essential for the continued development of mature and competent human beings (Kahn et al. as quoted by Cavanagh 1991: 1254). Conflict can also be seen as part of the process of testing and assessing oneself and may thus be viewed as positive in the sense that it gives one an opportunity to make full use of one's reasoning capacities (Deutsch as quoted by Cavanagh 1991: 1254). Conflict provides an opportunity to bring about change and avoid stagnation. It can benefit group behaviour because cohesiveness is usually promoted during times of conflict (Blake and Mouton as quoted by Cavanagh 1991: 1254). Conflict stirs us to use our skills of observation and memory. It shocks us out of sheeplike passivity; it causes us to take note of things and make plans, and it leads to reflection and ingenuity (Dewey, in Hein and Nicholson 1990: 328).

Conflict is not viewed as something negative, as was the case in earlier years. Any organization in which people interact with each other has a potential for conflict. Conflicts are normal and inevitable consequences of social and organizational life (Coser, as referred to by Cavanagh 1991: 1254). However, when conflict in an organization is severe and persistent, too much stress is created and the effect is a disruption of the functioning of the organization, a broken schedule, and general apathy among workers.

CAUSES OF CONFLICT

A potential for conflict exists because of the nature of the upbringing of many nurses and other employees. People may react with hostility towards one another because of basic insecurities and because of unfulfilled emotional needs which emanate from nearly forgotten childhood experiences. When people have to work together closely, as is generally the case with nurses who 'work as a team', the behaviour of some nurses is apt to provoke a hostile reaction from some of their teammates, although the 'instigator' might be totally unaware that her seemingly 'friendly' behaviour might excite other people.

Stress can be created by factors in the working situation such as too little or too much responsibility, lack of managerial support, lack of participation in decision-making, and the need to cope with rapid technological changes. These factors may all lead to the development of conflict situations.

When nurses have to work in close proximity to each other, such as in intensive care units where they constantly have to interact with one another and with the physicians, stress builds up and the potential for conflict is obvious.

When nurses hold beliefs, values, and goals which differ from those of the nurse managers, physicians, patients, visitors, and hospital administrators, the situation is ripe for conflict. For example, nurses' values might differ from those of physicians regarding ethical issues such as abortion, AIDS, and 'do not resuscitate' orders. The personal goals of nurses also frequently differ from organizational goals, particularly with regard to staffing, scheduling, and the general organizational climate within which nurses work (Swansburg 1990: 474).

Nurse managers are often responsible for conflict in as much that they are expected to initiate and institute organizational changes. Change may upset the power equilibrium, threaten vested interests, create stress, and thus invite conflict (Gillies 1989: 480). Leadership style can cause discord. Authoritarianism and dogmatism provide a breeding ground for staff dissension and conflict (Cremer 1980: 24).

Nurse managers are themselves also subjected to considerable stress in their managerial role. They are subjected to the following pressures, among others:

- cost containment;

- improving the standard of patient care;

- collective bargaining;

- consumer awareness and involvement;

- increased accountability; and

- more demanding performance evaluations (Swansburg 1990: 475).

Off-the-job problems which affect the nurse's work performance and which often lead to disciplinary problems and conflict include (Swansburg 1990: 475):

- marital discord;

- alcoholism;

- mental stress; and

- financial problems.

Role ambiguity or confusion, and disagreement between the worker and her supervisor concerning job responsibilities, almost always leads to conflict. 'The greater the number of positions within a workforce, the more common are disagreements about expected role behaviour' (Gillies 1989: 481). Thus, within a given organization, the greater the number of hierarchical levels, the greater is the potential for interpersonal conflict (Gillies 1989: 481).

THE NATURE OF CONFLICT

A negative aspect of conflict is often encountered in nursing when a person in a supervisory position does not want to listen to the conflicting viewpoints of her subordinates. This may lead to hostile and disruptive behaviour and destroy initiative and creativity (Baker and Morgan 1986: 25).

Another negative consequence of conflict is the formation of 'us' versus 'them' cliques, with the result that teamwork is effectively disrupted. Each side becomes concerned with getting the most it can and plays down the other side. It is very difficult to resolve the conflict once it has progressed to this stage. When such a stalemate has developed, the conflict easily escalates and an environment of distorted communication, suspicion, and hostility prevails.

When conflict is not recognized it tends to go underground. It then becomes less direct, more destructive, and eventually more difficult to confront and resolve. New ideas do not appear frequently in this atmosphere and the new exploration of old ideas is also suppressed (Schmidt and Tannenbaum, in Hein and Nicholson 1990: 329).

When conflict is handled properly it can be healthy. When the two opposing parties have buried the hatchet and come to understand each other's viewpoints, a broadening of understanding of the problem develops and the interaction between the parties is perceived as stimulating and interesting.

THE FUNCTION OF CONFLICT

1. The expression of conflict allows the emergence of divergent beliefs and interests. When these divergent views are confronted it may lead to a synthesis, with the organization adapting itself to the real situation. Organizational peace is established in this way.

2. When an organization focuses creatively on the differences between workers, dynamic and lasting contributions are created (Skolik, in Hein and Nicholson 1990: 328).

3. A moderate level of interpersonal conflict may have the following constructive consequences:
   - an increase in motivation and the energy available to do tasks;
   - an increase in innovation because of the greater diversity of viewpoints and the heightened sense of necessity;
   - each party develops a greater awareness of her identity and

position because the parties are forced to articulate their views and to support their arguments (Walton in Hein and Nicholson 1990: 329).

EFFECTS OF CONFLICT

Conflict has an effect on the psychological health of the employees as well as on the general efficiency of the organization. When the employees in an organization experience consistent levels of unhealthy conflict, the trust and respect among them is diminished. The result of this is that relevant information regarding the work at hand is not shared readily, leading to lower productivity (Hein and Nicholson 1990: 330).

When conflict is not expressed directly it will be expressed indirectly — often in ways that create new conflict (Walton, as quoted by Hein and Nicholson 1990: 330). It takes emotional energy to suppress conflict, but it takes even more emotional energy to confront it. Conflict is therefore often handled in an indirect manner. Indirect conflict, however, has a longer life-expectancy and leads to greater costs (Walton, as quoted by Hein and Nicholson 1990: 330), but in indirect conflict one does not have to expose one's feelings.

When conflict is repressed, the hurt and angry/aggressive feelings drain energy away from productive work. Energy may be directed at getting back at the other person or party, and little time and energy is left for devotion to the task at hand (Hein and Nicholson 1990: 330).

The organization which can identify conflict behaviour and confront it before it is suppressed is the more successful one. Such an organization will have to be flexible and able to modify its norms, thereby assuring its continued existence under conditions that have changed (Hein and Nicholson 1990: 330).

STYLES/MODES OF RESOLUTION

There are several ways in which conflict can be resolved. These include avoidance, accommodation, compromise, collaboration, and competition.

Avoidance

In a study by Cavanagh (1991), it was found that the most commonly used conflict-management style among staff nurses and nurse managers in a number of English hospitals was avoidance. This style is associated with individuals who tend to negate their own concerns as well as the concerns of the opposing group (Cavanagh

1991: 258). This is a powerful technique and may be used purposefully to frustrate the other party. One party often withdraws when other methods of resolution have failed.

Avoidance does not solve the problem, and an escalation of the conflict usually develops. There are, however, times when it is necessary to pursue a strategy of withdrawal — ie when the time for discussion is inappropriate, when there is too much hostility, when data are lacking, or when there is no agreement between the parties on what the problem really is (Booth 1982: 452).

Withdrawal or avoidance frequently occurs when there is a great power difference between the two parties, and where the less powerful party is convinced it is unlikely that her concerns can be met. This sometimes occurs when there is a conflict between nurses and doctors, or between nursing auxiliaries and the chief nurse administrator. Alienation occurs when one person decides that it is useless to continue trying to communicate with another and therefore refuses to interact, or leaves the scene. This is often found to so among nurses who resign (Booth 1982: 452).

Individuals who tend to use this style when conflict looms tend not to take a stand or voice their opinions freely. It can lead to important issues being decided by default rather than by having the necessary input from all the staff members concerned (Cavanagh 1991: 258).

Accommodation

This is a co-operative interaction where one party or individual is prepared to give up her own needs for the sake of the other. The non-assertive party feels it is more important to maintain harmonious interpersonal relationships than to express her needs and opinions firmly. Usually this person or party needs the acceptance or approval of others. This person/party will also apologize, if necessary, to get the conflict resolved. Needs, opinions, and wants are usually expressed in a roundabout way (Cavanagh 1991: 1255).

This style is appropriate when the person was wrong, where the opponent is more powerful, when the issue is more important to the other party, when it is important to preserve harmony, or when it is necessary to collect social credits for later, more important issues (Marriner 1982: 29).

Compromise

This style is used by individuals who realize that, in conflict situations, every party cannot always be satisfied. Both parties are thus prepared to give a little and take a little to expedite matters, and expedient, mutually acceptable solutions are sought. The parties or individuals are essentially assertive people who will not always be prepared to put aside their viewpoint for the sake of a quick solution to a conflict. They will assert themselves and adopt another style when the issue at stake is regarded as too important to reach a quick compromise. Compromise leads to a lose–lose atmosphere since both parties have to give up something and are only partially satisfied. It is thus only used when both parties have equivalent power, when the goals are only moderately important, and a quick solution is sought for a limited period (Cavanagh 1991: 1256; Marriner 1982: 29).

Collaboration

When this style is used, there is a mutual willingness between the opposing parties to seek an effective solution which will satisfy both. This is termed a win–win situation, since both parties are concerned about the interests of the other, but are not prepared to give up their own positions simply to appease the desires of the other party (Cavanagh 1991: 1256). Finding an agreeable solution often involves innovative thinking, the weighing of insights from different perspectives, the resolution of hard feelings, and the exploration of alternatives until there is consensus on the final solution. This approach may, unfortunately, take more time than the results are worth.

Competition

This is a power-orientated, unco-operative mode where one individual or party is aggressive and pursues her own goals at the expense of the other. A win–lose situation is thus created (Marriner 1982: 29). This type of conflict resolution is very similar to forcing an issue. When this type of conflict resolution style is used too often, morale is damaged severely and commitment to the organization's goals diminishes markedly. It is appropriate when a quick or unpopular decision is needed, when the person forcing the decision is very knowledgeable about the issue/situation and thus able to make a sound decision, and when one must protect oneself against other aggressive people (Marriner 1982: 29).

Two–dimensional model of conflict resolution

The foregoing five styles of conflict resolution are based on a two-dimensional model. This model compares the degree to which an individual attempts to satisfy his own needs and concerns (assertiveness) with the degree to which an individual attempts to satisfy the needs and concerns of others (co-operation). An individual's conflict management style can thus be described in terms of assertiveness and co-operation: accommodating behaviour is unassertive and co-operative; avoiding behaviour is unassertive and unco-operative; collaborating behaviour is assertive and co-operative; competing behaviour is assertive and unco-operative, and compromising behaviour is placed intermediately between co-operativeness and assertiveness (Cavanagh 1991: 1256–7).

Specific strategies for the management of conflict

Stress listening

When a nurse manager is confronted by an angry sister or nurse who bursts out into a tirade of strong language and half-expressed ideas, the situation is potentially one where tempers can fly within seconds. It is the nurse manager who can turn such an angry confrontation into a productive meeting by employing the strategy of stress listening (Powell 1986: 27). The following points must be remembered when this strategy is used:

1. Sharing anger must be avoided. The nurse manager who reacts sarcastically or angrily to the barrage of words hurled at her becomes caught up in the outbreak herself. The nurse manager should master her emotions by staying calm, matter-of-fact, but sympathetic. This does not mean that she must be aloof or impersonal (Powell 1986: 27).

2. Respond constructively. The nurse manager should try to channel the angry sister's strong emotions into a productive channel. She should therefore convey, by both her verbal and non-verbal responses, that she is giving the problem and the employee her serious attention, and she should make use of the following tactics:

   - Avoid smiling and small talk. A comment, such as 'take a deep breath' to try to calm down the angry person is bound to put him/her on the defensive, adding to the frustration already present (Powell 1986: 27).

   - Maintain continuous eye contact. Continuous (not obtrusive) eye contact will signal to the angry person that her anger is important and noted.

   - Prevent interruptions such as phone calls.

   - Do not hide behind a desk.

   - Seek an informal seating arrangement to encourage communication.

   - Seat the employee.

   - Maintain a serious manner.

   Anger should be treated with respect to get results. If an angry person sees that a problem has the nurse manager's sympathy and understanding, it is easier to find a solution (Powell 1986: 28).

3. Ask questions. The strain of the angry outburst may cause the 'facts' to be poorly described and often to be disguised by emotional interpretations. To search for the cause of the anger, ask short, simple questions in a calm manner. Do not 'correct' any misinterpretations. Instead, guide the employee to an understanding of the problem step-by-step by asking leading questions after listening carefully to answers (Powell 1986: 28).

4. Separate fact from opinion. An angry person often finds it very difficult to separate the actual reasons for stress from her personal opinion about it. Single questions, asked calmly and punctuated by brief dispassionate summaries, will have a calming effect which would direct the anger away from the emotional interpretation and towards a more objective exploration of the facts (Powell 1986: 28). Anger usually stems from a personal evaluation of facts which may be correct but is often incorrect.

5. Avoid hasty responses. 'Haste is the supervisor's worst enemy in stress listening' (Powell 1986: 27). The nurse manager should wait until she understands the whole story, including the personalities involved, before making any decision. Even if the supervisor must respond directly to the employee's outburst, it must still be a planned response, not an impulsive one.

6. Encourage the employee to find a solution. If the nurse manager can present a solution to the problem or analyse it from the angry employee's perspective, the employee will be reassured that her viewpoint has been understood. Suggested solutions should be expressed from the employee's perspective using, if possible, her own reasoning.

7. Help the employee find a solution. Direct the employee with such leading questions as: 'what would you do?' or 'what ideas do you have?' to try to help her find her own solutions. Do not cut short or sidetrack the employee and do not offer paternalistic advice or make embarrassing comments. Let the employee do the interpreting, but point out alternatives when they appear.

When the above tactics are followed, the employee's self-esteem is not challenged and the angry outburst is used to stimulate constructive responses (Powell 1986: 28).

Managing defiance

When an employee defies the management of the nurse manager, she employs a strategy which is aimed at getting the manager to respond in a manner which suggests managerial guilt, lack of self-discipline, and incompetence. The following steps are recommended (Murphy 1984: 68):

1. Distinguish between defiant behaviour and normal on-the-job mistakes, or a hesitancy to accept organizational changes.

2. Identify the defier. Avoid generalizing the defiance to several people. There is usually one central figure responsible for defiance.

3. The manager must prepare herself emotionally and intellectually. She should remember the following opening words for approaching the defiant person: 'I understand you're upset, but...' and 'this is neither an appropriate way or an appropriate setting to discuss this issue. Please join me now for a discussion.' These words must be delivered in a low, calm but firm voice (Murphy 1984: 68). The manager must stay calm at all costs and must restrain herself emotionally.

4. The manner in which the manager communicates with her subordinates should demonstrate to them what is appropriate behaviour. She must, however, do her best to share information of mutual professional interest with them and explain up-coming changes in policy timeously.

5. When challenged, the manager must respond immediately and with the necessary resolve. If possible, move to a private setting; for example, if defiance occurs in a meeting a short break should be called.

6. After the initial incidence of defiance has been handled, a private session or two should follow with the employee to evaluate the behaviour, to probe for underlying reasons, and to teach (Murphy 1984: 69).

Defiant behaviour must be controlled by a manager in a mature, forthright fashion.

Managing defensive people

Explosions of defensive behaviour are often seen among nurses who feel that they are being ignored and that their wishes and needs do not count with nurse managers. The nurse manager may thus be faced by an individual who explodes by firing emotionally charged accusations at her. What should her approach be to such a person? The following six steps should be followed to try to bridge the differences between the two (Silber 1984: 57):

1. Listen actively to what the other person is saying to you. Ask questions to clarify issues where necessary. Allow the defensive person to talk and unwind emotionally until she is completely finished (Silber 1984: 57).

2. Defensive people are psychologically hungry for positive feedback in a one-to-one encounter. You should therefore give them feedback on what you understand from their outburst so that they will realize that you fully understand their needs, their wishes, their ideas, and their complaints. The feedback that you give must show that you recognize their feelings and are empathetic towards them. Empathy, however, does not mean agreement. Defensiveness can be dealt with by truly listening for, and giving feedback on, the emotional meaning of the words used. You must show that you are genuinely willing to work with the other person to improve the situation or relationship (Silber 1984: 58).

3. When emotions have dissipated you should share your point of view of the problem and your knowledge and understanding of the situation. This must be done factually and objectively. No advice should be given and no accusations should be made (Silber 1984: 58).

4. It is now the other person's opportunity to give you feedback on her interpretation of your viewpoint. If there are any misunderstandings or confusions, they must be clarified. To solve the problem(s) and reach an acceptable solution, the information must be differentiated and defined in specific terms.

5. It is now possible for the two individuals to look for common bridges of agreement that can lead to an acceptable solution. Both parties' expectations have been clearly expressed and discrimination between wants or wishes and what must or should be done can be made. Thus a mutual understanding of the issues concerned can form a foundation for trust which can revive the damaged relationship.

6. Finally, one must consider whether the defensive nurse/doctor/ sister had a valid point of view and a better approach to the issue than you had. If this is so, an apology or expression of regret will be the appropriate route to follow. A well-meant apology among professionals can soothe the most turbulent emotions.

Before the interview is ended, the two individuals must decide how a difference of position must be handled in future so that the person need never again charge into the office to cross swords with you again (Silber 1984: 58).

GUIDELINES FOR MANAGING CONFLICT CONSTRUCTIVELY

The following general rules and principles regarding conflict management will stand the nurse manager in good stead:

1. Clear guidelines should be formulated on what is appropriate behaviour to follow when intervening in a conflict situation before any conflict arises — eg do not lose your temper, give each party/person time to state their case, do not allow the two parties to interrupt each other.

2. A supportive environment where people feel free to express their feelings, where they feel free to make unpopular suggestions, and where they can become creative in seeking solutions which will end the conflict, is imperative for conflict resolution.

3. The conflict should be handled in a non-combative way which will produce a win–win solution. When conflicts are conducted as open warfare, people become very hostile towards one another, blaming each other, and no real resolution is possible in such an atmosphere.

4. Choose the correct time for managing the conflict. Postponing confrontation for too long may cause the conflict to escalate. However, although one party may want to confront the other party immediately, the other party may not be prepared for it at that moment, with the result that unnecessary defensiveness and resentment may develop on the part of the unprepared party.

5. Do not hesitate to confront people if their behaviour warrants it. Tell people what you think about the behaviour they exhibit, what is wrong with it, and how it should be corrected.

6. One should focus on the issues at stake, not on the personalities of the people engaged in the conflict. When attacks are launched on the personalities of people engaged in a conflict, the potential for escalation of the conflict is high.

7. Communication must be fostered. Conflicting parties tend not to listen actively to each other; they are more concerned in preparing a defence to the other party's viewpoints. When the two parties do not listen constructively to each other, no agreement can be reached.

8. In a situation of conflict it is necessary for each person/party to understand the perceptions of the other. Although one party may not agree with the other party's perception of the problem, it is still necessary to understand that perception fully in order for communication to be opened up.

9. Mutual interests should be emphasized. The wise nurse manager will try to reconcile the interests of each party rather than the positions of each party, because frequently their interests are similar — eg the improvement of patient care. It is only the

methods for achieving the mutual goals which form the stumbling block. When mutual interests are identified, this will serve as a building block for overcoming the conflict.

10. It is necessary to separate issues because conflicts often involve a number of issues at any time and trying to resolve all of them at once can complicate the process. The different issues should thus be separated into components and only those issues that are important to both parties should be confronted. Some of the other issues may be more important for one party than the other and accommodation will often be found on the part of each party regarding such issues, with the result that the important ones can be more easily resolved.

11. Examine all solutions and accept the one most acceptable to both parties (Swansburg 1990: 479).

12. A premature resolution should be avoided because when a solution is selected before all the options have been examined, it may not be the best one in the long term. One person may still feel dissatisfied, with the result that the conflict will most likely surface again sooner or later. When time is at a premium, it is better to agree to a temporary solution and to agree that this solution will be examined and its success evaluated after an agreed time period (Baker and Morgan 1986: 27–9).

13. The manager must not become defensive or reprimanding or monopolize the conversation. These responses only serve to increase the frustration.

14. When confronted by a defiant person, follow the steps for managing defiant behaviour.

15. When confronted by an emotional outburst, give the person concerned time and use empathetic listening so that she can unwind completely.

16. Indicate, by your behaviour, that you trust and care for your employees, that you are willing to consider viewpoints that differ from your own, and apologize genuinely when you are the one who is at fault (Silber 1984: 58).

GENERAL RULES FOR THE MANAGEMENT OF CONFLICT BETWEEN TWO PARTIES

When one wants to diagnose and resolve a conflict between two conflicting parties it is useful to have a clear understanding of all the differences between the concerns of the parties and the sources of these differences. It is useful to ask:

- What are the areas of agreement between the parties?
- What is the nature of the differences between the concerns of the parties?
- What are the reasons for the differences?

The first step in resolving the conflict is to focus attention on areas of agreement, such as:

- both parties agree that there is a problem;
- both parties agree that the status quo is unsatisfactory;
- both parties agree that something should be done.

In the second step, the nature of the differences should be considered. There may be disagreement over facts, goals, methods, or values. It is far easier to resolve differences over facts than differences over values.

Thirdly, the nurse manager should explore the reasons for the differences, eg:

- parties might not have the same facts;
- parties might have different pieces of information;
- parties might have different perceptions of events;
- parties might define the problem in different ways;
- parties might have different views regarding their own power and authority.

Strategies for conflict resolution include the following:

- Win–lose — eg use of the power of one's position, use of mental or physical power, use of majority rule.
- Lose–lose — eg use of compromises, bribes, resorting to rules, arbitration by a third neutral party.
- Win–win — eg use of problem-solving, reaching consensus, focusing on goals.

NEGOTIATION

The nurse manager is faced with the challenge of incorporating the negotiating process into every aspect of her practice. The art of negotiation is a set of learned and acquired skills which requires a conscious use of some rules, coupled with an imaginative personality.

There are two basic types of negotiation: co-operative (ie everybody wins) and competitive (ie one party wins, the other loses).

There are three criteria that must be met for negotiation to take place:

- the issue must be negotiable;
- the negotiators must be interested in giving as well as taking during the process;
- the negotiating parties must trust each other, as well as the negotiating process (Smeltzer 1991: 26).

There are three rules for effective negotiation:

1. A knowledge of human behaviour is essential.
2. Strategies for negotiation must be understood.
3. The needs of both parties must be met during the process.

The normal behaviour of individuals may change during the negotiation process because of the stress created. Thus behaviour often becomes more routine and less creative. The human needs and feelings which come into play during the process may cloud the issues so that the negotiating process becomes blocked and the application of specific strategies may be needed to get the process back on track.

Principles of negotiation

One or both parties would like to change the relationship between them during the negotiating process. It is thus imperative that the following principles must be adhered to to maintain relationships:

- Maintenance of your own identity and insight into your own motives, values, perceptions, and skills.
- The other party's values must be understood without judgement.
- The issues to be negotiated must be potentially solvable.
- Flexibility must be exhibited when analysing and reacting to issues and behaviours.
- Skills must be used to repair damaged relationships (Smeltzer 1991: 27).
- It is wise to understand the background, needs, goals, personal interests, and feelings of those whom you are dealing with.

Steps in the process

1. Prepare for negotiation — ie introduce the issue(s).
2. Give a general overview of what is to be accomplished during the process.

3. Orientate everyone briefly on why negotiation is required on particular issues.

4. Define or redefine the issues to be addressed.

5. A logistical plan for when each issue will be worked on must be developed.

6. Discussions must be encouraged during the conflict stage.

7. Aspects on which a compromise must be reached must now be addressed.

8. Agreement in principle must be reached in the settlement stage.

9. The agreement must be restated and summarized.

10. Compliance with the agreement must be monitored after settlement is reached (Smeltzer 1991: 27–8).

Rules for negotiating

- It is important to appear in attire in which you feel comfortable and presentable.

- The language that you are using should be appropriate for the occasion. When selling an idea, it should be explained in a positive way — that is what it will solve, why it will work, and what it will improve.

- The attitude that one conveys is important. A positive attitude which conveys that one expects to achieve good results will have the potential for acceptable compromises. No energy should be wasted in questioning other people's motives while negotiating. When one is searching for hidden motives instead of concentrating on what is said and on the proposals which are put forth, the outcome is rarely successful. An attitude of confidence, which comes from careful preparation and positive beliefs about the right to pursue a certain solution, should guide the negotiating process. One should be in control of one's attitude at all times.

- Agree on terminology. It is impossible to reach a meeting of minds unless everyone is talking the same language.

- Both parties should listen actively to each other's suggestions and ideas. Encourage the other party to explain further, asking about the exact benefits of the idea, and giving feedback on how you see the idea benefiting the situation and on the obstacles to its implementation. Furthermore, one needs to probe and find out how the obstacles could be overcome and to suggest ideas to this effect.

- It is necessary to be assertive during the process. An apologetic attitude will not achieve anything.

- The correct information and facts should be brought to the negotiating table; one should focus on one's strengths and negotiate within a realistic range.

- Questions can be used to gain control over the situation or change the tone of the process. Questions can be used to call attention to a specific point, to give information, to initiate a thinking process, or to cause the discussion to reach a conclusion.

- Encourage full expression of positive and negative feelings within an accepting atmosphere.

- Key themes in discussions should be identified and restated at regular intervals.

- The parties should be encouraged to provide frequent feedback on each other's comments. Each party must truly understand the other's position (Sullivan and Decker 1992: 481).

- Each party's self-respect should be protected. The conflicting issues must be dealt with, not the personalities of individuals.

- The creation of a defensive environment must be avoided by communicating ideas clearly, not overreacting to the stress created, not rejecting alternatives prematurely, and by the disclosure of real feelings.

- Strategies to overcome deadlocks in the process include calling a caucus among a party's members, summarizing ideas, changing the subject, asking hypothetical questions, diagnosing differences, and talking about the past and future needs of both parties. It may even help to change the environment by moving from one room to another (Smeltzer 1991: 28).

- At an agreed interval, the progress made should be followed up.

- At the closure of the process, positive feedback should be given to the participants regarding their contributions and co-operation in solving the conflict (Sullivan and Decker 1992: 481).

RULES FOR THE PREVENTION OF CONFLICT

1. Establish clear rules, policies, and guidelines in your organization, and make them known to every employee.

2. Appreciate the efforts of people and be genuine in your praise for work well done. People must feel that they are worthwhile to the organization where they are employed.

3. Create a supportive climate where people are free to try out new ways of doing things. This energizes people to make suggestions, and it promotes creative thinking which, in turn, leads to better solutions to problems. Relationships are also strengthened when employees work in such an environment (Swansburg 1990: 479).

4. Avoid power play where your decisions or plans are apt to create conflict because the employees do not agree on implementing them. Rather seek agreement by trying to serve some interests of both parties (Swansburg 1990: 479).

5. The manager who has the necessary self-esteem recognizes the contribution she has to make and possesses the ability to value the input of others.

6. The manager should be able to identify with the values of others. This creates an atmosphere of open relationships with an expectancy of success (Webb 1985: 17).

7. She should be able to quickly identify the traits of responsibility and trustworthiness in others, producing warm and open responses (Webb 1985: 17).

8. Nurse managers should behave assertively, especially in situations which hold high priority for them.

9. If the nurse manager wants a satisfied staff who can focus on job productivity, it would seem well worth the effort to provide active support and open communication (Clark 1979: 23).

10. Feedback about behaviour is constructive, but not feedback about personality traits. She would be wise not to give advice, but to enlist the other's help in finding solutions and identifying tasks to be completed. Desired behaviours should be stated, those that do not meet a level of satisfaction should be pinpointed, suggestions from employees on how to change unsatisfactory behaviour should be supported, and a system of rewards for attaining certain levels of competence should be built into the managerial organization (Clark 1979: 24).

CONCLUSION

Conflict situations in nursing are rife and research indicates that the handling of conflict is one of the manager's responsibilities which she likes least. Nevertheless, it is essential that conflict be identified and managed constructively in order for an organization to prosper and to produce work of a high quality. The nurse manager who follows the guidelines given here might find that she becomes more adept at handling the conflict in her particular work situation.

References

Baker, M. K. and Morgan, P. J. (1986). Building a professional image: handling conflict. *Supervisory Management,* February 1986, pp. 24–9.

Booth, R. Z. (1982). Conflict resolution. *Nursing Outlook,* September/October 1982, pp. 447–53.

Cavanagh, S. J. (1991). The conflict management style of staff nurses and nurse managers. *Journal of Advanced Nursing,* volume 16, pp. 1245–60.

Clark, C. C. (1979). Assertiveness issues for nursing administrators and managers. *JONA,* July 1979, pp. 20–4.

Cremer, L. M. (1980). Dealing with conflict — the role of the ward sister. *Curationis,* volume 3, number 1, pp. 22–5.

Gillies, D. A. (1989). *Nursing Management. A Systems Approach.* Second edition. Saunders: Philadelphia.

Green, C. P. (1986). How to recognize hostility and what to do about it. *American Journal of Nursing,* volume 86, number 11, pp. 1230–4.

Hein, E. C. and Nicholson, M. J. (1990). *Contemporary Leadership Behaviour: Selected Readings.* Third edition. Lippincott: Philadelphia.

Marriner, A. (1982). Comparing strategies and their use in managing conflict. *Nursing Management,* volume 13, number 6, pp. 29–31.

Jacobsen-Webb, M. (1985). Team building: key to executive success. *JONA,* volume 15, number 2, February 1985, pp. 16–19.

Powell, J. T. (1986). Communication. Stress listening: coping with angry confrontations. *Personnel Journal,* May 1986, pp. 28–9.

Silber, M. (1984). Managing confrontations: once more into the breach. *Nursing Management,* volume 15, number 4, pp. 54–8.

Smeltzer, C. H. (1991). The art of negotiation. *JONA,* volume 21, number 7/8, pp. 26–9.

Sullivan, E. J. and Decker, P. J. (1992). *Effective Management in Nursing.* Third edition. Addison-Wesley: New York.

Swansburg, R. C. (1990). *Management and Leadership for Nurse Managers.* Jones and Bartlett: Boston.

PART FIVE:

CONTROL

CHAPTER 24

PERFORMANCE APPRAISAL AND PRODUCTIVITY

Rosemaré Troskie

CONTENTS

INTRODUCTION

Performance appraisal involves determining the worth of a person's work performance using different measures. Good management requires accountability and requires the acceptance of responsibility for delegated work. Evaluation of work performance is an essential control measure.

To use evaluation as an instructive instrument, feedback should be given to the person who has been evaluated. This will address her developmental needs. Evaluation implies that measurable norms have been set. In nursing, the employee's training requirements, scope of practice, and job requirements are norms that could be used to evaluate job performance. As evaluation involves generalization, describing judgement in terms of measurement, one should guard against subjectivity. This is especially important when dealing with a 'once-off' instance of good or poor performance (Troskie 1990: 19–20).

Performance appraisal could be described as a systematic process whereby an employee's strengths and developmental needs can be evaluated, and where various methods can be used to enhance the employee's productivity. Merit rating is linked to performance appraisal. In South Africa, merit rating was introduced to improve the productivity of civil servants and was subsequently adopted by employers in all sectors. Each employer decides on the incentives he or she will use. These incentives could be monetary, or could involve recognition through promotion, or the delegation of more responsibilities or authority.

REASONS FOR EVALUATION

1. The main reason for performance appraisal is to improve work performance, thus enhancing the productivity of an employee. Unsatisfactory workers are informed of the areas that need improvement and satisfactory workers are also encouraged to improve. Guidelines are given on how to improve work performance.

2. People who are ready for promotion are identified, special skills are observed, and training needs are noted.

3. Evaluation also serves to determine whether goals have been achieved and whether standards within the organization have been adhered to.

4. Productive employees can be remunerated in accordance with their achievements. This remuneration or merit pay could

enhance the employee's self-motivation. In theory, according to Geis (1987: 133), merit pay reinforces excellent work. In practice, however, the objective of consistent improved performance is not always achieved and a system of merit pay may even lead to frustration and may hinder work performance.

5. Problem areas in the work situation can be detected and eliminated. When the problem areas and reasons for their existence have been identified, steps can be taken to overcome them. Reasons could be a lack of practice, training, knowledge, or motivation (Bernhard and Walsh 1990: 199–200).

6. Personnel research is enhanced as information related to the work performance of personnel becomes known. One can determine whether personnel turnover is more prominent amongst poor performers or not.

7. Personnel can be placed according to their abilities, and reasons for not performing up to standard can be determined (Hellriegel and Slocum 1989: 759).

8. Events in an organization can be controlled, results achieved by individual employees and groups can be compared, and formal and informal guidance towards professional development can be administered (La Monica 1990: 307). Evaluation is important for setting and attaining organizational and personal goals.

9. A review of an individual's performance should also reduce costly turnover and absenteeism by increasing the commitment of employees to the institution.

10. Evaluation should also help to decrease or eliminate grievances and win employees over to management's side by instilling a team spirit (Riley 1983: 32).

11. The developmental and training needs of nurses can be identified.

12. Evaluation could form the basis for termination of employment when consistently poor appraisals follow on real and consistent efforts to remedy the problem (Tappen 1989: 464).

13. In order to improve coaching and developmental planning the manager and employee should agree on personal and professional development goals at the beginning of the year. These objectives are not the normal job performance objectives, but are additional ones. Personal development goals relate to such skills as communication, planning, time management, and human relation skills, while professional goals relate to growth and development within each employee's current job (Deets and Tyler 1986: 51–2).

PRINCIPLES OF PERFORMANCE APPRAISAL

1. Evaluation should be carried out in accordance with set standards and objectives related to job requirements. The objectives that the employee should pursue should be based on the job description for the specific post.

2. The performance that is evaluated should be directly related to the standards and objectives that are included in the job description (which are also known as the *key performance areas*). According to Bornman (1992) the employee and her supervisor should sit around a table, decide on the employee's key performance areas, and set certain objectives to meet the requirements within these areas.

3. The supervisor should work with the employee over a long period of time. Too wide a span of control does not contribute towards effective evaluation. The direct supervisor is therefore the appropriate person to evaluate the employee (La Monica 1990: 307).

4. A representative sample of the employee's performance should be monitored. Isolated cases of unusually good or bad performance should not influence the evaluation, but one should attempt to assess the norm (Gillies 1989: 538).

5. The evaluation should be based on *job related behaviour* (Hellriegel and Slocum 1989: 765). The appraisal should focus on employee behaviour and results rather than on personal traits or characteristics such as enthusiasm or personality.

6. People who participate in evaluation should be taught how to use the system (McConnell 1984: 112–3). They should be trained to identify satisfactory job performance, how to complete the relevant forms, and how to give feedback.

7. Feedback should be given immediately after evaluation and it should focus primarily on positive aspects. This will result in a willingness to discuss the negative areas where a plan for improvement should be developed.

8. The employee should be given recognition when she performs well. Recognition, and not criticism, is the key motivator for improved performance. It is thus recommended that the employee and the supervisor who is carrying out the appraisal consult a list of job skills and mark those areas where the employee excelled or did well. These marked skills should be discussed during the feedback session, before discussing and setting goals for improvement. It is unwise to dwell on an

employee's developmental needs because the supervisor always reflects some of her biases when evaluating another person and there are very few employees who are able to truly accept negative judgement (Riley 1983: 33).

9. Attainable, measurable, and realistic goals should be set by both the reviewer and the employee. Active participation in goal-setting by the employee will ensure increased motivation to reach the goals. It is essential to set time-limits for the achievement of goals.

10. Feedback should be explained carefully so that the employee understands what has been said. This can be done by giving factual and accurate information. Respect the employee by listening to the explanation given for conduct under discussion, and indicate that you understand her viewpoint (Warfle and Hopper 1987: 115)

11. One of the most common sources of dissatisfaction among employees regarding performance appraisal outcomes occurs when an employee who was above average on certain skills does not receive a promotion while another employee who was above average on another set of skills satisfies the reviewer's criteria for promotion. It is thus imperative that the key performance areas of each job — ie those areas which are more heavily weighted than others regarding importance for appraisal — should be identified and made known among employees long before evaluation takes place.

12. To become proficient in doing an formal appraisal of an employee, the supervisor must practice by evaluating the employee on a day-to-day or continuous basis. This evaluation should at times be written down and shared with the employee.

13. It is essential that performance appraisals accurately reflect the employee's actual performance on the job. If the ratings are inaccurate, promotions will be seen as unfair, necessary training may not be implemented, and employee morale and motivation will be reduced (Sullivan and Decker 1992: 351).

14. The organization should have a mechanism whereby employees may appeal against the results of an appraisal.

FREQUENCY OF EVALUATION

The frequency of evaluation is a matter of some debate and varies from annual evaluation to continuous evaluation. Most authors, however, agree that evaluation should be carried out as soon as the orientation period has elapsed and then at regular intervals. Since many employers prescribe a trial period of three months before permanent employment, the first evaluation usually occurs after a three month period. It is assumed that the employee will socialize into the service, get into the routine, and accept the responsibilities prescribed in the job description during the trial period.

After the trial period the supervisor should evaluate the employee and give feedback on the areas that are satisfactory as well as the areas that need development (Troskie 1990: 276–8). Evaluation will only be effective if it is a continuous process. Even if the official form is only completed every three months the employee should be observed continuously.

Continuous evaluation will ensure that good practices are reinforced and that areas that need development are developed to ensure a satisfactory work pattern.

COMPONENTS TO BE EVALUATED

The nurse's job comprises a variety of activities. The multi-dimensional nature of the nurse's job requires a variety of performance dimensions to be evaluated, for example: initiative, job knowledge, communication skills, interpersonal skills, responsibility, and leadership abilities.

The appraisal instrument might focus on employees' traits, results of work performance, or their behaviour in executing their daily work (Sullivan and Decker 1992: 352). Most appraisal systems assess a combination of traits, results, and behaviours. The main objective which must be achieved by the performance appraisal will usually dictate which components will be used in the instrument.

When an appraisal is carried out for the purpose of promotion, results of work performance and behaviour should be evaluated. When appraisal is carried out for the purpose of determining training or developmental needs, the behaviour and the individual traits of the employee should be noted. The kind of evaluation used to determine merit, however, depends on the nature of the job, as well as the way in which the work is organized in the organization (Szilagyi and Wallace 1990: 522).

Traits or personal characteristics, such as initiative, ability to handle stress, integrity, and responsibility are often used in appraisal instruments because these traits are relevant to a variety of positions in the organization. Ratings on instruments reflecting *only* personal traits or characteristics may give rise to much discontent among employees. Court findings have not been favourable regarding organizations using these traits as the only dimension for appraisal when legal problems have arisen from low rating on such traits (Sullivan and Decker 1992: 354).

Although an appraisal instrument comprising objective, quantifiable results of performance is the ideal for evaluating work performance, it is unfortunately not easy to quantify such aspects as provision of quality care.

The use of behavioural criteria has gained some ground in recent years, but such criteria are time-consuming to develop and are usually only applicable to a narrow range of jobs.

A combination of the types of criteria mentioned above are usually included in the more recent types of appraisal instruments.

COMPILING THE EVALUATION INSTRUMENT

The instrument should be compiled in a way that is easily understood and can be used by both the employer and employee. Criteria for evaluation should be understood and agreed upon by both parties. The development of a reliable and valid instrument takes time but could have positive results. To ensure that the instrument is valid, the objectives for key performance areas should be included. The reliability of the performance appraisal is the extent to which it measures the level of work performance in accordance with the expectations laid down by the job description (Jerning and Young 1985: 35). The language should be simple and comprehensible to ensure that everyone interprets the terms in the same manner. The instrument should be simply-made and clear instructions should be given on how to use it.

Bias must be prevented and objectivity promoted as far as possible. Most supervisors display a degree of subjectivity by evaluating a subordinate according to their own expectations, resulting in ratings which are either too high or too low.

Avoid emotive words as they have a negative influence on the validity and the reliability of the instrument. Eliminate adjectives and adverbs such as 'manipulative', 'untidy', 'disorganized', 'reliable' (Gillies 1989: 542).

To evaluate effectively, the evaluator should know the work performance that should be evaluated as well as the knowledge and skills of the employee. The evaluator should have the ability to communicate the results of the evaluation, and must be willing to spend enough time doing evaluations and discussing them with the employees to achieve good results.

Stalker et al. (1986) describe the development of an appraisal instrument with the help of the computer. A tool was used that measured the performance of a clinical nurse with 70 indicators of behaviour which could be rated from 1–4 with a fifth column for 'not applicable'. The item scores for 256 completed forms were analysed by the computer. If an item was not applicable 70% or more of the time, or if the distribution of scores on an item did not follow a normal curve, the item was eliminated. In this way 32 of the 70 items were eliminated.

A factor analysis was then used to group clusters of items which belonged together. Ten factors emerged, with 44 items having a factor loading of 0.40 or greater. The four best performance indicators were selected for each performance category (Stalker et al. 1986: 13).

The categories of performance were (Stalker et al. 1986: 14):

- responsibility to patients;
- assessment of patients;
- implementing patient care;
- teaching/counselling patients and families;
- recording skills;
- leading staff;
- teaching/counselling staff;
- evaluating staff;
- self-development;
- research aptitude.

The rating scale for the 40 items is a seven point one. Because there was a belief that some types of nursing performance were of greater importance than others, the scoring of different categories was weighted. The categories which scored the highest were: responsibility to the patient, assessment of the patient, implementing patient care, teaching/counselling patients and families, and leading the staff. This instrument proved to be reliable and valid for appraising the performance of a certain category of nurse (Stalker 1986: 17).

METHODS OF EVALUATION

Evaluation can be formal or informal. To evaluate the real work performance of an employee both methods should be used. Informal evaluation takes place mainly while the employee is performing her work in the group. It can also be done during a ward round, or while a procedure is being performed. Participation during a meeting can be evaluated. The reaction of others can be monitored — for example a patient's reaction to treatment (Douglass 1992: 201).

Formal evaluation can be carried out as follows:

Essay report

The evaluator writes her own opinion without predetermined guidelines. This method of evaluation is not always reliable as a considerable amount of subjectivity is involved. The report should be based on the job description. The evaluator will have to make a number of brief observations or evaluations of the employee's behaviour over a lengthy period of time, otherwise patterns of behaviour will not be identified.

The reliability and usefulness of the report will depend on the evaluator's ability to express herself in writing. Expressing themselves in prose is, however, not the strong point of most nurses. The writing ability of the evaluator alone could thus make for an unreliable report, not because the evaluator intended it but because her writing is vague to the extent that the report's meeting could be ambiguous. Essay evaluation should thus only be used in combination with other evaluation formats.

Critical incidents

Critical incidents can be recorded by both the employee and the supervisor. The incident should be confirmed by giving the time, date, and people involved. The importance of the incident and its relationship to the employee's responsibilities should be described. To be identified as a critical incident the incident should have made a definite difference in the work setting, and it can only be defined as a critical incident when it involves behaviour or an action which is out of the ordinary. The results may be positive or negative. The incident should be linked to set standards (Douglass 1992: 201).

Noting these events may aid the formal appraisal carried out at the end of the year. The supervisor will, however, have to make the recording of critical incidents one of her regular activities. It is important to write down the action that took place and not only the supervisor's interpretation — eg 'Susan was rude to the patient'. Ideally the good critical incidents that were observed should be shared with employees, and they should be praised for their outstanding performance. Negative incidents should be shared with the view of improving behaviour and performance and warning employees that performance was unsatisfactory as soon as possible.

Ranking

The employee is measured against the performance of her co-workers in terms of whether she does her work just as well, better, or poorer than her colleagues. The evaluator ranks the nurses in order from highest to lowest, even if she does not feel there are real differences between them. Ranking might also take into account the different aspects of the job which are to be evaluated. Thus a nurse may be ranked highest with regard to assessment of patients' problems on admission, but lowest on giving adequate information to patients on discharge. The major problems with this type of evaluation are that the nurses must all be of the same category to be ranked against each other, it takes considerable time to do the ratings, and they can only be used with small numbers of staff.

Graphic rating scales

A Likert-type graphic scale measurement is used to measure work performance — for example, on a scale from 1 to 5, where 1 is equal to minimal work performance and 5 equals maximum work performance. The evaluator must indicate where she feels that the employee's conduct should be placed on the scale.

Unfortunately there is considerable scope for error because one rater might assign a number 3 to a specific type of conduct, while another might mark the same conduct as 4 or 5 on the form. The scale could therefore be made a little more reliable by adding words to the numbers, for example, 'poor or unsatisfactory (1)'; 'fair or below average (2)'; 'good or average (3)'; 'very good or above average (4)'; 'excellent or outstanding (5)'.

Even the meanings of the above words ('average'; 'fair or below average') might not be clear to all evaluators. An effort is sometimes made to be more descriptive regarding a number's meaning. Troskie (1990: 73–4) uses the scale below to evaluate newly-qualified nurses:

- Level 1 = Supervision and instruction are needed. Was not introduced to the theory and principles.

- Level 2 = Supervision is needed. Understands theory and principles, but has had limited practice.

- Level 3 = Safe, but practice is needed. Able to perform without supervision, but needs practice to perform efficiently.

- Level 4 = Completely competent. Can perform efficiently without supervision.

In addition to the above scales, behaviour expectations scales (BES) have been developed as well as behaviour observation scales (BOS).

The development of behaviour expectation and observation scales is done in the following sequence:

1. The basic task dimensions of a job are identified.

2. Critical incidents which will describe effective and ineffective behaviour that is relevant to the chosen dimensions are described.

3. Several groups of expert judges are asked to judge the relationship of each critical incident to a dimension and then to rate the

behaviour in the incident in terms of how effective it will be in achieving the objectivity associated with the task dimension.

4. Items for which there is disagreement are thrown out. The result is a pool of very specific items describing effective and ineffective behaviours for a particular job (Szilagyi and Wallace 1990: 543).

An example of a behaviour expectation scale is given in figure 24.1.

Figure 24.1: A behaviour expectation scale

4 — You could expect this nurse to accommodate a visitor's wishes within reason.

3 — You could expect this nurse to consider the visitor's request sympathetically.

2 — You could expect this nurse to explain the reason for her refusal.

1 — You could expect this nurse to refuse point blank to admit visitors outside visiting hours,

---

An example of a behaviour observation scale, is depicted in figure 24.2.

Figure 24.2: A behaviour observation scale

1. Arrives at work on time.	Almost always 1 2 3 4 5 Almost never
2. Does not document the patient's condition.	Almost always 1 2 3 4 5 Almost never
3. When unsure about the doctor's request, discusses it with the professional nurse in charge.	Almost always 1 2 3 4 5 Almost never

---

Forced choice comparison

The evaluator selects the descriptive statement that best describes the employee, or the statement that describes her least well, from a number of descriptions. Both positive and negative items are grouped, which forces the evaluator to choose from both in order to describe the employee's behaviour. The following is an example that could be used:

Choose the description that is best suited to describe the employee as well as the one which is least likely to describe her:

(1) is respected by peers

(2) tends to complain about work

(3) immediately reports any change in a patient's condition

(4) cannot handle an emergency (Gillies 1989: 542)

Criterion reference skills

Criterion reference skills are directly related to the job description and include communication skills, interpersonal relationships, and supervision and teaching skills. The steps in the nursing process are usually referred to. The supervisor and the employee must agree on the criteria for evaluation (Douglass 1992: 202).

Checklist and weighted checklist

A checklist contains all nursing activities expected of the employee. The appraiser marks the 'yes' or 'no' column to indicate whether a task has been carried out. A space may be provided to comment on any aspect of performance. The frequency or degree of performance is not addressed (Douglass 1992: 201–2). According to Andrews (1985) the checklist comprises several descriptive statements, and only those applicable to the specific employee are marked. The grand total of the statement is used as the appraisal mark.

The weighted checklist includes both effective and ineffective descriptive statements concerning work performance. The statements are classified from 'excellent' to 'poor' (Andrews 1985: 318).

Management by objectives

The job description should be used as a basis for appraisal. Performance standards should be described in behavioural terms. The behaviour expected of the employee should be clearly indicated. Both appraiser and employee should participate in the evaluation. Then they discuss the outcome and set short-term objectives to improve performance. This is a less subjective method of evaluation.

The objectives that should be met during the evaluation period are determined by both the appraiser and the employee. At the end of the period they jointly decide to what extent the objectives have been met. The employee is given the opportunity to develop creative, critical thinking to find better methods to perform the job. Employees are guided to do their own appraisals using predetermined norms.

Self-evaluation

Self-evaluation is an important component of evaluation, as nobody knows the potential of the employee better than herself. The accuracy of evaluation can be enhanced by setting criteria for evaluation. Self-evaluation is always formative as the person involved strives towards maximum development.

Peer group evaluation

People at the same level of employment evaluate one another and compare their performance. The problem is that they sometimes refrain from giving negative feedback. O'Loughlin and Kaulbach (1981) describe the peer review system which was instituted in a hospital. The process involved five stages, namely:

1. Review of the charts, kardex, and the care plans of the patients cared for by the nurse being evaluated.

2. An interview with the patients.

3. Observation of the nurse.

4. Summary of findings by the review group.

5. Presentation of the findings and recommendations to the reviewed nurse.

The nurse who was to be evaluated was told in advance of the date, but not who the appraiser would be. The three appraisers were also chosen at the same time, in order for them to observe the nurse prior to the date of the formal evaluation (O'Loughlin and Kaulbach 1981: 23).

On the day of the review, two evaluators reviewed the charts, kardex and care plans, while the third interviewed the patients to determine their satisfaction with the nursing care that they had received. The three reviewers then met and completed the professional skills appraisal tool, which was a list of minimum standards regarding nursing care for primary nursing. The tool comprised 76 items grouped under the following headings (O'Loughlin and Kaulbach 1981: 24–5):

- technical competence;
- communication skills;
- organizational skills;
- originality;
- judgement;
- assertiveness/forcefulness;
- achievement;
- human relations.

The reviewed nurse usually carried out a self-evaluation as well using the above tool. A discussion was then held where the evaluations were discussed. A senior professional nurse, area supervisor, or nursing service manager was usually invited to attend the discussion.

The two authors reported that the nursing staff were still hesitant at that stage about accepting the use of this system for performance appraisal.

Key performance areas

The Transvaal Provincial Administration, under the auspices of Dr Bornman (1992), instituted a method of appraisal similar to that described by Cocheu (1986: 91–105). The system had six objectives:

- a uniform approach in the organization;
- management by objectives, modified to suit the service;
- active employee participation;
- periodic review and update;
- differentiated performance levels;
- employee development (Cocheu 1986: 94–5).

The system required a rating scale that would encourage employees to set challenging objectives. Cocheu (1986) used the terms 'exceeded', 'achieved' and 'below' to indicate the extent to which employees met specific expectations. Each level of performance was defined to give the appraiser a guide for assigning ratings.

The next step was to plan the performance of the employee. Both the supervisor and the employee defined important elements in the employee's job. Bornman (1992) used the term *key performance areas* and Cocheu (1986) *key result areas* to describe these elements. For the purpose of this discussion the term *key performance areas* will be used. These key performance areas represent the specific areas for which the employee is held accountable for producing results. For each key performance area, the specific end result which the employee plans to accomplish should be indicated.

Objectives are then drafted by the employee and the supervisor. These should be based on the goals of the organization. After coming to an agreement as to which objectives are attainable, the objectives are prioritized according to their relevance for organizational goals. The time in which the objectives should be achieved is specified, as well as the methods to be used to attain them.

Progress reviews are carried out after specific periods ranging from three to six months. At these reviews the strengths and the areas that need development are determined. Objectives are reviewed and adjusted if necessary.

Part of the appraisal is directed at performance factors. The performance factors used in the public sector are job performance, knowledge and insight, interpersonal relations, and leadership. Critical incidents are used to verify performance in these areas (Cocheu 1986: 102).

Job performance factors to be evaluated are responsibility, organization, and productivity. Examples of skills which are evaluated to assess responsibility are a sense of duty, loyalty, and correctness; those skills used to assess organization are planning and adaptability, and those used to assess productivity are work speed, quality, and drive. Examples of skills evaluated under knowledge and insight are initiative and the ability to identify the core of a problem. Examples of skills evaluated under interpersonal relations are tact, adaptability, and ability to handle conflict. Skills that are evaluated to assess leadership abilities are self-confidence, ability to discipline personnel, and the exercise of controlling measures with regard to personnel's conduct and activities.

At the final appraisal review the extent to which objectives were achieved is evaluated as well as the development that has taken place. The supervisor and the employee have the opportunity to make comments to defend their appraisals.

PROBLEMS IN PERFORMANCE APPRAISAL

Many performance appraisal programmes are unsuccessful in achieving their original goals. The following are some of the problems experienced:

1. Effective performance appraisal takes time and energy. It cannot be left until the last minute. When it becomes a one-way process where the employee does not participate, the manager will not get the co-operation of the employee, and work performance will not improve.

2. Incomplete data-gathering, using a limited number of appraisals, can create a false image. Appraisal must be done regularly and completely. Often an inappropriate method of evaluation, concentrating only on mistakes, is used. The inability to distinguish between present and past performance can also lead to unfair appraisal.

3. The most important problem in performance appraisal is subjectivity in the appraiser's judgement. Two people can observe and judge an employee in totally different ways.

4. The halo effect. This implies that the appraiser evaluates all the dimensions of the employee's work performance at the same level. It happens when the appraiser bases her judgement on general impressions. Another reason can be that the appraiser's knowledge of the employee's work performance is influenced by only one aspect of her work. When appraisal is conducted on the basis of personality and traits the halo effect is more prominent. The rater who erroneously thinks that if a person is friendly and good-natured she will render good nursing care without question, may assess an employee as 'friendly' and then rate

her highly on all aspects of her job performance whether the rating truly reflects performance levels or not.

5. Clarity of standards. The concepts used in the evaluation instrument should be clear and should be understood by the appraiser. The employee should be informed about what is expected of her in the job. Terminology should be defined — for example, what is good, satisfactory, and poor.

6. Not being acquainted with the employee. Appraisers who do not acquaint themselves with employees cannot evaluate them fairly. The appraiser then tends to evaluate the employee as satisfactory (Andrews 1985: 325).

7. Differences between appraisers. A person's own values and norms often determine her actions and can influence an evaluation. When one supervisor evaluates an entire group this effect will not be as prominent because everyone will be evaluated according to the same norms. When different people are involved in the evaluation, the evaluation could differ from one person to another. Clarifying the rating scales could limit this factor (Andrews 1985: 325).

8. Strict or lenient appraisal. When a supervisor evaluates a subordinate according to her own standards rather than the standards set for the evaluation, the subordinate could be evaluated too strictly or too leniently. This 'similar-to-me' error also occurs when the evaluator permits one aspect of the individual's behaviour to influence all the others. It thus follows that if the evaluator is extremely tidy, the subordinate who appears to be somewhat disorganized or untidy in one area of her work, or in her general appearance, will be likely to receive low ratings on all the aspects of her performance which are evaluated.

9. Ego-involvement. Sometimes a supervisor's ego causes a subordinate to be appraised more highly than is deserved. This is an error of judgement which should be guarded against (Andrews 1985: 325).

10. Sometimes the evaluator will assess an employee as 'average' because the evaluator does not want to be criticized (Andrews 1985: 325).

11. The 'horns effect'. An employee is appraised at a lower level because of one of the following reasons (Gillies 1989: 546):

    • an employee who has consistently shown performance that has been above average makes a mistake shortly before the final evaluation and this influences the evaluation negatively;

- an employee's performance is above average but she tends to differ from the supervisor;

- an employee performs excellently but does not conform with the supervisor's ideas of, for example, acceptable dress and demeanour;

- an employee performs better than average but associates with colleagues who perform poorly.

PERFORMANCE APPRAISAL WITH MERIT RATING

When performance appraisal is associated with merit rating, the following aspects should be kept in mind.

According to Herzberg, money alone does not motivate but it can keep employees' morale and productivity at an acceptable level. Other motivators should be used to supplement it. Employees will experience greater job satisfaction and will exhibit a better relationship with their employers if they are remunerated adequately for their performance (Jernigan and Young 1985: 59–60).

Other motivators include recognition, success, promotion, and responsibility. If a task is performed to perfection and the supervisor acknowledges it by giving praise, the employee feels valued. Giving the employee more responsibility increases her self-confidence in her own abilities. Promotion that is not necessarily accompanied by increased remuneration could also be a motivator that promotes higher productivity (Jernigan and Young 1985: 60).

The system of monetary remuneration should be used with great deliberation and fairness. If the system is not accepted as fair, it will not be successful. Ambiguity in the requirements for remuneration brings about many obstacles (Jernigan and Young 1985: 60).

The key to successful monetary remuneration rests in effective and acceptable performance appraisal.

Problems with merit pay administration

Three main problems have been identified by Geis (1987: 132). These problems are the following:

- pay and performance are perceived as unrelated;

- secrecy of merit pay leads employees to believe that inequity in increases exists;

- the sizes of the increases are too small to be effective.

The economic state of the country often prevents employers from rewarding outstanding performance with a pay increase. The amount of money available, rather than performance, determines salary increases (Geis 1987: 134–5).

REASONS WHY PERFORMANCE APPRAISALS FAIL

1. Judgements about personalities serve as the basis for evaluation. Personality traits are often the criteria used to evaluate employees. Words like 'adaptability', 'initiative', 'reliability', and 'attitude' have a strong personality connotation. Semantic problems also occur when using these criteria. It is therefore essential that these criteria should be clearly defined in order for everyone who participates in the evaluation to interpret them in the same manner (McConnell 1984: 109–10).

2. Appraisers are often not competent to evaluate. Often the people doing the evaluation are not able to make personality judgements as it is difficult to distinguish between the causes and the results of behaviour. This can result in conflict and interpersonal problems being labelled as unacceptable behaviour. It is, however, not the behaviour that should be changed — rather, the conflict should be resolved (McConnell 1984: 110).

3. Appraisers do not feel comfortable in their roles. Making permanent records of an evaluation of an employee's performance is a serious matter as it could influence her whole career. This causes the appraiser to evaluate people at a higher level than they deserve, or else everyone is evaluated on the same level to prevent extreme evaluations. Resistance to carrying out the performance appraisals is also a cause for failure of the system, and often no follow-up is done (McConnell 1984: 111–2). The appraiser often finds it difficult to evaluate the employee because she is not familiar with the system.

4. The appraiser has the wrong attitude. The appraiser is too sensitive to the psychological reaction of the employee because:
   - most employees see themselves as average;
   - the appraiser believes that the employee will not like her if she is evaluated as below average;
   - evaluation is a time-consuming activity;
   - when differences in performance are identified, it results in jealousy, rivalry, and hostility.

5. The employee has the wrong attitude (Metzger 1988: 63).
   - The employee feels that if she is an average worker she will not get opportunities for promotion, or she feels that being evaluated as below average will give her a stigma that will stay with her throughout her work-life.

- The employee believes that being recommended for further study, identifies her as a borderline case.

6. Sometimes employees are only evaluated once a year, when the form has to be filled in. This results in the employee being unaware of areas that needs developing. Filling-in forms is often done when pressure is put onsupervisors by management (Geis 1987: 135).

Sullivan and Decker (1992: 316) recommend the following measures to be considered to overcome some of these obstacles:

- The nurse manager needs to be rewarded for doing performance appraisal conscientiously.

- The nurse manager's superior needs to present a good model of how an appraisal should be performed.

- The nurses who have been rated highly should be rewarded: pay increases should not be 'across-the-board', and promotion should be tied to outstanding performance.

PERFORMANCE APPRAISAL INTERVIEW (REVIEWING SESSION)

Giving positive feedback is an essential skill for nurse managera. The instrument that can be used to give feedback is a *performance appraisal review*. This interview is carried out to determine to what extent the objectives that were set have been achieved. During the interview, the results achieved are measured against agreed objectives as set out by the employee and supervisor. The value of this system is that performance is planned systematically and the employee is more willing to co-operate because she participated in the planning phase. The interview should not contain elements of surprise, so the employee should also receive feedback during the whole evaluation period (Hellriegel and Slocum 1989: 765).

The objectives of this interview are to:

- inform employees of possible areas that need development and to decide on methods to develop those areas;

- ensure that employees identify their strengths and experience the appreciation of management;

- take the employees' future performance into consideration and to motivate them to achieve new objectives;

- give the employees the opportunity to air their views.

The results of poor performance appraisal interviews

Often the evaluation process meets the requirements but the interview is not well planned. Some services do not involve the employee in this final phase of evaluation, and make decisions only on the supervisor's evaluation. In the absence of input from the employee, the validity of the evaluation is questionable. Inefficient interviews often also have the following effects:

- A demoralized workforce may develop because employees do not know how they are performing.

- High personnel turnover is experienced because of insufficient recognition.

- An apathetic attitude, or complacency, may develop depending on the outcome of the evaluation.

- Misunderstanding, hostility, and even sabotage may be experienced when an employee feels that the evaluation is unfair.

- Good performers are discouraged by the interview and their productivity diminishes, especially when general comments are made and specific incidents are not mentioned. Appraisers often think that good performers can handle criticism well and put more emphasis on negative aspects.

- Poor performers are not touched by the interview and do not know where they should improve because the interviewer does not emphasize the areas that need improvement.

- When interviews are only conducted annually there are more negative feelings because feedback on both good and bad activities are given too long after they have actually occurred. Employees cannot handle a great amount of criticism at one time (Zima 1983: 253–6).

Characteristics of a good performance appraisal interview

Successful performance appraisal interviews that motivate an employee to improve her work performance should, according to Zima (1983: 258), have the following characteristics:

- a high level of participation of the employee in the development of the evaluation process;

- a helpful and constructive attitude rather than a critical approach by the supervisor;

- solutions to problems that could obstruct the employee's work performance should actively be sought;

- objectives that should be achieved in the future must be set co-operatively between the employee and the supervisor.

According to Malinauskas and Clement (1987: 170) the skills that the interviewer should acquire are the following:

- Verbal skills. These are necessary to give feedback to the employee. The terms used in discussing the employee's performance should have a positive connotation — for example, concentrate on 'developmental needs' rather than 'shortcomings'. Use descriptive rather than evaluative words since judgmental terms lead to defensiveness. Be supportive by conveying empathy — for example 'we all make mistakes like that. That is quite understandable.'

- Listening skills. The supervisor can detect how the employee feels about the evaluation through listening. Paraphrasing indicates that the supervisor has been listening and understands what the employee has said. The employee can also correct any misunderstandings. Ask open-ended questions which give the employee the opportunity to clarify certain issues. The interview should be a two-way process where both people have the opportunity to air their views and to defend their conduct. Listening skills deal primarily with emotions.

- Non-verbal skills. Body language plays an important part in the interview. The supervisor should first of all be aware of her own body language and secondly be aware of that of the person she is interviewing. Tone of voice, and how something is said, often determines whether the listener believes what is being said. Both content and emotions can be conveyed by body language.

Checkpoints to determine the causes of performance problems

A systematic analysis of the facets of the problems in an employee's performance is necessary to determine their causes. Zima (1983: 258) proposed the following points to be checked:

- Shortcomings related to skills and knowledge. Employees who do not have the necessary skills and knowledge will not be able to perform adequately. Performance objectives and the individual's training needs and experience should be investigated. Discussions with other supervisors and the observation of actual work performance could contribute towards discovering the shortcomings of personnel.

- Organizational obstacles could obstruct an employee when performing a task. Obstacles could include a lack of time, an incorrect priority list, and defective apparatus. Workflow analysis, and discussions with supervisors, employees, and patients can also help to identify shortcomings.

- Behavioural obstacles. Interpersonal factors can get in the way of effective work performance. Interdepartmental conflict is a serious obstacle that can result in disruptive competition, mistrust between members, non-participation, and poor co-ordination.

- Wrong use of motivation or incentives. When an employee's potential is underutilized, the employee's post should be analysed to see if there are sufficient challenges.

Planning a performance appraisal interview

Plan the contents of interviews so that all subjects have been covered. The following can be done to ensure that everything is at hand:

1. Keep all records. To enable the supervisor to give positive feedback on an employee's work performance, all incidents and situations that could display the employee's work performance should be recorded. Both good and bad aspects of work performance should be recorded to prevent hearsay evidence. The supervisor should study the job description of the employee as well as all records before the interview. All the objectives that were set for the employee should be taken into account. The employee should be aware of the evaluation criteria, and should have time to prepare herself to give feedback on her performance. The evaluation form, together with all the information at hand, should be studied carefully and an assessment of the evaluation should be made.

2. Study the employee's job description. The aspects that should be addressed can be identified if the responsibilities of the employee are compared with the objectives set at the beginning of the evaluation period. Checking what is expected of the employee can contribute towards identifying strengths and areas that need development.

3. Give the employee notice of the interview beforehand. At least one week's notice is necessary. It is good practice to give the employee an indication of what will be discussed. The supervisor should determine in advance how effective the employee's work performance is, what the reasons are for her performance, and if necessary what can be done to improve performance. This preparation will ensure that the most important aspects are covered during the interview.

Conducting the performance appraisal interview

- Create a climate conducive to the success of the interview and bring about rapport with the employee.

- Use the guidelines as set out in the evaluation form to ensure that all the necessary aspects are covered.

- First discuss the strengths and give the necessary support.

- Do not address more than two areas that need development at a time, listen to what the employee has to say about them, be sparing with criticism, and get the employee's opinion on key issues before making a judgment.

- When the supervisor gives her evaluation she should concentrate on work performance standards, not personality traits. The supervisor should be very specific as to what 'good' and 'poor' performance mean to ensure that the employee knows clearly where improvement is needed.

- Give the employee the opportunity to disagree with the evaluation. The discussion should be guided towards specific incidents and methods of improving work performance.

- Listen carefully to what the employee has to say and respond to it. A good practice is to repeat periodically what has been said and acknowledge what the employee is saying.

- Solve problems before the interview ends.

- Plan together for improvement, and decide on a date to evaluate progress. Assure the employee of support from the supervisor or management in attaining the new objectives.

- After the interview, the supervisor should monitor the employee's progress and good performance should be rewarded.

- Communication after the interview is just as important as during the interview.

- Recognition by remuneration (merit pay, praise) when objectives have been achieved motivates employees to be successful (Hellriegel and Slocum 1989: 765–6).

Some 'do nots' during a performance appraisal interview

- Do not discuss personalities, keep to the work.

- Do not play essential criticism down — the employee should become aware of its importance.

- Do not use the 'sandwich' method where recognition alternates with critique: the recognition will not be noticed by the employee.

- Do not criticize the employee for issues that are beyond her control. This will result in justified criticism not being accepted.

- Do not argue over the evaluation, just give the evaluation with the necessary explanation (Hellriegel and Slocum 1989: 765–6; Douglass 1992: 203).

Evaluating the interview

The interview should be evaluated to determine whether:

- a relaxed atmosphere was attained;
- the employee was at ease;
- the evaluator was at ease;
- the employee participated in the interview;
- there was two-way communication;
- the employee's self-evaluation was requested;
- feedback on the employee's work performance was given;
- the evaluation was based on predetermined criteria (and if not why not?);
- the critique was constructive and, if not, what was negative;
- all the areas of performance were covered (and, if any were not, why not?);
- specific examples were given when criticizing an issue;
- comments were aimed at work performance;
- the employee was asked to propose methods for improvement;
- objectives and programmes to meet them were set jointly;
- the employee was not compared with other personnel;
- salaries and remuneration packages were left out of the discussion;
- the 'sandwich' technique was avoided;
- the interview left positive impressions, and what these were;
- there were any negative aspects, and what these were.

PRODUCTIVITY AND PERFORMANCE APPRAISAL

Productivity is a complex and multidimensional matter, basically seen as a calculated ratio between input and output. The main issue remains effective utilization of available resources (Ibielski 1991: 128). The more input that needs to be invested to get the same expected outcome, the lower the productivity.

Productivity should be seen as a ratio rather than a constant, so management should determine in advance what the minimum acceptable performance for each employee should involve (Ward and Price 1991: 415).

Effectiveness refers to the successful achievement of expected outcomes and the economical use of resources. These two variables are an integral part of productivity (Ward and Price 1991: 415).

HOW TO IMPROVE PRODUCTIVITY

1. Improve the methods of work performance so that the job can be done in a shorter time. Provide personnel with the necessary equipment to assist them in functioning effectively. Time saved can be used to eliminate overtime and mistakes, and can improve the quality of patient care (Ward and Price 1991: 415).

2. Non-nursing tasks should not be done by nurses. Prevent unnecessary paperwork or meetings. Include staff in compiling an evaluation instrument; ensure they get feedback after evaluation (Pritchard, Roth, Jones and Roth 1990/1991: 57–63).

3. The workload should correspond with the number and the categories of personnel. If there is an imbalance between the personnel and workload, there is an increase in personnel turnover and absenteeism (Gupta 1991: 357).

4. When the health care personnel work as a team instead of working in segmented units, unnecessary meetings and overlapping are prevented. Duplication of information is eliminated and a more horizontal authority structure is established. More responsibility and job enlargement increases the productivity of personnel (Gupta 1991: 358).

5. The development of a sound patient classification system to determine the number of hours of nursing care that each patient requires is a prerequisite for determining the number of nursing personnel which an institution or unit should have. It is thus necessary to calculate the staff complement that a service needs since it is one of the main input factors regarding productivity.

6. Careful analysis should also be made of the type or types of nursing care modalities which would render the most effective service with the existing nursing staff members.

7. Try to streamline nursing documentation. Eliminate duplication of documentation where possible. Bedside flow sheets, with appropriately labelled sections which the nurse should complete whilst working with the patient, should be used more.

8. Health education should be carried out in groups as far as possible, and video-presentations should also be incorporated, as well as clear informative booklets that patients can take home with them.

9. The use of equipment and supplies must be controlled conscientiously. Inventory control should remain an important feature in this control function.

10. Nursing staff should become knowledgeable about economic aspects of their profession such as marketing, productivity, cost-containment, accountability, and human resource management.

11. The contributions of professional nurses should be maximized through participative management and other decentralized decision-making structures.

12. People are more productive when they find their jobs meaningful. To enhance the importance of the job the following should be considered: task identity, variety of skills, significance of task, autonomy, and feedback coming from the job itself (Guthrie et al. 1985: 18).

CONCLUSION

Performance appraisal and productivity are inseparable. Personnel should be aware of the standards and criteria against which productivity will be measured. The evaluation process is a continuous process of assessing the employee's performance. Both the supervisor and the employee should participate in the process. Each participant in the process should know how the evaluation should be done. Feedback and repeating the evaluation are essential components of performance appraisal.

According to Stahl (1983: 46) appraisal of employees' performance should be directed towards:

- developing standards of satisfactory performance

- identifying employees' strengths and weaknesses and providing effective counselling;

- refinement and validation of personnel appraisal techniques;

- establishing an objective basis for personnel actions such as selection, placement, promotion, and salary advancements.

The main problems experienced in developing an appraisal system are objectifying standards and determining what to appraise as well as ensuring that the performance reported is representative and not exceptional (Stahl 1983: 48).

References

Andrews, Y. (1985). *Die Personeelfunksie*. Haum: Pretoria.

Bernard, L. A. and Walsh, M. (1990). *Leadership. The Key to the Professionalization of Nursing*. Second edition. Mosby: St Louis.

Cocheu, T. (1986). Performance appraisal: a case in points. In *Performance Evaluation, an Essential Management Tool*, edited by C. S. Becker. ICMA: Washington.

Deets, N. R. and Tyler, D. T. (1986). How Xerox improved its performance appraisals. *Personnel Journal*, April 1986, pp. 50–2.

Douglass, L. M. (1992). *The Effective Nurse Leader Manager*. Fourth edition. Mosby: St Louis.

Geis, A. A. (1987). Making merit pay work. In *Performance Evaluation, an Essential Management Tool*, edited by C. S. Becker. ICMA: Washington.

Gillies, D. A. (1989). *Nursing Management: a Systems Approach*. Second edition. Saunders: Philadelphia.

Gupta, Y. P. (1991). Emerging productivity and cost control in the hospital industry. *National Productivity Review*, Summer 1991, pp. 351–65.

Guthrie, M. B., Mauer, G., Zawacki, R. A. and Couger, J. D. (1985). Productivity: how much does this job mean? *Nursing Management*, volume 16, number 2, pp. 16–20.

Hellriegel, D. and Slocum, J. W. (1989) *Management*. Fifth edition. Addison-Wesley: Menlo Park.

Ibielski, D. (1991). Productivity must not be inhuman. *National Productivity Review*, Spring 1991, pp. 127–8.

Jerning, D. K. and Young, A. P. (1985). *Standards, Job Descriptions, and Performance Evaluations for Nursing Practice*. Appleton-Century-Crofts: Norwalk.

La Monica, E. L. (1990). *Management in Nursing*. Springer: New York.

Malinauskas, B. K. and Clement, R. W. (1987). Performance appraisal interviewing for tangible results. In *Performance Evaluation, an Essential Management Tool*, edited by C. S. Becker. ICMA: Washington.

McConnel, C. R. (1984). *Managing the Health Care Professional*. Aspen: Rockville..

Metzger, N. (1988). *The Health Care Supervisor's Handbook*. Aspen: New York.

O'Loughlin, E. L. and Kaulbach, D. (1981). Peer review: a perspective for performance appraisal. *JONA*, volume 11, number 9, pp. 22–7.

Pritchard, R. D., Roth, P. L., Jones, S. D. and Roth, P. G. (1991). Implementing feedback systems to enhance productivity: a practical guide. *National Productivity Review*, Winter 1990–1, pp. 57–66.

Puetz, B. E. (1985). *Evaluation in Nursing Staff Development: Methods and Models.* Aspen: Rockville.

Riley, M. (1983). Employee performance reviews that work. *JONA,* volume 13, number 10, pp. 32–3.

Stalker, M., Kornblith, A. B., Lewis, P. M. and Parker, R. (1986). Measurement technology applications in performance appraisal. *JONA,* volume 16, number 4, pp. 12–17.

Sullivan, E. J. and Decker, P. J. (1992). *Effective Management in Nursing.* Addison-Wesley: Menlo Park.

Szilagyi, A. D. and Wallace, M. J. (1990). *Organizational Behavior and Performance.* Scott Foresman: Illinois.

Troskie, R. (1990). *'n Kritiese Evaluering van die Bevoegdheid van die Nuutgekwalifiseerde Verpleegkundige.* D.Litt. et Phil verhandeling, Universiteit van Suid-Afrika. UNISA: Pretoria.

Ward, M. J. and Price, S. A. (1991). *Issues in Nursing Administration — Selected Readings.* Mosby: St Louis.

Warfle, D. M. and Hopper, L. (1987). Managing employee performance. In *Performance Evaluation, an Essential Management Tool,* Edited by C. S. Becker. ICMA: Washington.

Zima, J. P. (1983). *Interviewing: the Key to Effective Management.* SRA: Chicago.

CHAPTER 25

RISK MANAGEMENT

S. Koch

CONTENTS

INTRODUCTION

Risk management is a relatively new field. The interest that has developed in this aspect of nursing and patient care may be attributed to several factors. These include the following (Dienemann 1990: 61):

- the current emphasis on quality assurance;

- rising insurance premiums resulting from successful malpractice claims;

- AIDS; and

- radiation.

Directors of health services today demand programmes to protect the resources and assets of their organizations.

In health services, a risk involves the possibility of harm or financial loss to the institution. When a patient or employee sustains injuries in a hospital and claims compensation, the hospital could suffer financial losses as a result. A comprehensive quality control programme should include the control of risks to patients, hospital employees, and other members of the health care team.

Risk management in the health service developed from a need to counter rising costs caused by increased insurance premiums which institutions had to pay as a result of successful malpractice claims.

RISK MANAGEMENT AND QUALITY ASSURANCE

In some institutions quality control and risk management programmes and committees are combined. Both risk management and quality assurance, however, are merely different approaches to the same general problem. Both techniques aim to improve the quality of patient care, but the motivation behind them is different.

Risk management is seen as a technique for reducing financial losses — for example those losses resulting from malpractice claims. Quality assurance, on the other hand, is seen as a process for monitoring and improving the quality of patient care in hospitals.

GREATER ACCOUNTABILITY

In spite of limited funds and resources, nursing professionals are expected to provide high quality nursing care. Nursing professionals can be, and often are, held accountable for negligence, but the authorities have to bear the financial burden of malpractice and negligence claims against the hospital.

Successful claims against nursing staff have been divided into eight categories, because most claims fall into one of these categories (Dienemann 1990: 62; Swansburg 1990: 514–18). The categories are:

- administration of medicine;

- accidents related to assistance during operations;

- falls;

- burns;

- electric shock;

- nosocomial infections;

- mistaken identity; and

- misinterpretation of signs and symptoms.

THE PURPOSE OF RISK MANAGEMENT

The purpose of risk management is to establish a programme to identify and correct shortcomings in the care of patients. In this way malpractice claims can be prevented.

There is a very real possibility that incidents may take place in health services. Consumers of health services are aware of this. An incident is any occurrence which does not comply with the routine functioning of a hospital or the routine care of a particular patient. It may be an accident, or a situation which holds serious implications for the patient or staff member involved. When an incident with negative consequences occurs, some consumers claim compensation. Swansburg (1990: 511) reports that statistics from one insurance company show that 85% of the compensation claims it pays are related to events that occur in hospitals.

Health care services, including hospitals and nursing institutions, are generally regarded as business concerns, and many consumers are ready to exploit an incident with negative consequences. Many incidents are preventable, and public awareness of this fact has led to an increase in claims for compensation.

Swansburg (1990: 512) states that the objectives of a risk management programme are:

- the protection of the assets of a hospital against claims for indemnity;

- control over injuries;

- to be as effective and economical as possible.

THE CLASSIFICATION OF RISKS

Risks can be divided into five categories:

- prevented risks;

- normally prevented risks;

- managed risks;

- unprevented risks; and

- unpreventable risks.

Referr to Richards and Rathbun (1983: 24) for further details.

RISK MANAGEMENT PROGRAMME

It is important that a risk management programme for nursing services should be linked to the existing organizational programme. Familiarity with the organizational programme and communication with the risk manager will lead to co-operation and the smooth functioning of the risk management system as everyone will be working towards the same objectives.

Dienemann (1990: 62) states that an institution's risk management programme should include the following:

- a declaration of intent;

- the structure of the risk management committee;

- an interrelationship between risk management and quality assurance, on-the-job training, patient advocacy, professional health and safety, fire safety, and security programmes;

- reporting of incidents and risk detection policies, procedures, trends, and the results of analyses;

- risk financing plans, including recommendations concerning what kind of insurance cover is needed and the level of this cover;

- a claims management programme;

- a mechanism for the annual evaluation of the risk management programme.

A copy of the risk manager's job description will help the nurse manager to understand the unique and important role of this person. The risk manager is central to the design of a risk programme for the nursing profession. Dienemann (1990: 62) states that many risk managers are nursing professionals with concomitant experience in quality care.

Components of a risk management programme

The identification and control of risks are two important components of a well-designed risk management programme, according to Dienemann (1990: 63–9).

Risk identification

- Risk identification is achieved through routine reporting of incidents. It is essential that nursing staff are trained in this regard so that they know what to report. The routine reporting of incidents should be part of the programme.

- Those who are reporting an incident must not report their own view of why the incident occurred or of what could have prevented it. Only the incident itself must be reported; it should be reported timeously, and the events leading up to it should be reported in the actual sequence in which they occurred.

- Incident reports provide a good indication of what is needed and form an important subsection of risk management programmes.

- Incidents should always be reported immediately and in writing. All health institutions have standard forms for this purpose. Policy regarding the immediate reporting of incidents should be strictly followed. The head of an institution should be informed by telephone about the occurrence of a serious incident even before the written report reaches him.

- Each incident should be evaluated to determine its degree of seriousness. After the incident report has been completed, a decision must be made on how to use this information to prevent the recurrence of the incident.

- Trend analysis. This kind of analysis includes routine analysis of particular aspects of importance — eg in incidents involving falls the aspects to analyse would include, for example, the patient's age and diagnosis, the type of unit involved, and any sedatives taken. A computer can be handy here. Quarterly or annual summaries will facilitate the drawing up of a profile of incidents.

Risk control

The second component of risk management is risk control. A proactive risk management system, in which steps are taken to rectify problems that have been identified, helps to prevent risks.

When a change in policy is needed to prevent the occurrence of specific accidents, it requires specific and open communication channels in order to notify all employees as soon as possible of the change.

When an incident has occurred, it is wise to be open with those involved. Inform them that you are aware of the incident and intend taking the necessary steps to rectify the matter.

Potential problems and threats of legal action should be reported immediately — not only to the head of the institution, but also to the risk manager (or anyone specifically responsible for risk management). The risk manager will analyse the situation and inform all those involved in the incident of her analysis. The patient will be visited in order to gain his perspective. Family members concerned will be asked for their account of the incident and will be assured that a repetition of the incident will be avoided. It is important to maintain communication and good relations with the parties involved and to handle the matter professionally in order to prevent legal steps from being taken.

Risk management activities

According to Swansburg (1990: 512), the risk management process entails:

- identification of actual risks;

- analysis of risks in terms of possible losses;

- development of risk control and risk financing techniques;

- monitoring the risk control programme for effectiveness, and modifying it if necessary.

Sullivan and Decker (1992: 455) state that risk management demands a team approach. It should be a daily and continuous process of detection, training, and intervention.

The programme requires high commitment, including commitment from the chief executive officer and the head of nursing services.

Sullivan and Decker (1992: 455) maintain that a risk management programme should include the following activities:

- identification of possible risks of accidents, injuries, or financial losses;

- reviewing current monitoring systems (incident reports, audits, committee minutes, oral complaints, patient questionnaires) of the institution, evaluation of their completeness, and establishing whether additional systems are required in order to provide the factual details which are essential to risk management control;

- analysing the frequency, degree of seriousness, and causes of incidents; planning risk intervention strategies required and estimating the possible losses associated with various kinds of incidents;

- reviewing and appraising risks relating to patient care procedures and new programmes;

- monitoring laws and codes relating to safety, consent, and care;

- eliminating or decreasing risks as far as possible;

- reviewing the work of other committees to determine potential risks and recommending preventative or remedial action. Examples of these committees are the infection control, medical audit, nursing audit, and safety/security committees.

- identifying the need to educate patients, families, and implementing suitable educational programmes;

- evaluating the results of the risk management programme;

- providing regular reports to top management and medical staff.

The establishment of a risk management programme begins with the top executives, who should also supply the resources. A risk management committee is then appointed. The members of the risk management committee are responsible for overall planning and decision-making in respect of risk management. The appointment of a risk manager is necessary in order to ensure the effective implementation of the risk management programme and to oversee its day-to-day management.

A risk management committee should be an interdisciplinary body including doctors, nursing professionals, chairpersons of related committees (eg infection control), a representative from patient accounts, legal council (ex officio), and representatives from insurance companies and training co-ordinators by invitation.

THE INCIDENT REPORT

Points to take note of when writing a report of an incident include the following:

- Reports must be in triplicate.

- The truth is important — the support of the hospital/authority can thus be obtained.

- Use clear and unprejudiced language; be brief and do not digress from the topic. Use the correct technical terms, for example 'inflamed', 'urinal', 'sitting position'.

- Make sure that all the copies are legible.

- Write the report as soon as possible after the event while the details are still fresh in your memory.

- Try not to use adjectives, for example 'the fat man'.

- The facts of the incident must be summarized objectively.

- The report should contain the specific details of the incident, medical follow-up (where applicable), and the sequence in which the events occurred. When deciding upon the content, take into account the people who are to read the report — eg nurse managers, the superintendent, or lawyers.

- The particulars and words used on the hospital's report form must be carefully chosen so that they cannot be construed as admissions of guilt or denials. Opinions should not be given.

Figure 25.1: An example of an incident report form

(adapted from NUA Workbook 1988: 105)

INCIDENT REPORT FORM

CONFIDENTIAL

Person involved   Hospital involved . . . .

Full name . . . .

	Ward Reason for hospitalization if known	
Patient ☐	Patient's condition *prior to* incident	
Reg. no. ☐	Normal ☐ Senile ☐ Disorientated ☐	
Dr in charge	Sedated ☐	
☐	Sedation given and time . . . . Other (give details)	
	Was a cot with sides used? Yes ☐ No ☐ Sides up ☐ Sides down ☐ Prescribed ☐	
Employee ☐ Visitor ☐ Other ☐	Department Position Residential address and telephone number Occupation Reason for presence at hospital	
Property involved ☐ Description	Equipment involved ☐	

PERSON INVOLVED IN INCIDENT

Date and time of incident . . . .
Short decription of incident by person involved. . . . .
. . . .
. . . .
. . . .
. . . .

Describe exactly what happened in your opinion, why it happened, and what caused
it to happen. If it was an injury, mention the part of the body that was injured and
the apparent nature of the injury; if property or equipment was damaged, describe
the damage. . . . .
. . . .
. . . .
. . . .
. . . .

Briefly describe your observations about the condition of the patient immediately
after the incident . . . .
. . . .
. . . .
. . . .
. . . .

Names and addresses of witnesses . . . .
. . . .
. . . .
. . . .
. . . .

Who informed the nursing professional in charge? . . . .

Date. . . . .

Time . . . .

Who informed the doctor? . . . .

Date. . . . .
Time . . . .

Was the person concerned seen by a doctor after the incident?

Yes □   No □

Date..............................

Time seen ....

Doctor's name..

Date of report.......................................

Signature of person who wrote the report ....

Rank ....

Any additional remarks ....
....
....
....
....

Doctor's report ....
....
....
....
....
....
....
....
....
....
....
....
....
....
....
....
....
....
....
....

Date of report...........................

Signature.........................

Amount of information needed and the structure of the report

- Note specific, relevant details, such as the names of the people involved, ages, room/ward numbers, reasons for hospitalization, places, and dates. Give the specific time — eg '17:00', not 'late in the afternoon'.

- The correct sequence of events must be reported.

- Sentences must be short but complete, for example: 'The patient fell backwards.'

THE ECONOMY OF RISK MANAGEMENT

To be financially feasible, efforts made in risk management must save more money than they will eventually cost. In most cases it is cost-effective to prevent injuries, but a thorough economic analysis will support an expensive quality control programme.

There are three contributions to the costs of risk-taking behaviour.

The first are the direct costs which are incurred as a result of an incident — eg the loss of skilled personnel's time as a result of litigation as well as the payment of compensation to an injured patient.

The second are the costs of the effort expended in preventing or controlling a risk before it leads to an incident — eg the costs of supplying sufficient and correctly trained staff for patient care, and the costs incurred by such practices as the use of disposable products to prevent the risk of infection.

The third are the costs of new risks arising from efforts to control existing risks. Richards and Rathbun (1983: 22) mention an example of complications arising from laboratory tests carried out on a patient because a malpractice claim was anticipated. The authors state that it would be difficult to defend a claim arising from an unnecessary medical test.

THE RISK MANAGER

Sullivan and Decker (1992: 456) describe a risk manager as someone who administers the risk management programme and who liaises between the administration, the risk management committee, and other relevant committees and departments.

The risk manager also acts as a communication channel between insurance company representatives, the institution's lawyers, and other parties. The risk manager reports to an executive officer and should fulfil a clearly identified role in the structure of the organization.

Risk managers do not have a typical profile and may have any background. Good communication skills and interpersonal relationships are necessary, as well as leadership and team-building skills.

Their duties may include the following (Sullivan and Decker 1992: 456):

- Scheduling meetings for the risk management committee.

- Revising incident reports daily, investigating if necessary, or referring to the appropriate physician, nurse manager, or committee to prevent a recurrence of the incident.

- Monitoring data-gathering methods such as the summarizing of incident reports.

- Periodically visiting patients who are exposed to high risks in order to promote awareness of the institution's concern for individuals, and to prevent negligence.

- Summarizing litigation periodically, as well as the costs incurred.

- Drawing up monthly incident report summaries.

- Developing a staff training programme in co-operation with the risk management committee members.

THE ROLE OF THE NURSE MANAGER

Nursing staff play a crucial role in the success of a risk management programme. A risk management programme needs the support of nurse managers. Their attitude influences that of the other staff. It also influences the participation of the other staff in the programme.

Sullivan and Decker (1992: 457) state that the high risk areas fall into five general categories: errors in administering medicine, complications in diagnostic or treatment procedures, falls, dissatisfaction of next-of-kin with patient care, and refusal of treatment or refusal to give signatures of permission for treatment. Nursing staff are involved in all these areas. A nurse manager is responsible for giving guidance and assistance to nursing staff in this regard.

In nurse management, the handling of complaints regarding incidents involving patients is an important responsibility. Guidelines for handling complaints include the following (Sullivan and Decker 1992: 462):

- listen carefully;

- do not speak until the other person has completed his or her version of the incident;

- do not get defensive — stay calm;
- ask about the other person's expectations of a solution to the problem;
- if appropriate, explain what can and what cannot be done to overcome the problem;
- agree on specific steps to be taken, and on specific deadlines.

Medical and incident reports are important when the conduct of the institution, the nursing staff, or the doctors is called into question. When reports are incorrect, or provide insufficient information, or have not been written at all, the chances of prosecution are greater — as are the chances of losing legal action. The nurse manager in charge of the nursing services of a health care institution must ensure that all categories of nursing staff know how to keep accurate records, as well as how to write accurate incident reports when necessary.

CONCLUSION

In this chapter the importance, aims, and activities of risk management were shown. The relationship between risk management and quality assurance was shown, as was the growing accountability of staff in health services. Risk management programmes were described and the roles of the risk manager and nurse manager were explained. The importance of the economics of risk management and control was mentioned, as was the importance of writing incident reports and the accurate reporting of events and details in these reports.

References

Dienemann, J. (1990). *Nursing Administration. Strategic Perspectives and Application.* Appleton and Lange: Norwalk.

Richards, E. P., and Rathbun, K. C. (1983). *Medical Risk Management.* Aspen: Rockville.

Smith, D. G. and Wheeler, J. R. C. (1992). Strategies and structures for hospital risk management programs. *Health Care Management Review,* volume 17, number 3, pp. 9–17.

Sullivan, E. J. and Decker, R. J. (1992). *Effective Management in Nursing.* Third edition. Addison-Wesley: Redwood City.

Swansburg, R. C. (1990). *Management and leadership for nurse managers.* Jones and Bartlett: Boston.

Workbook for Nursing Administration (1988). University of South Africa: Pretoria.

CHAPTER 26

QUALITY IMPROVEMENT IN A HEALTH SERVICE

Marie Muller

CONTENTS

INTRODUCTION

Nursing service managers are responsible for providing high quality nursing services. It is essential that these managers possess specialized knowledge and skills in quality assurance or quality improvement. Patients have certain expectations and rights regarding the quality of the health service they receive and they demand good service — particularly in view of the high costs involved. The public throughout the world is demanding that certain control measures be instituted in order to guarantee or assure good quality health services.

This chapter gives a general perspective on quality improvement in health services. The historical development of quality assurance will be described first, and the concepts of quality, quality assurance, and quality improvement will be explained. This is followed by some of the quality assurance models which are used throughout the world. The motives, and principles and process of quality improvement are described.

HISTORICAL PERSPECTIVE

Although Florence Nightingale played an important role in improving the quality of health services during and after the Crimean War (Dolan 1973: 166–78), the United States of America actually laid the foundation for formal quality assurance. The American College of Surgeons Program was founded in 1913. The purpose of this programme was to standardize medical procedures and to control the quality of the service provided.

The first standard for medical practice was published in America in 1917 (Ersoz, Jessee, Ladenburger, and Parsek 1988), stating minimum structural standards to guide physicians in health service practice. The first standard provides for the formal organization of medical staff. Specific membership requirements of the American College of Surgeons were prescribed in the second standard to ensure professional competence.

The third standard requires that rules and regulations which define health service practices by physicians be introduced and adhered to in hospitals. This standard includes regular evaluation of medical practice and forms the basis for peer group evaluation. The fourth standard requires that physicians keep accurate records, and the fifth standard sets out structural diagnostic requirements which hospitals should meet (Ersoz et al. 1988).

The first formal quality assurance programme was introduced by the American College of Surgeons and was called the Hospital Standardization Program (Paine 1983: 15).

These standards were used for several years until the American Joint Commission on Accreditation of Hospitals (JCAH) was established in 1951 to evaluate the quality of health services on a voluntary basis. An accreditation system was subsequently introduced. These post-war developments greatly influenced health services throughout the Western world. The focus at this stage was still principally on structural and process standards.

Structural standards refer to the physical and organizational structure within which nursing care is rendered — eg numbers of personnel, organizational and health policies, buildings, and equipment. Process standards refer to the actual rendering of care and consist of the elements of the nursing process — assessment, planning, implementation, and evaluation. (Product or outcome standards, on the other hand, refer to changes in health status, largely as a result of nursing and medical interventions.)

Since 1965, the Joint Commission on Accreditation of Hospitals (JCAH) began moving away from minimum standards and what was known as the era of *optimal achievable standards* began. This resulted in a complex process of certification and accreditation. This era has recently come to an end, and the trend in the 1990s is to focus on clinical and organizational performance as a whole, with the emphasis on providing individual patients with quality service — in other words, evaluation is aimed at the quality of the product (Schroeder 1987: 161).

A positive attitude towards quality had to be engendered, in contrast to a negative attitude such as 'What have I done wrong?' which has prevailed for the last decade or two. This 'good quality' approach changed the inspection mentality to a positive quality culture in health services, and resulted in a more decentralized approach. The accent shifted from prescription to the end-results of a service, in accordance with that service's chosen aims and indicators of quality (Ersoz et al. 1988).

The sharp increase in the costs of health services for patients, the greater expectations of the public concerning health care, their growing dissatisfaction with the quality of the health services provided by various health care institutions, and the increase in malpractice claims against health service practitioners, have forced hospitals in America to formalize their quality assurance activities. The activities involved in this formally structured process, however, became very expensive, mainly because of the numbers of personnel needed to perform them.

After the introduction of the Medicare and Medicaid schemes in America during the 1960s, the Professional Standards Review Organization was established there through legislation with the purpose of providing cost-effective quality health care.

In 1982 the Physician Review Organization (PRO) was established in America by legislation. Its aim was to improve the delicate peer-group evaluation system among physicians in order to bring about cost-saving measures in health services. The well-known Diagnostic Related Groupings (DRGs) were introduced in 1984 as a payment system where payment rates vary according to the type of case (American Hospital Association 1983: 111–3).

It is clear that America has played a leading role in the field of quality assurance, and its influence is still felt internationally.

The European model now views quality and its assurance from a wider perspective. Since 1948, when the National Health Service (NHS) was introduced in the United Kingdom, quality control has been seen as the responsibility of management at different levels of a health care organization. Quality assurance is controlled primarily by professional practitioners at a clinical level. No formal accreditation system is used, however (Shaw 1982: 218).

In European countries, quality assurance is seen primarily as the responsibility of the State, and no quality assurance is undertaken by institutions such as the Professional Standards Review Organization in America.

It appears that there is widespread reluctance to implement America's formal system. In 1979, the Netherlands established the National Organization for Quality Assurance, and quality assurance activities in health service institutions have been a legal requirement since 1985. The National Organization for Quality Assurance concentrates on the development of quality assurance methods and the training of health service staff to apply these methods (Coupe 1988: 24–5).

The World Health Organization's European Regional Office convened the Working Group on the Principles of Quality Assurance (hereafter called the European Work Group) in 1983, to investigate quality assurance in European health services. This group designed a strategy for quality assurance which it submitted to the various national authorities, and it recommended a three-dimensional quality assurance model (see figure 26.1) with a problem-solving approach (World Health Organization 1983: 1–21).

Although the Americans formalized quality assurance in their health service, the Japanese took the lead after the Second World War, with Deming's quality assurance principles and the utilization of quality control circles in management. The concept of quality control circles can be applied to quality assurance in general and the Japanese have implemented their systems in many services (Peters 1989: 25–6).

Several approaches to quality assurance have therefore been used and tested throughout the world. Since hospitals have been obliged to pay attention to cost control and quality control, quality assurance has became an essential factor in nursing, and leaders of nursing services have had to provide for quality assurance programmes in their management strategies. Since the 1970s, quality assurance programmes in nursing have increased to a surprising extent, and instruments designed in America have been tested and adapted in Europe and even in South Africa.

Figure 26.1: Schematic representation of the JCAH's new era quality improvement approach

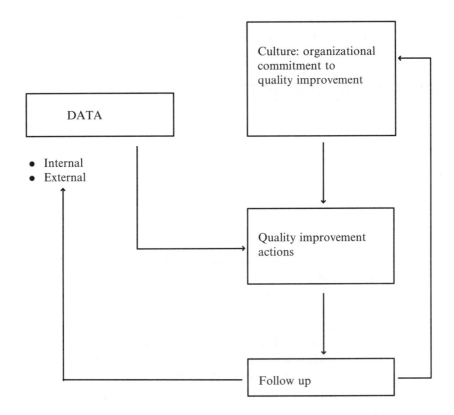

(Ersoz et al. 1988)

In spite of the accreditation system of the Joint Commission on Accreditation of Hospitals, currently known as the Joint Commission on Accreditation of Health Care Organizations (JCAH), users of health services in America are still dissatisfied with the quality of their health services, and users are intent on getting value for money. This has turned into a battle for survival as far as hospitals are concerned. Hospitals that wish to survive have to deliver proof of goal-oriented quality improvement, based on a complex and sophisticated system of monitoring and evaluating quality. The public demands that hospitals/health services must be accountable for the quality of services delivered by their personnel (Gillem 1988: 70–1).

In South Africa, quality assurance in the public sector is the responsibility of the hospital management and the State or provinces, and in the private sector it is the responsibility of the management of the health service, eg the board of directors. Each health practitioner is also responsible for the quality of his or her own professional performance. At present, quality improvement in South Africa is not as formalized as in Europe and America. Few formal quality improvement programmes apply in South African health services. Nursing professionals, however, are taking the lead in this respect.

EXPLANATION OF CONCEPTS

The concepts quality, quality assurance, and quality improvement are briefly explained below.

Quality

Quality refers to characteristics which are associated with excellence, and these characteristics form the criteria for assessing the quality of a specific service.

The characteristics associated with excellence can be seen from various perspectives. A patient views quality from the point of view of the care he receives and places a high premium on the provision of his immediate health requirements, such as empathy and the accessibility of the service. A professional practitioner views quality in terms of the knowledge and skill involved in professional practice. Management, on the other hand, attaches a financial/monetary value to quality (Bodo 1988: 262).

The Joint Commission on Accreditation of Health Care Organizations maintains that the provision of quality health services requires four essential components: optimum professional performance by all health practitioners, effective utilization of resources, minimum risks to the patient (such as possible injury and iatrogenic illnesses), and patient satisfaction (Ersoz et al. 1988).

The European Work Group accepts these components and agrees that quality health care should have the following characteristics (World Health Organization 1983: 5):

- professional performance (technical quality);

- resource utilization (effectiveness/adequacy);

- risk management (management of the risks associated with rendering a service, such as injuries and iatrogenic diseases);

- patient satisfaction with services provided.

This approach is similar to the opinion held by Douglass and Bevis (1983: 281–2) regarding quality health care, which can be summed up in the following four key words: safety, progressiveness, effectiveness, and acceptability. The authors explain (Douglass and Bevis 1983: 281–2):

- the service should ensure safety and comfort for the patient, the professional health practitioner, and others;

- care should be as technologically and therapeutically advanced as modern science allows;

- the service that is provided should be effective and economical as far as time, energy, and the utilization of other resources is concerned;

- the service should be legally and morally acceptable;

- it should be culturally acceptable to the users.

Quality therefore refers to the specific criteria which a service has to measure up to, and these criteria should be formulated according to the perspectives of the patient, the professional practitioner, and the management. The JCAH states:

> Do the right things right. To do right things, you must identify your customer's needs, convert those needs into agreed-upon requirements, then align your work process so you are capable of meeting those requirements. To do things right, you must execute your work processes in a way that meets those requirements. (Ersoz et al. 1988)

The characteristics associated with excellence can generally be explained in terms of the following:

- making the right decisions;

- professional, ethical, cultural acceptability;

- safety and the provision of a therapeutic environment;

- the service should be technologically and therapeutically advanced;

- effective results and effective utilization of resources;

- accessibility;

- appropriate risk management;

- patient satisfaction;

- management satisfaction;

- medical practitioner satisfaction;

- professional performance by appropriately qualified personnel.

The characteristics associated with excellence must be specified in a quality improvement programme, taking into account the particular circumstances.

Quality assurance

'Assurance' implies a guarantee of knowledge and competence by the practitioner, and an adequate service that provides value for money in accordance with the characteristics associated with excellence. Assurance further implies that certain formal quality control systems are in place. These systems are used to strictly monitor and assess the way in which standards are maintained, and to take remedial steps if necessary. Quality assurance is therefore a formal system that assures that the patient will receive service of a certain quality.

Quality improvement

Because it is not always practicable to provide a formal assurance of a specific level of competence and service, the JCAH has adopted an approach towards quality assurance in which the term 'assurance' has been replaced with the term 'improvement'.

Quality improvement still refers to a system in which the quality of the health service is formally monitored and assessed, and where deliberate steps are taken, or programmes are instituted, to cope with existing problems and to improve the quality of the service provided. Quality improvement also implies putting quality into practice, but with the assumption that quality can never be completely guaranteed. It means the pursuit of providing the best possible service, within the constraints of certain circumstances. The JCAH views quality assurance in a somewhat narrower or more specific sense with the focus on the specific needs and circumstances within an institution or health service, and not so much on the environmental issues and constraints influencing the health service.

Quality improvement also implies a certain attitude held by practitioners and management; it should be a way of life — a constant striving towards providing a better service.

Quality improvement, therefore, is a planned programme in which the quality of service is objectively monitored and evaluated, opportunities for improvement are identified, and a mechanism is provided for taking remedial steps to bring about and maintain improvements (Sanazaro 1986: 27). It implies a constant commitment to health care service of a high quality.

Quality improvement models

A model provides a scientific basis for quality improvement — ie a basis for putting quality into practice. Various models for quality improvement are briefly described below.

Systems model

The systems model is probably one of the most well-known approaches towards quality improvement. According to Gillies (1989: 72) the function of any system is to convert information, energy, or materials into a planned outcome or product for use within the system, outside the system, or both. The systems model is a cyclical process, consisting of:

- inputs — eg information and resources needed;

- the execution process: the way in which resources are employed to reach objectives;
- outputs: these represent the results achieved or the product produced;

- feedback: the results compared with predetermined criteria — the achievement of objectives. This information is utilized as input resources (see figure 26.2).

Figure 26.2: Schematic representation of the systems model

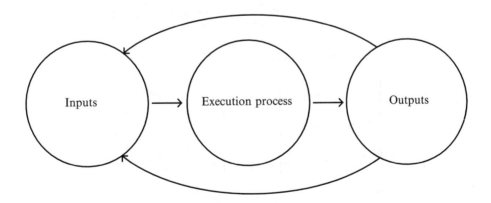

In the systems model the external environment plays a significant role, which may influence the quality of inputs and the execution process, as well as the outputs. Important variables in this regard are the socio-economic situation, the political climate, and the education system.

Internal environmental variables also determine the success of the systems approach. Human resources are important here — particularly in respect of knowledge, skills, management style, and communication, which may have an influence on the results. In a health care system, complex human factors such as patients, health practitioners, and management manpower, determine how the health service will be rendered.

The process to be followed in quality improvement is analogous to the steps of the systems approach. The quality improvement process consists of certain inputs — ie manpower and resources — the process of utilization of the inputs in rendering care, and the output or results achieved, which is then referred back as part of the input for another cycle of the quality improvement process.

European quality assurance model

The European Work Group designed a national three-dimensional quality assurance model (see figure 26.3) which accommodates components which it associates with a quality health service: professional performance, effective resource utilization, risk management, and patient satisfaction. The provision of a service takes place on four levels: the self-care level, and the primary, secondary, and tertiary levels. Quality assurance levels include the

Figure 26.3: Schematic representation of the European Work Group's three-dimensional matrix model

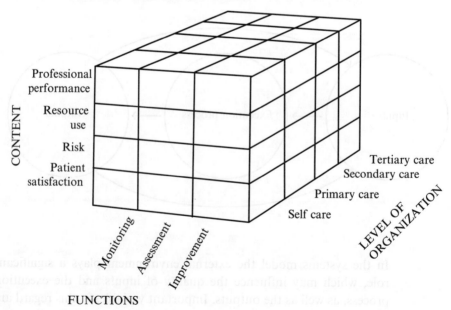

(Adapted from World Health Organization 1983: 14)

monitoring of health care, analysing the data, identification of problems regarding care, and correcting the problems where possible, taking into account the changes which occur in organizational behaviour from time to time (World Health Organization 1983: 10–16).

Quality improvement model of the Joint Commission on Accreditation of Health Care Organizations

The Joint Commission on Accreditation of Health Care Organizations currently rejects quality assurance models since it believes that quality health care cannot be guaranteed. Instead, it uses a quality improvement model focusing on the improved functioning of the organization as a whole (Ersoz et al. 1988). This quality improvement model consists of five pillars (see figure 26.4), based on the organization's values, in an effort to improve the functioning of the organization as a whole in line with the total quality management approach (Ersoz et al. 1988).

1. Identification of client needs. The first step in this pillar model is to identify client needs. The organization must define the nature and extent of the services to be provided, and the needs must be set out at departmental as well as nursing unit level. The patient's needs should be understood at each level of service provided, and a concerted effort should be made to provide for these needs.

2. Complete involvement. The involvement of all professional practitioners is a precondition for quality improvement. This includes the 'unrecognized quality experts' — ie those who are involved in actual patient care and who are, in fact, specialists in the field of providing a health service. These specialists are not always consulted when problems are being solved or when remedial steps are being taken (Ersoz et al. 1988).

3. Measurement and evaluation. The actual measurement and evaluation of the quality of the service is the third step in quality improvement. Priorities in this respect depend on the needs of clients and the department concerned. Practitioners should stipulate and establish priorities for evaluation themselves (Ersoz et al. 1988).

4. Systematic support. The next quality improvement pillar, namely systematic support, includes consistent organizational support in order to achieve quality improvement. An organization should demonstrate its commitment to the strategic aim of achieving a high quality service through its policies, and its financial and other organizational procedures. Without support from the organization, even the best idea will not have the desired results (Ersoz et al. 1988).

5. Continuous improvement. Continuous improvement of quality is the last pillar on which this model is based. 'The quality journey is a continuous search for a better way' (Ersoz et al. 1988), which implies continuous efforts to improve the service provided.

This pillar model presents an all-embracing approach, in which the health care organization as a whole is involved in quality improvement. Authority is distributed and all those involved are accountable for the quality of the service.

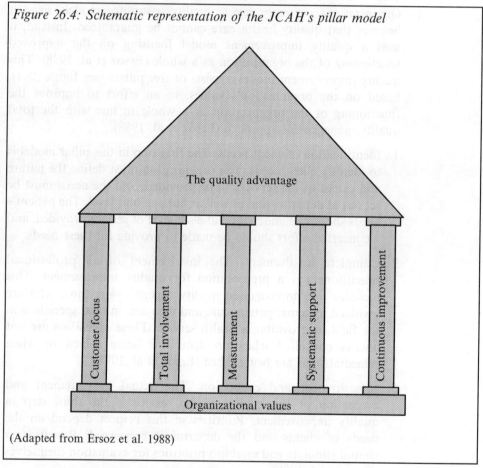

Figure 26.4: Schematic representation of the JCAH's pillar model

(Adapted from Ersoz et al. 1988)

Professional nursing quality assurance model

Several nursing models or theories have been published. Florence Nightingale (1880) initiated these models.

Nursing theories offer conceptual and theoretical frameworks which delineate the nature of nursing and address the question 'What is nursing and how does it work?' from a theoretical viewpoint. These nursing theories form the basis for quality improvement as seen from the nursing perspective.

Before the quality of nursing can be assessed, it is important to first explain the nature of nursing. In America a particular nursing theory forms the basis of a quality improvement programme in a nursing service. Standards are formulated, and are based on the nursing theory concerned. The quality of nursing is then formally evaluated. Remedial steps are again based on standards, as formulated by the selected nursing theory.

In South Africa, nursing is not usually based on any specific theory, and only specialized nursing models (obstetrics and psychiatric nursing) are available. Nursing standards are usually based on those found in American and European professional literature, or else they may be based on those standards taught by South African nursing training institutions.

Before a quality improvement programme can be devised it is important that nursing staff first consider the question 'What is nursing and how should it be practised?' This could offer guidelines and a scientific framework for assessing the quality of nursing.

Several nursing quality assurance models are available in the literature and these may be used for putting a high quality service into practice. Some of the better-known models are described below.

The Norma Lang model

Norma Lang (1976) developed the first American nursing quality assurance model in 1974. It consists of five steps (see figure 26.5):

Figure 26.5: Schematic representation of Lang's quality assurance model

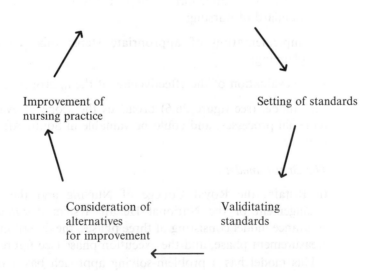

Declaration of values

Improvement of
nursing practice

Setting of standards

Consideration of
alternatives
for improvement

Validitating
standards

- statement of values: social and professional values and scientific knowledge serve as primary inputs;
- the setting of standards: process/structure/product;
- determining the degree of realism and validity of the standards and how they are actually put into practice;
- selection of the most appropriate alternative for improving nursing practice;
- improvement of nursing practice.

This model is relatively simple, and Bruwer (1986: 262–3) believes that it is suitable for South African nursing practice, especially during the developing phase of quality assurance.

Laing and Nish model

The American Nursing Association accepts the Norma Lang model, to which Laing and Nish (1981: 22–4) have added eight steps:

- description of the values regarding patient care which are adhered to in an institution;
- choose criteria and establish standards for the structure, process, and outcome of nursing care;
- confirmation of the chosen standards and criteria by the nursing personnel of the institution;
- evaluation of actual meeting of standards;
- analysis of factors influencing results;
- selection of appropriate steps necessary to maintain a high standard of nursing;
- implementation of appropriate steps: this requires careful planning;
- re-evaluation of the effectiveness of the appropriate steps.

This model (see figure 26.6) broadens the scope of evaluation and remedial processes, and could be valuable in South African nursing practice.

The British model

In Britain, the Royal College of Nursing and the top nursing management of the National Health System designed a quality assurance model consisting of three phases: the describing phase, the measurement phase, and the execution phase (see figure 26.7).

This model has a problem-solving approach based on the three levels of Britain's health service system: district, organizational, and

Figure 26.6: Schematic representation of Laing and Nish's quality assurance model

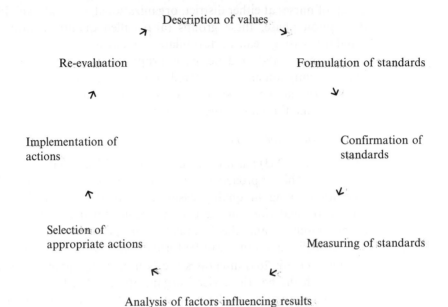

(Adapted from Laing and Nish 1981: 23)

Figure 26.7: Schematic representation of British quality assurance model

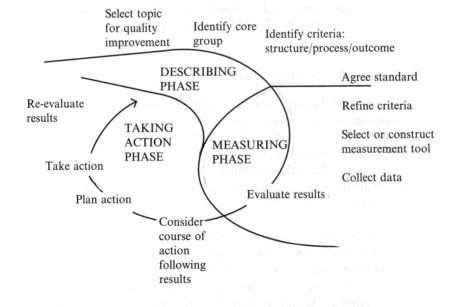

(Adapted from Kitson 1988: 30)

local level. Problems influencing quality nursing are identified by a group of nurses at either district, organizational, or local level. In the description phase, these groups (also called quality assurance or standard setting teams), formulate standards for specific topics, declare them valid, and design appropriate criteria. In the second phase, quality nursing is measured and assessed on the basis of these service criteria. The supervisors concerned then take remedial steps based on the findings of the second phase (Kitson 1988: 29–32).

South African approaches

Bruwer (1986: 263) has introduced a South African quality assurance approach. This approach consists of a development phase, which includes training in quality assurance, an analysis of the actual process of rendering nursing care, strategies for the implementation of programmes, and the formulation of policy, in this sequence, before quality assurance can be formalized (see figure 26.8).

Bruwer (1986: 263) integrates the Norma Lang quality assurance model with the health services' organizational structure on the one hand and the values of the institution and the nursing department regarding patient care on the other hand. In this approach, standards are formulated, the quality of care is assessed, and the necessary remedial steps for quality improvement are taken.

Muller (1986) uses a simplified process of quality improvement consisting of the formulation of standards, the evaluation of performance, and remedial action (see figure 26.9).

Although these models imply that certain standards can be formulated, the focus of the evaluation is on professional performance.

Reasons and motives for quality improvement

The World Health Organization's European Work Group has investigated the reasons for quality assurance programmes in health services. The Work Group found that the desire for quality assurance is based on professional, social, and pragmatic factors, as well as public accountability, and an endeavour to improve management functions and to facilitate innovations (World Health Organization 1983: 3–6).

1. Professional motives. One of the characteristics of professionalism is the pursuit of excellence and the desire to regulate one's own performance. Health practitioners are therefore eager to become formally involved in quality assurance (World Health Organization 1983: 3). Professional motives play a key role in the establishment of quality improvement programmes.

Figure 26.8: Schematic representation of Bruwer's quality assurance model

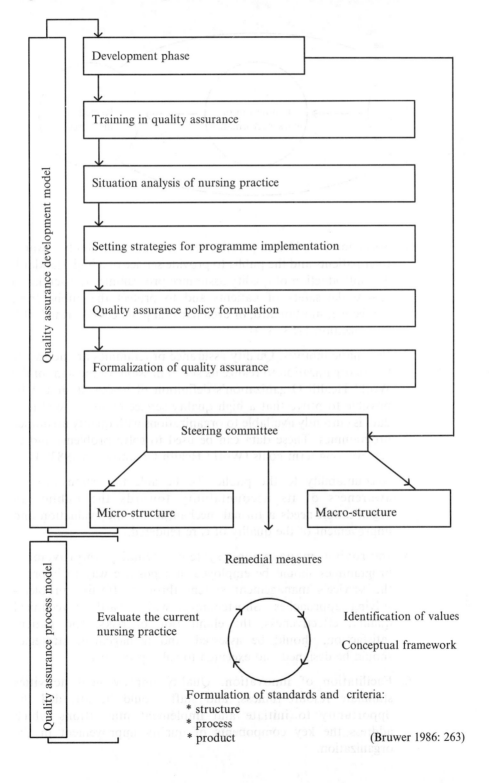

Figure 26.9: Muller's (1986) model of quality improvement

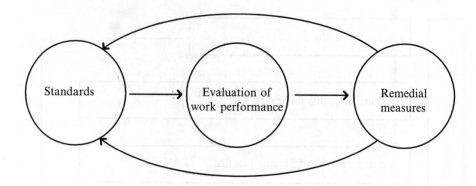

2. Social motives. Health practitioners have a responsibility towards their patients and the public to provide service of a high standard. The introduction of quality assurance programmes is essential to ensure the safety of patients and to protect the public from ineffective, substandard, or even harmful practices (World Health Organization 1983: 3–4).

3. Pragmatic motives. Quality assurance programmes are necessary for an organization to realize its stated mission. In the light of the World Health Organization's definition of health, it should be possible to prove that a high quality service exists. A wealth of data is currently available to organizations with quality assurance programmes. These data can be used to solve problems and to achieve long-term goals (World Health Organization 1983: 4).

4. Accountability to the public. To be able to demonstrate an awareness of its accountability towards the public, an organization needs a formal mechanism for the evaluation and improvement of the quality of care rendered.

5. Improving management systems. Quality improvement programmes should be employed in a positive way to improve the service's management system through effective problem-solving approaches. Shortcomings with regard to technical quality, effectiveness, the elimination of risks, and patient satisfaction, should be assessed, and management strategies should be designed and executed to solve problems.

6. Facilitation of innovation. Quality improvement activities stimulate resourcefulness, and staff should be afforded the opportunity to initiate and implement innovations which address the key components of quality improvement in the organization.

THE PRINCIPLES OF QUALITY IMPROVEMENT

Several principles for quality improvement have been described in publications. Edward Deming's general principles, the European perspective, and the JCAH's approaches are briefly described below.

Deming's approach

William Edwards Deming, an American statistician and consultant, was approached shortly after World War II by Japanese industrial leaders to help build up their economy. He succeeded in helping the Japanese to bring about a quality assurance culture. Japan's products eventually dominated the world market, which is sufficient proof that Deming's approach succeeded in that particular case (Gillem 1988: 71).

Deming (1986: 72–8) stresses that a business has internal as well as external clients, and the primary aim of a business is to provide for the needs of these clients. He developed management principles in which high quality service became a lifestyle. These principles can be applied equally successfully to hospitals and other health services.

Deming believes that health services should shift their focus from quality assurance to quality improvement. Although these quality improvement principles were originally only applied to production businesses, certain American private hospitals have been implementing the following fourteen principles since the 1980s (Gillem 1988: 71).

1. Principle one: the introduction of long-term goals for service improvement. This first principle centres on management's leadership role in quality improvement. The manager cannot simply delegate this responsibility to a committee. Top management should demonstrate dynamic management for continuous improvement of the quality of the service. Long-term goals are a prerequisite and should be made known to all the employees — professional and non-professional alike. Institutions that fail to formulate their goals for the future, or to make them known to employees, will not survive in the business world.

2. Principle two: adopt a new philosophy. Everyone should adopt a new philosophy, namely '... doing things right the first time' (Gillem 1988: 72). Professional practitioners and non-professional workers should develop a positive attitude towards their work, and doing things right the first time should become a matter of routine. Costs should be considered from a long-term investment viewpoint, which would encourage quality of service and lower costs over the long term.

3. Principle three: inspection should no longer be a means of achieving quality. Regular inspection, in the form of formal evaluation, is inclined to focus on negative performance and tends to demoralize health practitioners. Performance evaluation should be aimed at improvement of skills and effective application of new technology for the improvement of productivity and quality. The health service should develop information and evaluation systems to improve the quality of service rather than concentrating on yesterday's mistakes.

4. Principle four: when equipment and supplies are purchased, health services should not just consider the purchase price but should consider all the costs involved and involve sellers as part-owners or as shareholders in the organization. Aspects such as installation costs, durability, and service by the seller, all contribute towards total costs. Deming maintains that inspection costs are lowered if sellers are involved as shareholders in the organization and all those concerned are committed to providing quality service. Long-term planning of manpower, particularly health manpower, should include efforts to retain personnel. Hospital managers should consider the total costs of training and personnel development as an asset which has a positive influence on productivity and quality of service.

5. Principle five: constantly improve each activity which is inherent in the planning and provision of a high quality service. To bring about good quality service in a hospital, each employee should know how to make these improvements and should obtain the necessary authority to do so. Each employee should, therefore, know the hospital's mission and definition of good quality service. A decentralized approach to management is thus advocated, where every employee is given the authority to constantly strive to bring about the necessary changes in their everyday activities in order to improve the services they render.

6. Principle six: training and personnel development. Deming points out that continuous education and personnel development are indispensable for good quality service. In hospitals, however, these are the first areas to suffer when there is a need to economize because of budgeting problems. The value of training and personnel development should not be underestimated. A formal personnel development system should be in place to determine personnel needs in a scientific manner and to meet these needs appropriately. The focus should not be on how the work ought to be done, but on how it can be improved. Personnel should be regarded as the organization's most valuable asset.

7. Principle seven: the establishment of leadership for the improvement of top level management. Deming believes that organizational management greatly contributes towards poor performance. Quality improvement depends on improvement of the top level management. When leadership behaviour at the top is improved, it inevitably leads to improved managerial behaviour lower down the hierarchy with the result that employees are put in a better position to improve the quality of the services they render.

8. Principle eight: eliminate fear. Deming maintains that the hierarchical post structure in a hospital makes subordinates fearful of making suggestions for improvement: '... professional role guarding and fear rob the professionals, the institution, and ultimately the patient, of better quality' (Gillem 1988: 75). He thus advocates that the traditional hierarchical structure should be changed to a flatter one in order to provide a leadership that understands the purpose and methods of quality improvement.

9. Principle nine: break down barriers between departments. According to Deming, hospital departments often function in isolation from each other and teamwork is replaced by competition, which is detrimental to the quality of service. When competition is emphasized at the expense of team work, resources are not used or shared as they should be. A concerted effort to break down these barriers requires leadership and a participative management approach.

10. Principle ten: eliminate slogans, warnings, and targets for personnel. Deming rejects slogans and general warnings such as 'improve quality' or 'provide better care' and believes that slogans like this, and indirect warnings, result in counterproductive behaviour. These slogans imply that the worker's performance is not up to scratch and in fact point to management's inability to improve quality by creating formal systems.

11. Principle eleven: eliminate work standards that prescribe numerical quotas for the day. If the achievement of short-term quantifiable objectives is always the aim, it is easy for the employee to lose sight of the need to continuously improve the overall level of quality. Deming points out the danger of the exclusive use of short-term quantification of objectives for achieving long-term goals. It is particularly important in a health service organization to focus on quality. When the management sends out a message that figures are important, employees will provide figures. But if the message is perceived as concern about quality service, the employees will react accordingly, and productivity will automatically follow.

12. Principle twelve: pride in doing the job. Deming believes that the evaluation of performance occurs in too isolated a manner and that individual job performance receives too much attention. Teamwork and the achievement of the group's mutual goals are much more effective for quality improvement. Management behaviour should not focus on individual motivation only; it should also promote group motivation to improve the service as a whole.

13. Principle thirteen: the introduction of a powerful training and self-development programme. Deming believes that good service begins and ends with adequate training and that it requires management to concentrate on the training needs of personnel. Intellectual stimulation will lead to resourcefulness, which has a positive influence on service. The value of motivated personnel in an organization is too often underestimated, in Deming's opinion. Motivation leads to higher productivity and high quality service.

14. Everybody in the institution should participate to accomplish a transformation from traditional management to modern management where employees at the bottom of the hierarchy are given sufficient authority to make and implement decisions regarding their work activities in order to deliver improved services. This also involves a change from viewing quality as something which must be improved only when problems crop up to something which must be improved continuously.

The European perspective

The European Work Group (World Health Organization 1983: 7–18) propagates the principles set out below for formalizing quality assurance in health services at the organizational policy formulation level.

1. Consider financial and legal implications. Each country's approach towards health service financing is different. Financial allocation for quality assurance is therefore a political decision that should be approached with sensitivity. The possibility of legal steps against practitioners and health service organizations where minimum standards are not achieved will necessarily have to be considered when national strategies are considered for quality assurance.

2. Obtain public support. The European Work Group believes that the mustering of public support for quality assurance will enhance professional motivation in this regard. The European Work Group warns against politicizing quality assurance in

health services. Medical practitioners react negatively when their involvement in quality assurance is made obligatory by legislation, as was the case in the American Professional Standards Review Organization's programme (World Health Organization, 1983: 7–8).

3. Stimulate professional curiosity. It seems that getting professional health practitioners — particularly physicians — involved in quality assurance activities is a problem. The European Work Group believes that the announcement of quality assurance results would stimulate their curiosity and encourage their involvement. Data systems should be utilized to the maximum to demonstrate the results of changes in practices to the practitioners.

4. Training for students. Formal aspects of quality assurance — philosophy, knowledge, skills, and activities — should be taught to all health service practitioners.

5. Develop support resources. When quality assurance in the health services is accepted by a country as a goal, the necessary support should be developed and made available to four target groups: the public, policy-makers, managers of health service institutions, and students. Professional accountability for quality assurance must be reinforced among all health workers.

6. Develop support between institutional managers. The European Work Group stresses the fact that quality assurance is the responsibility of management and that it is management's task to encourage it. The design and operation of data gathering and processing systems can be promoted if co-operation exists in this regard.

7. Although the development and implementation of quality assurance programmes could initially cost the organization money, it holds long-term advantages for the country as a whole. Health is one of the cornerstones of a country's economy, and national legislation for quality assurance is therefore justified and necessary. Health service institutions should be forced in some way to engage in quality assurance programmes.

8. Quality assurance activities. The European Work Group suggests a multifaceted approach towards quality assurance activities in health care. These activities should include monitoring quality, solving problems, and improving care at all levels of the health service, following a three-dimensional approach, as illustrated in figure 26.3.

Quality assurance activities

The quality of care should be monitored in a scientific manner, and standards and norms should be set by the professional practitioners themselves. The methods used for identifying problems are the choice of every organization, with the proviso that problems are, in fact, identified.

The European Work Group stresses the fact that quality assurance should take place at all levels of a health service: at the self-care, primary, secondary, and tertiary care levels. This quality assurance focuses on the professional performance of each health practitioner, the way in which resources are utilized, risk identification and prevention, and patient satisfaction with the care (compare figure 26.3).

Training of professional health practitioners is a quality assurance activity which requires a national strategy. One of the greatest stumbling blocks in putting quality assurance into practice is the lack of knowledge and skills of management and other health practitioners. For that reason, quality assurance should form part of student training. Planning and development of education strategies for the public and politicians, in order to obtain their support for quality assurance in health services, should not be forgotten.

When a country does not have a formal system of quality assurance in its health service, the necessary financial assistance must be provided for the essential requirements of research and development. National and local budgets should make provision for research in quality assurance.

The development of information systems for monitoring quality assurance is a time-consuming and complicated process. The European Work Group suggests that, to develop cost-effective systems, research should be co-ordinated at national level, with international consultation where necessary. The usefulness of a specific system is based on the country's philosophy and approach towards quality assurance. The monitoring of structural, process, and product standards will determine the nature of the information system. The European Work Group warns against a system that does not produce accurate results, which often causes negative feelings towards quality assurance as a whole. Quality assurance activities should also include remedial measures to improve the service.

Personnel development programmes should be introduced on the basis of needs as they are identified by monitoring results of quality assurance programmes. These personnel development programmes should focus on changing the attitudes of individuals, which is probably one of the most difficult quality assurance activities. The European Work Group recommends the consideration of reward systems and stresses that the success of quality assurance lies in change in the organization. Strategies to change the organization should be made available at national level and the necessary training should be provided.

The perspective of the Joint Commission on Accreditation of Hospitals

The JCAH emphasizes the commitment of all those involved as one of the most important principles of quality assurance and warns against stumbling blocks such as a lack of clarification of the values held regarding the provision of nursing care, an atmosphere of fear, and a lack of information and information systems for gathering, processing, and reflecting valid data.

The JCAH propagates the following organizational principles, as set out by Ersoz et al. (1988):

1. The organization's mission in respect of quality assurance and improvement should be clearly spelt-out and made known to the employees.

2. Organizational culture should place a high premium on quality assurance and should stimulate a communication network in the organization which demonstrates participative decision-making and effective problem-solving in order to foster commitment to quality assurance.

3. Strategic planning in an organization should aim to improve the quality of patient care and should offer proof of integrated financial, strategic, resource, and programme planning.

4. Organizational change should take place when recommendations by the quality assurance committee, based on quality evaluations, necessitate it.

5. Leadership skills should be present, at management level as well as clinical level, and programmes should exist to develop these skills on a continuous basis.

6. Organizations should have a continuous quality assurance programme, and the management should implement recommendations of the quality assurance committee based on the evaluation of job performance, in a positive way.

7. Effective personnel management should be seen as part of the quality assurance process in order to improve the standard of service provided.

8. Facilities, equipment, and the necessary technology should be obtained, in line with the organization's mission and objectives, to bring about quality service.

9.   An organization should aim for optimum integration and co-
     ordination between the different departments to bring about the
     effective application of conflict management and to strive for
     quality service at all times.

It is clear that, in many respects, Deming's principles correspond
with those of the JCAH.

Although there has recently been a shift in emphasis in American
health services from quality assurance to quality improvement, there
are nevertheless certain principles which apply to both these
approaches. It is clear that a formalized system should exist which
requires a co-ordinated approach and commitment from all those
involved.

THE PROCESS OF QUALITY IMPROVEMENT

The three-step quality improvement approach is discussed below.
The three steps are:

- the setting of standards;

- the evaluation of job performance based on these standards;
  and

- taking remedial steps.

Standards as the basis of quality assurance

A standard is a description of the characteristics associated with
excellence — the criteria used for measuring and assessing excellence.
A standard is therefore a valid and explicit description of the desired
quality of job performance and contains criteria or indicators for
assessing the quality of nursing tasks.

There are three types of standards, as developed and described by
Donabedian (1969): structural, process, and product standards.

Structural standards

A structural standard is a standard that concerns the composition of,
and the resources in, a health service which go to make the provision
of a service possible — in other words, the support structure. In a
nursing service, structural standards would include all those
infrastructure factors that make nursing possible. Some examples
of structural standards are standards relating to hospital equipment,
the size of service units, and supplies needed. Structural standards
refer to the physical set-up in which, and through which, service
takes place. The question 'What is needed?' is a question about
structural standards.

Process standards

A process standard applies to the way in which a task should be executed — those aspects or factors focusing on the actual way the practice is conducted (clinical nursing, management, training, research). It applies to the actual nursing interactions that are carried out. In clinical nursing, a process standard usually follows a scientific approach to the nursing process — ie assessment, planning, implementation and evaluation. The process standard therefore implicitly describes the 'what and how' of clinical nursing, management, training, or research.

Product standards

The product standard refers to the results that have to be achieved. In clinical nursing, product standards describe the desired health changes in the patient — for example, control of pain or healing. In nursing training, the product standard describes the performance expected of the student. In management, financial standards would be more appropriate. The product standard should preferably have a quantifiable value, for example an infection figure of less than 2%.

Evaluation of the quality of service

Evaluation refers to the formal way in which information is gathered and assessed in relation to set standards and criteria. It is important that specific norms exist for assessment. The acceptable level of performance is predetermined, and, wherever possible, is expressed in figures. These figures are then used for assessment.

Various methods exist for evaluating the quality of nursing, and a combination of methods is recommended for extensive evaluation. Evaluation requires measurement, and measurement requires instruments. To evaluate the quality of nursing, nursing service managers have to develop instruments for evaluation based on set standards.

The different methods used for evaluation are briefly described below, as well as the process of evaluation and the kind of evaluation instruments needed.

Self-evaluation

In self-evaluation the nursing professional assesses her own quality of nursing using the standards that have been set. Self-evaluation is the way in which the nursing professional determines her own level of competence. The effectiveness of this evaluation depends upon the individual's personal goals, her perception of herself, and her self-confidence and assessment abilities. Self-evaluation is a personal matter used for personal and professional development. The results of this evaluation are not made known generally, but are dealt with by the individual herself.

Auditing

Auditing is an evaluation method for assessing the quality of nursing, as reflected in hospital documents. Since complete and accurate documentation of all nursing tasks is a professional and an ethical requirement, it is assumed that the nursing professional does indeed document all nursing tasks and that the quality of the nursing can be assessed in this way.

There are two methods of scientific auditing: continuous and retrospective auditing. Continuous auditing is carried out on a daily basis by the nursing professional and the supervisor, while retrospective auditing is carried out formally on completion of the patient's health treatment — eg after the patient has been discharged. It is important that the auditing instrument is based on the specific kind of nursing practised, as well as the standards set in the nursing service.

Direct observation

Direct observation is used during the execution of nursing tasks. It is often employed during student training, where the supervisor or lecturer observes and assesses nursing interactions step-by-step. This method of evaluation is time-consuming and requires that suitable instruments be developed. The focus is on the immediate execution of tasks, not on the total results of the health treatment.

Peer group evaluation

This is a process in which a person's conduct or job performance is evaluated by the members of the professional group to which that person belongs. The evaluation method consists of critical debate, is more informal, and provides direct oral feedback. A requirement of this evaluation method is that the group should possess professional maturity, and the focus should be on performance and not on personalities. Group feedback could be perceived as threatening, and constructive group evaluation skills are required, with clear rules and criteria for debating and evaluating, as well as the application of appropriate group leadership by the group leader or facilitator.

Personnel evaluation could also be regarded as a kind of peer group evaluation, except that the supervisor gives feedback on a one-to-one basis.

Incident monitoring

Negative incidents that are harmful to the quality of nursing are monitored and evaluated. Incidents such as the administration of the wrong medication or incorrect identification and treatment of a patient, are recorded and assessed according to a laid-down policy and a specific system. A record of negative incidents is compiled in writing and evaluated by an individual or group.

Patient satisfaction

In this method the patient's view of the quality of the service provided is assessed. Patient satisfaction can be continuously assessed during informal rounds or through direct communication with the patient during health care or treatment. Patient satisfaction could also be tested formally and in writing by requesting the completion of an evaluation instrument or through an interview. The patient completes a questionnaire and assesses the quality of the service received according to his own judgement and expectations. It may be difficult for a patient to assess the nursing alone, and often total health care or treatment is evaluated by one specific instrument. In this case questions are not only asked about the quality of the nursing — they are asked about the quality of the food or the treatment by administrative staff.

The development of evaluation instruments

Evaluation of the quality of the nursing requires the development of valid instruments and monitoring systems for gathering certain information. In the first place, this information should be accurate, and it should reflect the true picture of the attribute under consideration.

It is important that evaluation instruments and monitoring systems are based on the standards that have been set. For this reason the setting of standards is a prerequisite for the development of instruments — standards form the basis for developing appropriate instruments, and therefore determine the validity of the evaluation.

Standards are expressed in terms of measurable criteria and measurable gradings or evaluation scales are subsequently formulated. These gradings can be descriptive, or numerical, or both.

Examples of descriptive gradings include:

- poor – good – excellent

- safe – unsafe

- complete – incomplete

- accurate – inaccurate

Numerical gradings attach a numerical value to a criterion.

It is important that the evaluation scale used is clearly set out in order to increase the reliability of the measurements. The method used to produce the final calculation should also be clearly set out.

Requirements an evaluation instrument should meet

Evaluation instruments should be valid, reliable, and practicable.

1. Validity. The validity of an instrument refers to whether it measures what it is supposed to measure according to the standards that have been set. It is not realistic or practical to endeavour to assess all nursing tasks. To ensure valid evaluation, it is important to assess those nursing tasks that really matter — ie those that have a meaningful influence on the quality of nursing.

2. Reliability. The reliability of the evaluation instrument refers to whether the same result would be obtained if exactly the same circumstances were evaluated again, or whether the same result would be obtained when two different people evaluate those same circumstances. The accuracy of the measuring and grading is important here; an objective point system or grading system is important. This is not easy since two evaluators may have different opinions on the quality of the task and may allocate different points or grades for the same task. The instrument should therefore provide a grading scale which is described in clear terms and which does not lend itself to different interpretations.

3. Practicability. The evaluation instrument should be easily understood and suitable for the purpose for which it was designed. To increase the workability of the instrument, it is advisable to give guidelines as to how the instrument should be used, what the grading scales mean, and what each criterion means. If these aspects are clearly understood, the instrument will be more reliable.

Gathering of data

Data gathering is a crucial step in evaluating the quality of nursing. Sufficient data must be gathered to obtain a true reflection of the quality of the nursing. If there are too few data, this will give a distorted image, but gathering too much data is expensive and wasteful. The principles for data gathering that are set out below should be followed:

- determine the target group — eg patients, nursing professionals, or documents;

- work out the profile and calculate the population size of this target group, for example 500 patients per month;

- determine the distribution of this target group, for example divided into departments (medical, surgery, paediatrics), units, or sections;

- take a random sample to ensure a balanced representation from each group or section;

- the selection of a random sample must be objective and must be unbiased — for example, draw every fifth document for auditing;

- sufficient data should be gathered to obtain a true reflection of the quality of the nursing;

- gathering too much data should be avoided (enough data have been gathered when adding more data continues to reveal the same trends or information);

- if the amount of data to be gathered is difficult to determine, take at least 10% of the total population to begin with, and reduce this to 5% if there are signs that too much information is involved;

- the type of information to be gathered is determined by the standards that have been set;

- to ensure that objective assessment and reliability are obtained, the data should preferably be gathered by two evaluators working independently.

Data analysis and interpretation

The analysis and interpretation of the data should reflect the quality of nursing and should therefore be carried out very carefully. The final evaluation of the quality of the nursing is converted into figures and should preferably be undertaken by two independent evaluators, who can then compare their findings. If there is a difference, the evaluators should discuss the differences, their analyses, and their interpretations.

The interpretation of data is based on norms, expressed in figures; for example an infection figure of 2% in a unit. When this norm is exceeded, it means that the quality of the nursing in preventing infection in the unit is not as it should be. When data are interpreted, it is also important to analyse factors which could have influenced the results — for example the personnel profile, or other exceptional circumstances.

Evaluation of data

The final evaluation of data should be carried out by a group. A team approach in the evaluation of quality health service increases the reliability of the results. It is unreliable to base an assessment of the quality of nursing on only one evaluation method, such as auditing.

Remedial steps

The third step in the quality improvement process is the taking of remedial steps. This is accomplished through personnel development programmes, based on the formal results of evaluation. Deficiencies and shortcomings are addressed and the knowledge and skills of the nursing professional are improved. Continuous training is important to ensure personal and professional development of the nursing professional. Positive changes in behaviour should take place and should be reflected by the results of evaluation.

CONCLUSION

Approaches towards quality assurance have changed internationally with an emphasis on quality improvement, which fosters a more positive attitude among health practitioners. Several considerations are associated with quality improvement, and different countries have different approaches. The formalization of quality improvement in South Africa has not gained sufficient momentum at this stage. The quality improvement process is complicated, and all health practitioners in health service organizations should be involved in its implementation to improve the quality of the service provided.

In the next chapter we describe how a quality improvement programme can be put into effect in a nursing service.

References

American Hospital Association (1983). *Dynamics of Utilization Management.* AHA: Chicago.

Bodo, T. L. (1984). Quality care assessment and assurance. *Journal of Nurse-Midwifery,* volume 29, number 4, pp. 261–5.

Bruwer, A. (1986). *Gehalteversekering in Verplegingsdienste.* D.Cur thesis.University of Port Elizabeth.

Coupe, M. (1988). QA and psychiatry; reflections on the Dutch experience. *Health Service Management,* volume 84, number 3, pp. 24–7.

Deming, W. E. (1986). *Out of the Crisis.* Centre for Advanced Engineering Study. Massachusetts Institute of Technology: Cambridge.

Deming, W. E. (1988). Transformation of the western style of management. *Productivity South Africa,* volume 14, number 3, p. 22.

Dolan, J. A. (1973). *Nursing in Society. A Historical Perspective.* Thirteenth edition. Saunders: London

Donabedian, A. (1969). *Medical Care Appraisal — Quality and Utilization. A Guide to Medical Administration.* American Public Health Association: New York.

Douglass, L. M. and Bevis, O. (1983). *Nursing Management and Leadership in Action.* Fourth edition. Mosby: St Louis.

Ersoz, C. J., Jessee, W. F., Ladenburger, M. and Parsek, J. D. (1988). *The Essentials of Quality Assurance for Physicians, Nurses, and Clinical Support Services.* G-7 International Academy of Health Care Management: Wiesbaden. (Study Course Manual).

Fitch, H. (1986). JCAH standards for quality assurance: the basics. *Nursing Management,* volume 17, 10 October, pp. 68–9.

Gillem, M. (1988). Deming's 14 points and hospital quality: responding to consumer's demand for the best value health care. *Journal of Nursing Quality Assurance,* volume 2, number 3, pp. 70–8.

Gillies, D. A. (1989). *Nursing Management. A Systems Approach.* Saunders: Philadelphia.

Jernigan, D. K. and Young, A. B. (1983). *Standards, Job Descriptions, and Performance Evaluations for Nursing Practice.* ACC: Norwalk.

Kitson, A. (1988). Raising the standards. *Nursing Times,* volume 84, number 25, pp. 28–32.

Laing, M. and Nish, M. (1981). Eight steps to quality assurance. *The Canadian Nurse,* volume 77, number 10, pp. 23–5.

Lang, N. M. (1976). *The Overview of Quality Assurance, Definition and Purpose of a Quality Assurance Plan: A Model for Quality Assurance in Nursing.* Mosby: St Louis.

Muller, M. E. (1986). *Kwaliteitversekering in 'n Kardio-Torakale Verpleegeenheid.* MA.CUR. thesis. University of South Africa: Pretoria.

Muller, M. E. (1992). *Verpleegdiensstandaarde vir Privaathospitale.* Academica: Pretoria.

Nightingale, F. (1980). *Notes on Nursing. What It Is and What It Is Not.* Churchill Livingstone: London.

Peters, M. (1989). Quality and productivity. The Deming perspective. *Productivity South Africa,* volume 15, number 2, pp. 25–6.

Sanazaro, P. F. (1986). The principles of quality assurance in health care. *World Hospitals,* volume 22, number 1, 27–9.

Schroeder, S. A. (1987). Outcome assessment 70 years later: are we ready? *The New England Journal of Medicine,* volume 6, number 3, pp. 160–2.

Shaw, C. D. (1982). *Quality Assurance: What the Colleges are Doing*. King's Fund Centre: London.

World Health Organization (1983). *The Principles of Quality Assurance*. EURO Reports and studies, number 94. WHO Regional Office for Europe: Copenhagen.

CHAPTER 27

THE IMPLEMENTATION OF A QUALITY IMPROVEMENT PROGRAMME IN A NURSING SERVICE

Marie Muller

CONTENTS

INTRODUCTION

A quality improvement programme is a planned, wide-ranging programme which strives to provide patients with excellent nursing service. This service is achieved by the objective monitoring and evaluation of the quality of the nursing, as well as by taking appropriate remedial steps to improve the quality when necessary. A quality improvement programme is therefore a formal, valid, and reliable method of measuring the quality of nursing, in order to improve its standard.

A quality improvement programme can be implemented in a nursing service using either a centralized or a decentralized approach. The centralized approach requires the establishment of a central quality improvement committee, which co-ordinates and controls the quality control activities. The decentralized approach implies that each nursing unit, section, or department puts its own quality improvement programme into effect, according to its needs. In a decentralized approach control is delegated to unit level, while the quality improvement activities are co-ordinated at a central level for the sake of cost-effectiveness.

Bruwer (1986) recommends that the formal implementation phase of a quality improvement programme should be preceded by a development phase. The purpose of the development phase is to prepare the personnel for formal quality improvement and to put the infrastructure for quality improvement in place. This development phase may take several years. In the formalization phase the quality improvement programme is formally put into effect; formal monitoring and evaluation of the quality of nursing takes place, and remedial measures are instituted where the quality is found to be inadequate. It is important not to focus on clinical nursing only but rather to try to improve the functioning of the health care organization as a whole. There should be a general quality improvement programme in the health service, and the nursing service's programme should form one of its branches.

THE QUALITY IMPROVEMENT COMMITTEE

Formal quality improvement is never an automatic process. It is essential to set up a committee with formal authority to execute quality improvement activities. For this reason it is recommended that a professional nurse should be appointed and given authority to improve the quality of the nursing. In America, this post is referred to as the 'quality improvement co-ordinator'.

The setting-up of a quality improvement committee, under the chairmanship of the quality improvement co-ordinator, is the first step towards implementing a quality improvement programme in a nursing service.

Principles for setting up the committee

The following principles apply to the quality improvement committee:

- the quality improvement committee can adopt a centralized and/ or decentralized (unit- or department-based) approach;

- a quality improvement planning committee is set up to do preliminary investigations and planning before the actual quality improvement activities can take place;

- involvement by all personnel members is important, with acknowledgement of the clinical and non-clinical specialists at all levels of the nursing service;

- all the nursing units or departments (for example surgical, medical, intensive care, obstetrics) should be represented on the planning committee. Representation must be proportional to the sizes of the different units or departments — ie big departments should have more representatives than smaller ones;

- committee members should be selected or democratically elected, in line with the composition, circumstances, climate or managerial attitude prevalent in the nursing service.

The composition of the committee is important and will determine the success of the quality improvement programme at this stage. The level of motivation of the committee members is the most important factor since resistance to change may be anticipated and expected. Formal monitoring and evaluation of the quality of nursing is often perceived as threatening and should be dealt with sensitively and with professional maturity.

Responsibilities of the quality improvement committee

Formal responsibilities should be allocated to the quality control committee before a quality improvement programme can in any way gain momentum. The activities of the quality improvement committee can be divided into two phases — the development phase and the formalization phase.

DEVELOPMENT PHASE

The committee's activities in the development phase form the foundation of the formal quality improvement programme, and therefore determine the success of the formalization phase. This committee's responsibilities and activities focus on the development of the quality improvement programme, and prepare the nursing personnel for the implementation of the formalized quality improvement programme (see figure 27.1).

Figure 27.1: Development phases of a quality improvement programme

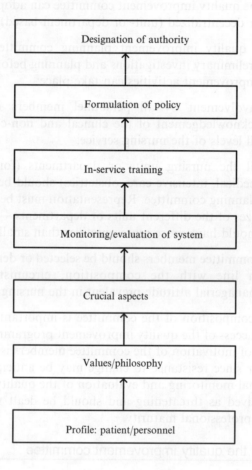

Profile analysis

A quality improvement programme should be appropriate for the nursing service that is using it. This requires a profile analysis of the patients and the personnel.

A patient profile should be drawn up to obtain a true reflection of the nature and extent of the nursing undertaken in the nursing service. A statistical analysis is made of the patients: this looks at the number of patients, their health/sickness profile, the intensity of nursing required (intensive care, long-/short-term nursing); the division of patients into different departments — eg obstetrics, paediatrics, the division of the available number of beds into different units, the sizes of the units, and the division of patients into different diagnostic categories. This information affects the nature and strategy of quality improvement in the nursing service.

It should be borne in mind that the patient profile is subject to change, and that revision will in all probability be necessary at some stage. Without revision, the quality improvement programme will become outdated.

Next, it is necessary to analyse the personnel profile. The number of nursing personnel, the professional and academic profile — especially as far as employees' knowledge and skills regarding quality improvement activities are concerned — should be determined. This information could affect the duration of the development phase in the quality improvement programme.

Value analysis

The committee should analyse values in the nursing service, department, or unit. Quality improvement is always linked to values, especially values relating to people (patients, family members, colleagues, other personnel) and to nursing itself. Nursing professionals' human relations are analysed as these form the foundation of their relations with patients and other personnel. It is also necessary to examine their values as far as nursing and the quality of nursing are concerned.

Formulating a philosophy of quality improvement

After the analysis of values is completed, a quality improvement philosophy is formulated, which guides all subsequent quality improvement activities. The committee formulates the quality improvement philosophy. This could be an extension of the existing philosophy which is formulated for the nursing service or the institution as a whole.

Identification of 'crucial aspects of nursing'

A quality improvement programme should be goal-oriented and meaningful. It is impossible to monitor and evaluate all nursing interactions in a nursing service; it would simply be neither realistic nor cost-effective. It is therefore necessary to identify those 'crucial aspects' which determine the quality of nursing in the nursing service, department, or nursing unit. These 'crucial aspects of nursing' form the centre of the quality improvement programme.

Crucial aspects of nursing are those interactions that have a significant effect on quality. Crucial aspects also refer to those interactions that occur most frequently; in other words, those actions that occur often or affect many patients (or nursing professionals) — for example the administration of medication, the admission and discharge of patients, or specific monitoring actions in the unit.

Crucial aspects also refer to high-risk nursing interactions, or interactions that often cause problems. Here again the administration of medication is important, since medication always implies a high risk. Accidents that have a high risk of happening frequently in a unit should be identified (eg patient falls in a geriatric unit) together with those that have an important bearing on how the quality of nursing care is evaluated. Then there are certain interactions that often elicit complaints (from the management or medical practitioners, for example). Risk factors necessitate the establishment of risk management in a nursing service. Risk management consists of monitoring systems for evaluating, preventing, and rectifying risks.

The committee members are therefore responsible for identifying crucial aspects of nursing, which will direct the quality improvement programme. The crucial aspects of nursing care which need to be monitored could either be those which are commonly found in the nursing care of all types of patients in the institution (general aspects), or they can relate to the delivery of nursing care in a particular unit where patients with specific diseases are treated. These aspects would relate to the nursing care of a patient suffering from a particular illness — eg aspects of the treatment and nursing care of diabetic comas in patients suffering from diabetes.

Examples of general crucial aspects of nursing in a nursing service are:

- admission and discharge of patients;

- transfers of patients between units and services;

- administration of medication;

- dealing with intravenous transfusions;

- carrying out physicians' instructions and prescriptions;

- identification of patients;

- documentation/record-keeping of nursing tasks;

- infection control.

Specific and unit-based crucial aspects of nursing can be identified by unit personnel. Examples of crucial aspects of nursing in a medical intensive care unit are:

- mechanical ventilation of patients;

- haemodynamic monitoring of patients;

- prevention of acute complications;

- administration of medication;

- dealing with emergencies (specifically according to the unit's patient profile, such as ventricular fibrillation, or diabetic coma).

A quality improvement programme is based on the most crucial aspects of nursing. For this reason it may be necessary to list the aspects which have been identified according to their priority, using decision-making strategies such as the nominal group technique (see chapter 9). Selection of five or ten aspects is more than sufficient for the implementation of a quality improvement programme.

Formulating standards and criteria

Next, the committee members are responsible for formulating standards based on the crucial aspects of nursing that have been identified. This requires the analysis of existing standards and criteria and studying the available literature on the crucial aspects of nursing in order to identify all the different patient care aspects which must be considered when executing particular nursing activities, as well as what is considered to be safe and correct nursing practice regarding a particular nursing activity. A measurable 'threshold level' is set for each standard and can be used to determine whether the standard has been met or not.

In most cases a 100% compliance or threshold level is indicated — ie if the nursing action falls short of 100% it is not considered to have attained the prescribed standard. Achievement of 100% compliance may, however, be unrealistic for certain criteria due to such factors as patient characteristics and the availability of resources.

Below is an example of an identified crucial aspect of nursing in an intensive care unit: haemodynamic monitoring.

Standard:

Constant, safe haemodynamic monitoring of patients with a Swan Ganz catheter is carried out accurately and recorded, with appropriate haemodynamic reduction/manipulation, following the physician's instructions.

Measurable threshold values:

- accurate measurement of haemodynamic pressure: 95%;

- accurate and timeous recording of pressure: 95%;

- appropriate and timeous haemodynamic manipulation: 90%;

- bleeding complications or pneumothorax: 2%;

- infection resulting from Swan Ganz catheter: 2%.

A quality improvement programme is intrinsically a complex activity. The variables used to measure the crucial aspects of nursing should be written in clear, unambiguous words so that they cannot be interpreted in different ways by different evaluators. Just as only certain nursing actions are selected for evaluation, so only certain crucial interactions in a nursing activity are selected for evaluation — eg when evaluating the activity of giving an injection, crucial aspects could be seen as:

- using a sterile syringe and needle;

- administering the correct dosage of the medicine; and

- injecting on the correct bodily site.

When too much monitoring is required, personnel become discouraged and reluctant to monitor incidents thoroughly. This may have a negative effect on the validity and reliability of the results and fail to give a true reflection of the quality of the nursing.

GENERAL METHODOLOGY FOR FORMULATING NURSING STANDARDS

Muller (1990: 49–55) investigated and described the methodology for formulating nursing standards. The formulation of standards is a systematic process which may be approached from different angles and includes, among other things, the involvement of experts in nursing and following a specific work method.

Approaches to the formulation of standards

When a nursing service manager or a quality improvement committee endeavours to formulate standards, the approach they take should be carefully considered. There are two main approaches: *general* and *specific*.

In the general approach, standards are set for general use, whether at national, regional, or local level. In a nursing service, general standards would apply to all the nursing professionals in the service — nursing documentation standards are an example. It is best, here, to adopt an integrated approach using structural, process, and product standards. General standards, therefore, have a wide-ranging approach which benefits the nursing service as a whole — even at a national level.

The specific approach, on the other hand, is aimed at formulating standards applicable to specific nursing interactions in a particular discipline and/or nursing unit. These standards are used at a unit or departmental level, as decided upon by the nursing professionals concerned. Specific standards are reflected in procedure manuals, and even in nursing care plans.

The involvement of specialists

The formulation of standards is a participative process which should involve specialists. They could be involved either in the formulation or in the verification of standards. Participation motivates people to implement those standards.

Working methods

The formulation of standards is a process that requires one to follow particular methodological steps in order to establish valid and usable standards. A committee of specialists should be made responsible, in the first place, for research — reviewing the existing standards and studying the available literature in order to gauge the required level of nursing practice. The committee of specialists draws up preliminary (draft) standards, based on existing and researched standards, as well as on the value analysis of human relationships and attitudes towards nursing. In other words, the committee members involved in the preliminary formulation of standards and criteria should study the relevant literature about the relevant nursing practice, in order to carry out the necessary cognitive analysis of variables.

This phase of formulating standards is called the *development phase of the formulation procedure,* as suggested by Lynn (1968).

Preliminary or draft standards are thus drawn up, supported by justifications outlining the reasons for their existence, having the required measurement criteria, as well as acceptable threshold values for each criterion. When these criteria have been confirmed, the standards are submitted to selected nurses for verification and refinement. These nurses are selected according to the following criteria:

- superior ability as demonstrated by appropriate experience and academic qualifications in relevant subjects;

- specialist knowledge in the methods used for formulating standards;

- nurse practitioners who will be involved in the implementation of standards after the initial quality improvement evaluations have been carried out.

Standards should never be enforced by one person, or even by a committee. The set standards should go through a process of refinement in order to confirm whether they are realistic and valid.

Having submitted the preliminary or draft standards to the selected nurses mentioned above for refinement, final standards and criteria are set by the committee and submitted for debate and verification by as representative a sample of the original nurses as possible so that final confirmation of standards and criteria can take place. This phase is called the *quantifying phase* (Lynn 1986).

In an institutional or regional context, confirmation of standards can take place through consensus decision-making. When national standards are formulated, however, verification or ratification of standards should be more scientific, as suggested by Lynn (1986). A formal quantification phase is completed, with each standard and criterion being assessed by selected nurse experts. A four-point ordinal grading scale is recommended to quantify the content validity of each standard and criterion.

The specialists allocate a grade (on a scale of one to four) to each standard, as suggested by Muller (1990: 53). A grading of one means that the standard is irrelevant or not appropriate at all, a grading of two implies lack of clarity, a grading of three implies that the standard is appropriate but requires reformulation, and a grading of four implies that the standard is complete, clear, well-formulated, and highly appropriate. The standard is consequently accepted, rejected, or reformulation is recommended.

Nursing service standards serve as guidelines for the maintenance of high quality nursing and are essential for the formalization of a quality improvement programme. It is important, however, that the standards be accepted by the employees who have to implement them.

Development of a monitoring and evaluation system

Next, the committee members are responsible for the development of appropriate monitoring and evaluation systems, based on the standards as appropriate for each crucial aspect of nursing that has been identified. Monitoring refers to a planned, systematic process of continuous and appropriate data-gathering, which is then used to evaluate the quality of nursing.

To develop and implement a quality improvement programme, a monitoring system is necessary. For example, in an intensive care unit for haemodynamic monitoring, a monitoring system for Swan Ganz catheters should be developed which provides for the assessment of the accuracy of measurement, recording, reduction/manipulation, and the detection of the presence of complications (bleeding, pneumothorax, infection).

A document should be provided for each crucial aspect of nursing to record the monitoring of each criterion. It is important that the monitoring system be simple and clearly understood at this stage.

The monitoring system of the quality improvement programme does not replace the normal system of documentation; it is specially developed as an additional incident-monitoring system to evaluate the quality of nursing. If the administration of medication has been identified as a crucial aspect of nursing, for example, the normal documentation for the administration of medication will still be required, but when the wrong medication has been administered (according to the chosen criteria and threshold values) a specific incident form must be completed to report this.

An evaluation system should also be developed. Evaluation should be valid and reliable, so that the actual quality of nursing can be determined — the truth must be reflected. The validity of the monitoring and evaluation system is based on the formulated standards and associated criteria for each standard. The system should apply to each criterion and threshold value identified for each crucial aspect of nursing. Evaluation is also based on the threshold values determined for each criterion.

To reflect the quality of nursing is no simple matter. The accurate measurement of specific criteria is important to ensure reliability. Even the number of measurements needs to be carefully considered. For example, one needs to consider whether all patients with Swan Ganz catheters should be sampled for evaluation, or whether 10% would be sufficient.

The monitoring and evaluation of the quality of nursing also requires a communication network. Such a network is used for the gathering of data, which are passed on to a processing section or team, as well as for feedback of the results to the staff who are responsible for taking remedial steps. The use of computer systems could be considered. What is really important, however, is the network of interpersonal relationships between the nurse practitioners (where the nursing interaction takes place), the person gathering and processing the data for monitoring, and the person responsible for taking remedial steps. The formulation of a policy of ethics, for publishing the results, is another consideration because it might not be feasible to let the results of quality improvement activities be published if the reputation of the institution and/or its personnel could be harmed.

Gathering and processing data are complex processes. Important aspects in this respect are:

- What kind of data are needed?

- Where and by whom should the information be gathered?

- How much data/information should be gathered (for example, 5% or 10% of all cases)?

- When should the data be gathered?

- Who should receive the data?

- In what form should the information be delivered?

- Where should the data be processed?

- Who should process the data?

- How should the processed data be dealt with, and by whom?

The use of trial runs in this development phase is appropriate for testing the processes of data-gathering and data-processing. The better the nursing service is prepared for the formalization phase, the less traumatic and the more effective the implementation of the formal quality improvement programme will be.

IN-SERVICE TRAINING

The quality improvement committee is responsible for planning, implementing, and evaluating in-service training. During the development phase, the creation of the right climate for the implementation of a quality improvement programme is surely the most important consideration. Personnel should have a positive attitude towards formal quality improvement, although resistance to change is to be anticipated. An attitude of 'What have I done wrong this time?' should be discouraged, and a positive attitude of 'What have I achieved and where can I improve?' should be encouraged.

The development and the formalization of a quality improvement programme hold tremendous financial implications for an organization but this should be seen as a long-term investment. The staff are the most important resource in any health service and the planning and implementation of an intensive in-service training programme is therefore necessary.

In-service training in the following aspects of quality improvement is necessary:

- quality improvement strategies (centralized and/or decentralized strategies);

- identification of crucial aspects of nursing and determining priorities that may significantly affect the quality of nursing;

- formulation of standards;

- development and design of monitoring and evaluation systems (general research techniques and skills);

- validity and reliability measures in the formal monitoring and evaluation of the quality of nursing;

- data-gathering methods;

- analysis and interpretation of data;

- compiling/writing evaluation reports;

- development and use of communication systems;

- using the principles of group dynamics;

- decision-making strategies (eg consultation and consensus decision-making; democratic decision-making; negotiation);

- general risk-management skills, as well as use of resources;

- interpersonal and communications skills (creating a positive climate which is non-threatening);

- development/use of computer systems for quality improvement.

FORMULATION OF GOALS AND OBJECTIVES

The quality improvement committee must formulate goals and objectives for the quality improvement process during the development phase. This mustbe carried out in the early stages of the quality improvement process. The committee members should decide, in view of the nursing service's personnel profile, how long this development phase should take and formulate goals and objectives accordingly. International literature suggests a development phase of between two and five years. Examples of goals might be that the committee should endeavour to develop:

- a quality improvement culture within two years;

- general standards and criteria within one year;

- unit standards and criteria within two years;

- monitoring and evaluating systems within three years.

Clear goals will direct and motivate the quality improvement committee. It is necessary to be realistic, however, and the existing workload of the personnel on the committee should be considered.

FORMULATION OF POLICY

The formulation of policy by the quality improvement committee is usually developed during the formalization process. The following issues should, however, be addressed:

- the nature of data gathering (general and/or specific);
- the frequency of data gathering (eg monthly or weekly statistics);
- who is responsible for data gathering;
- the way information is dealt with, processed, and made known;
- ethical standards regarding the publication of evaluation results;
- who is responsible for remedial measures;
- costing and budgeting for quality improvement (budget allowances for additional nursing personnel who are constantly working on the quality improvement programme, as well as for computer analysis of results, typing and editing costs, etc.).

FORMAL DELEGATION OF AUTHORITY

When the preliminary quality improvement committee has completed all the groundwork for the formalization phase, it is time to consider the formal structures. Should there be a central quality improvement committee or is a totally decentralized approach going to be followed? A formal infrastructure for quality improvement should then be set up, a committee should be formed, rules of procedure should be formulated, and the hierarchy of the various committees set out. Formal allocation of responsibilities is necessary through rules of procedure and post descriptions, in order for the formalization phase to proceed.

THE FORMALIZATION PHASE

The formalization phase is the formal implementation of the quality improvement programme in the nursing service. It implies formal monitoring and evaluation of the quality of nursing, as well as formal reporting to the public. Formal evaluation and accreditation can be undertaken by an external organization (such as the JCAH in the United States of America), but in line with the quality improvement programme of the nursing service. The formalization phase aims to ensure that the quality improvement programme is planned, implemented, and evaluated formally (see figure 27.2).

Principles

- The quality improvement programme should correspond with the needs that were established on the basis of the patient and personnel profile of the health service — the so-called 'crucial aspects of nursing'.

Figure 27.2: Formalization phase of a quality improvement programme

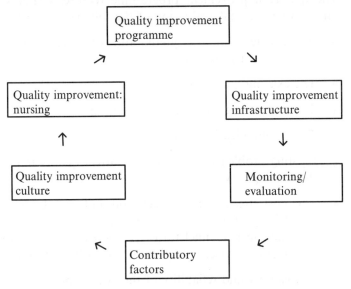

- Implementation of the quality improvement programme should be realistic, taking into account the infrastructure and financial position of the health service.

- An appropriate quality improvement infrastructure should be initiated and mobilized in the nursing service.

- Monitoring and evaluating systems should be wide-ranging and reliable: a combination of quality improvement activities should be carried out to obtain an authentic reflection of the quality of nursing. One-sidedness should be avoided — eg, quality nursing should not be based on the auditing of documents alone.

- The personnel involved in the monitoring and evaluation of quality nursing should demonstrate knowledge and skills in this respect in order to ensure validity and reliability in the evaluation of results.

- The factors that influence the quality of nursing should be critically analysed and reported — for example incidents such as strikes, emergencies, absenteeism among personnel.

- The quality improvement programme should be implemented in a positive way to engender a culture of 'What have we achieved?' rather than 'What have we done wrong this time?'

- The quality improvement programme should show positive results in the actual improvement of the quality of the nursing — this would prove the programme to be worthwhile.

Evaluation of the quality improvement programme

The quality improvement programme requires evaluation at least once a year. Formal evaluation of the following aspects is required:

- Achievement of the goals and objectives of the quality improvement programme.

- The existing quality improvement climate.

- The monitoring and evaluation system.

- The communication system.

- Existing problems or factors that affect quality improvement in the nursing service.

- The cost-effectiveness, direct and indirect: budgeting of the quality improvement system, as well as long-term results such as reduction in personnel turnover, increased work satisfaction in the nursing service, reduction of claims for restitution.

- The validity and reliability of the evaluation.

- The validity of the quality improvement system, according to the patient profile.

- Utilization of the evaluation results by the management, education section, and clinical practitioners for general quality improvement in the nursing service;.

- General professional development for the nursing professionals.

The formalization phase of a quality improvement system requires the participation and commitment of all nursing professionals in the nursing service. Quality improvement cannot be brought about by one person alone. It needs a formal process requiring valid and reliable monitoring and evaluation in order to obtain a true reflection of the quality of nursing. The formalized quality improvement system should be seen to be working and improving the quality of nursing; it should not merely be tolerated because it is fashionable.

CONCLUSION

The implementation of a quality improvement programme consists of a development phase and a formalization phase. It requires specialized knowledge and skills in quality improvement, of which the formal monitoring and evaluation of quality nursing are really crucial skills. It is not possible to assess every nursing interaction, so a quality improvement programme should be developed which will give a true, valid, and reliable reflection of reality. The quality of nursing in a nursing service is influenced by various factors throughout the organization and therefore the aim should be to improve the service of the organization as a whole, and not only the clinical nursing side. The quality improvement programme should be cost-effective and have positive long-term results.

References

Decker, S. M. (1985). Quality assurance: accent on monitoring. *Nursing Management,* volume 16, number 11, pp. 20–4.

Ersoz, C. J., Jessee, W. F., Ladenburger, M. and Parsek, J. D. (1988). *The Essentials of Quality Assurance for Physicians, Nurses and Clinical Support Services.* Study course manual. G-7 International Academy of Health Care Management: Wiesbaden.

Fitch, H. (1986). JCAH Standards for quality assurance: the basics. *Nursing Management,* volume 17, number 1, pp. 68–9.

Isaac, D. N. (1983). Suggestions for organizing a quality assurance program. *Quality Review Bulletin,* volume 9, number 3, pp. 68–72.

Kibbee, P. (1988). The emerging professional: the quality assurance nurse. *Journal of Nursing Administration,* volume 18, number 4, pp. 30–3.

Lynn, M. R. (1986). Determination and quantification of content validity. *Nursing Research,* volume 35, number 6, pp. 382–5.

Mason, E. J. (1978). *How to Write Meaningful Nursing Standards.* John Wiley and Sons: New York.

Matheson, G. W. (1983). Designing a quality assurance program: an approach that works. *The Hospital Medical Staff,* volume 12, number 4, pp. 11–17.

Muller, M. E. (1990). Navorsingsmetodologie vir die formulering van verpleegstandaarde. *Curationis,* volume 13, parts 3 and 4, pp. 49–55.

Muller, M. E. (1992). *Verpleegdiensstandaarde vir Privaathospitale.* Academica: Pretoria.

Sanazaro, P. F. (1986). The principles of quality assurance in health care. *World Hospitals,* volume 22, part 1, pp. 27–9.

Schroeder, P. S. and Maibusch, R. M. (1984). *Nursing Quality Assurance. A Unit-Based Approach.* Aspen: Maryland.

CHAPTER 28

INFORMATION SYSTEMS IN NURSING MANAGEMENT

S. W. Booyens

CONTENTS

INTRODUCTION

'It was estimated in 1981 in the United States, that hospitals spend between 7 to 10 billion US dollars annually to acquire and communicate information' (Lombard 1989: 14). This means that one third of hospital expenditure in the USA was related to the handling of information — eg information regarding personnel and patients (including all their records) — and communication with internal and external sources. Vast amounts of money could be saved (around 15% of hospital expenditure on the acquisition and communication of information) if only cost-effective communication systems could be installed in each hospital with over 200 beds (O'Keefe 1981: 11 as cited by Lombard 1989: 14). The information/data overload which confronts the nurse manager can only be effectively managed by making use of modern computer technology.

Historically, each organization has certain storage areas which are used for the placement of data. Examples of such storage areas are books, files, pieces of paper, ledgers, and the minds of people working in the organization. It is, however, very time-consuming and difficult to retrieve information because a particular file may be missing, a person may be busy and not available, and the time lag often results in incomplete or misleading information. Computerized information systems give accurate, up-to-date, and complete information on which decisions can be based (Scholes et al. 1983: 412).

The uses of computers in nursing administration vary but often include some of the following (Finkler 1985: 18):

- development and utilization of patient classification systems;
- budgeting for unit and departmental expenses;
- budgeting for the staffing of units;
- monitoring current staffing needs;
- preparation of reports;
- inventory control.

REQUIREMENTS FOR SUCCESSFUL IMPLEMENTATION

There are a number of factors which must be taken into account before a computer system is purchased and put into operation in an institution. The following aspects have been pointed out by nurses who had experience of this.

Choosing a system

1. It is important that software needs determine the type of hardware that will be acquired, and not vice versa.

2. Software needs must be evaluated carefully, keeping in mind the amount of finance available (including whether there will be enough money to train people to use the software), the amount of memory required, availability of graphics, whether the package is divided into modules which can be added on, whether it is user-friendly, and whether it will fulfil the needs of the institution (McNairn 1986: 45–7). The nurse manager would need a software package which incorporates a spreadsheet for budgeting and financial planning purposes, a database for filing, sorting, searching, and keeping records, a word processing facility to write, format, and store text for correspondence purposes, and a statistical facility to perform statistical tests. An application package would be useful for the ward sister in order to plan the nursing process for each patient and for working out the monthly duty roster for staff (McNairn 1986: 45–7).

3. Nurses must be included in committees when assessing what system is needed.

4. An integrated system must be planned beforehand.

5. Long-range plans must be included initially.

6. Committees must not be too large.

7. Ergonomic considerations such as the noise produced by printers, the production of static electricity, temperature and humidity controls, power sources, and control of dust must be taken into account.

8. It must be remembered that the reports and forms in use cannot all be maintained in the same format as that in which they were used in the manual system.

9. Adequate training must be provided.

10. Nurses must be able to articulate both the reason for requesting a system and its implications for nursing.

11. Nurses in training should be introduced to the computer technology which is being used in the hospital setting.

12. Nurses must be aware that they must be able to describe their own function in detail before it can be programmed.

13. Issues of confidentiality must be considered before the introduction of a system (Cox 1987: 181; Scholes et al. 1983: 380).

TERMINOLOGY

1. *Data*. Data require some processing before they can take on a useful and applicable format — ie before they can become usable 'information' (Murdick, as quoted by Hansen 1982: 5).

2. *Information*. 'Information is a sign or set of signs that predispose a person to take action' (Murdick, as quoted by Hansen 1982: 5). It is a finished product which can be used directly in decision-making and action (Hansen 1982: 5–6).

3. *Integrated system*. Any computer software system that combines two types of software — eg spreadsheets and word-processing.

4. *Operating system*. This system manages the resources of the computer itself and provides a special command language for directing the computer to perform useful tasks. An example of an operating system is MS-DOS (Finkler 1985: 21).

5. *Spreadsheet system*. This is an electronic software program containing vertical and horizontal columns and which is orientated towards 'number crunching'. It is used for computing and recomputing a complex series of calculations and for answering 'what if' questions (eg 'what will the forecasted budget for next year amount to if there is a 5% increase in the number of admissions?').

6. *Database system*. This is a software program which is devised to store data in a number of different files. A database is used as a record-keeping device, recording vast amounts of data — eg names and particulars of patients and personnel.

7. *Minimum Basic Data Set (MBDS)*. This is a small set of meaningful indices (also called a minimum patient data profile) which is used in a hospital information system (HIS) to arrive at decisions regarding patient care. It is usually designed for decisions regarding medical treatment programmes and incorporates the categories of patient identification, epidemiological variables, socio-economic status, admission details, diagnosis and management, outcome, and patient billing (Shipham et al. 1989: 12–14).

8. *Nursing Minimum Data Set (NMDS)*. This is a set of core nursing data which reflect a standardized set of meaningful indices portraying nursing practice — eg information derived from the practice of nursing itself, not from physicians' orders, hospital policy, or rules and procedures. It can be used by all nurses who require information regarding nursing. It is different from medical, health, and hospital information because it is founded

on configurations of the nurses' perceptions of patient needs, the patients' responses to treatment, and the nurses knowledge acquired through experience and education (Werley and Lang 1988: xvii).

9. *Patient census system.* This is a computer program system which monitors all patients occupying beds as well as all the available beds which could be occupied by patients (Werley and Lang 1988: 94).

THE UTILIZATION OF COMPUTER INFORMATION IN THE HOSPITAL

Computer information could be used for several purposes. These include staffing, scheduling, personnel administration, financial control, quality assurance, planning, and the production of reports.

Staffing

It is necessary to implement a computerized patient classification system before a computerized staffing system can be established. The steps involved are usually as follows:

1. A list of nursing care requirements for patients is drawn up. This list usually contains such items as bath and mouth care with assistance, complete bath and mouth care, non-routine positioning, life-support monitoring, special elimination measures, simple or complex dressing-change, etc. The items are grouped under headings such as: physical/hygiene measures, nutrition, elimination, activity level, monitoring, medications and IVs, procedures and treatments, psychosocial interventions, and teaching (Coetzee 1985: 45).

2. The nursing staff enter each patient in the unit on a form against the listed nursing requirements. The information on the forms is read off to the computer, making use of an optical sensor.

3. Nursing care requirements are weighted and an acuity score is calculated for each patient by taking into account the number of requirements of that patient and the weighting of each requirement. The weighting of each nursing care requirement is based on the relative time it will take a nurse to execute the nursing care needed.

4. The score for each patient is then classified into different acuity classes, eg 0–20 = 1, 21–40 = 2, 41–60 = 3, etc. Acuity classes normally vary from 1 to 5 where '1' means 'self care' and '5' means intensive care.

5. It is necessary to establish the number of nursing hours devoted to nursing care in each category. This can be done using time and motion studies which take into account direct nursing care, indirect nursing care, and personal time (Coetzee 1985: 45). When the hours of nursing care required per category have been established, factors such as the following should also be taken into account:

   • the number of beds in the unit;

   • the normal bed occupancy;

   • the characteristics of the patients, eg old/young, male/female, rural/urban, etc.

   • the nursing care standards operating in the particular hospital;

   • the architectural structure of the unit;

   • the amount of support from other hospital departments;

   • the educational levels and levels of experience of the nursing staff (Coetzee 1985: 45).

6. The computer is used to perform the necessary calculations.

7. The nursing department can then be supplied with the following information (Coetzee 1985: 46):

   • a patient acuity list for each unit;

   • patient acuity level — summary of the whole hospital;

   • patient acuity tendencies for each unit;

   • staffing requirements according to level of experience, work shifts for each unit, and work shifts for the whole hospital;

   • scheduled staffing for any unit for each day of the week;

   • average variance in staffing requirements according to level of experience;

   • reports which show the difference between the actual, scheduled, and required personnel per unit.

It is evident that many nursing administration hours can be saved by such a system. Other advantages of such a system are, according to Coetzee (1985: 47):

   • patient care needs are classified accurately and timeously;

   • daily personnel requirements are calculated quickly;

   • nursing staff can be distributed to units on a scientific and accurate basis which will lessen the underutilization or overutilization of personnel;

- trends in patient acuity levels can be traced, and management is thus forewarned about them;

- it is possible to answer questions on how variations in patient numbers and in intensity of nursing care required will influence personnel requirements and budgetary requirements.

Scheduling

Computer programs are also available which can handle the daily distribution of nursing staff in a unit. These programmes are usually based on the two basic factors which determine the number of personnel needed, ie patient census and patient acuity.

A software program designed for scheduling purposes may typically consist of four modules — ie a personnel provision module, a filing cabinet module, a scheduling module, and a module for generating managerial reports.

The *filing cabinet module* contains all the relevant information about each staff member — eg name, title, staff number, preferences regarding working shifts, number of hours to be worked per week, educational and experience levels, weekend rotation, and the other units where the staff member may be rotated to if the hospital has such a rotation policy (Coetzee 1985: 52).

The *personnel provision module* is used to predict the pattern of staffing for a particular unit based on the following parameters which must be provided by management:

- the average daily census of the unit;

- nursing care hours per patient per day;

- the number of productive hours per individual per shift;

- the number of days off per year;

- the projected distribution of staff for 24-hours during the day, late afternoon, and night — eg 42%, 38%, and 20%;

- the staff mix percentages, eg 30% registered personnel, 30% students, and 40% auxiliary nurses (Coetzee 1985: 51).

The programme does the necessary calculations and then produces the projected or proposed schedule pattern for a particular unit. Nurse managers can deduce from this pattern the personnel required per unit, the difference between what is needed and the number of personnel available, and the number of personnel who will be needed when patient acuity and patient census variations occur per unit (Coetzee 1985: 51).

The *scheduling module* is used to calculate and schedule the personnel who are available according to the needs of the different units. This module thus incorporates the data in the filing cabinet module as well as those in the personnel provision module. A scheduling list is produced for a four-week period per unit. It is also possible to get a print-out of a staff member's individual schedule for the four-week period.

The *managerial report module* produces the following reports (Coetzee 1985: 52):

- a summary of productivity report showing, among other things, the difference between the budgeted personnel needs and the available personnel for each unit, the required personnel–patient ratios, bed occupancy rate, and patient acuity;

- a cost analysis report showing an analysis of the costs of the basic salaries for personnel, the costs for additional payments for weekends and night shifts, and overtime costs;

- a utilization of service advantages report showing use and abuse of sick leave, the hours worked on weekends by each member of staff, and the unproductive use of time per individual per shift;

- a report showing the census tendencies for each unit and/or for the whole hospital on a daily, monthly, seasonal, and annual basis.

- a report consisting of a worksheet for use by the nurse manager for the daily adaptations for personnel provision. This report helps the nurse manager to make optimum use of available personnel in similar units before she resorts to using a pool of relief personnel (Coetzee 1985: 52–5).

Personnel administration

In the field of personnel administration, the computer is a real ally. The following information should be computerized (with the option of adding other relevant information when it becomes necessary):

1. Payroll information with automatic notices regarding annual performance evaluations and calculation of pay increases.

2. Reports of current registration with SANC and SANA.

3. Demographic, professional, and biographical data of each member of the nursing personnel.

4. In-service education and continuing education records (Cox 1987: 178–9; Lombard 1989: 15).

When the above information is kept in the form of a database system, it is possible to get a number of records or reports from the computer, for example:

- an alphabetical list of all the nursing personnel;

- a list of registered versus non-registered personnel;

- a list of personnel arranged according to the units in which they are working;

- a list of personnel who have been employed for longer than 10 years;

- a list of personnel with additional qualifications in nursing administration, nursing education, etc.

- a list of personnel living within a radius of five kilometers of the hospital;

- a list of personnel who attended certain in-service education sessions (Coetzee 1984: 39).

Financial control

Budgets are usually the first items to be computerized in health services. Most of the computerized budget systems are similar to the popular spreadsheet programs which are being produced for use with personal computers (Cox, et al. 1987: 178). The most important characteristic of the spreadsheet is its potential ability to produce a financial model of any situation. When data and formulated mathematical relationships are fed into the computer, 'what if' questions can be answered.

The nursing service manager is then able to see on the computer screen or printout what the financial implications would be if, for example, she were to do away with six nursing auxiliary posts at a certain salary scale and substitute them with one post for a registered nurse at a different salary scale (Coetzee 1984: 39).

With the help of the spreadsheet it is easy to see what the financial implications of anticipated changes would be. It is thus possible to view and interpret new approaches on the screen before implementing them in practice, and to steer away from certain proposed changes if they appear too costly. The nursing service manager is able to put her case for certain changes before management in figures; this strengthens her argument considerably and makes her audience more attentive.

Examples of the use that can be made of spreadsheet programs are:

- calculation of the time that nurses spend in direct nursing care, indirect care, and personal time while on duty;

- motivation for the purchase of new items;

- motivation for the writing-off of used items;

- calculation of the cost of medications and provisions with regard to patient census and patient acuity levels (Coetzee 1984: 39);

- calculation of salaries, overtime, uniforms;

- calculation of the cost of hospital, ward, and theatre equipment;

- calculation of staffing levels;

- calculation of ward stock, food, and other non-chargeable costs (Lombard 1989: 15).

When the budget is computerized it is also easy to make comparisons, for instance between different nursing units and different budget allocations (eg personnel, continuing education, supplies). When budgets are computerized, monthly reports are usually issued which reflect each budget allocation budgeted for, the amount budgeted, the amount spent, and the remainder. One can usually also get the picture for the same item during the previous year. This makes cost control and budgeting for the following year much easier than in the past (Cox et al. 1987: 178).

Quality assurance

The computer is a helpful tool when the data generated by the completion of checklists and auditing of reports need to be analysed and compared with aspects such as staffing levels, patient acuity levels, and bed-occupancy rates for quality assurance purposes.

The results of a quality monitoring study are entered into a computer. These include results from checklists and audits of documentation and/or questionnaires completed by patients. The computer generates quality scores for each unit included in the study. The quality scores are then merged with data on actual and recommended staffing and paid hours to produce monthly quality assurance reports.

The following reports can then be made available to the professional nurse in charge of reviewing and exploration with the staff on the unit in order to improve the quality of care in the unit:

1. Summary of quality scores, unit statistics, statistics on recommended and actual hours worked by staff category, and productivity indices.

2. Scores for the quality assurance objectives against the total number of hours actually worked per unit.

3. Scores for the quality assurance objectives against time spent per patient.

4. Acuity levels by day of the month.

5. Recommended staffing versus actual staffing.

6 Actual total hours per unit of workload per day.

7. Percentage distribution of total staff by shift against average patient acuity (Culpepper 1984: 86).

Planning

The nurse administrator is concerned with everyday planning and strategic planning. Her decision-making abilities are enhanced when she has the necessary information at her fingertips and when it is accurate and up-to-date. If the following information is computerized and available when needed it will assist her in her general managerial and planning function (Lombard 1989: 15):

1. Information regarding patient administration:
   - patient admission and classification system;
   - patient acuity — ie acuity measured as the bed-occupancy rate or midnight census of patients against the average number of patient days per ward/unit;
   - assessing the number of days each patient spent in hospital for which that patient will receive an account;
   - amount and types of surgery performed per patient day;
   - theatre occupancy rates.

2 Information for nursing management:
   - job descriptions and job gradings;
   - performance appraisal system;
   - staff scheduling system;
   - quality assurance programmes;
   - infection statistics;
   - injuries on duty;
   - recruitment and retention programmes;
   - attrition rates and attrition analysis;
   - annual leave, sick leave, and absenteeism patterns;
   - disciplinary and grievance procedures.

Reports

There are many typing requirements in nursing administration — eg letters, job descriptions, policy and procedure manuals, and statements.

The nurse manager must also compile a number of reports — eg annual reports, and administrative reports. The micro-computer emerges as a valuable friend in this area. A great deal of time is saved by making use of the drafting, editing, and word-processing capabilities of the computer. The graphics component can be used to communicate data in a way which will make the understanding of essential relationships easier, using line graphs, bar graphs, and pie charts. It promotes the visualization of relationships that the author wishes to bring across to the readers of the report (Cox 1987: 180).

PROFESSIONAL STANDARDS AND ETHICAL DILEMMAS

There are a number of professional and ethical dilemmas which the nurse manager must take cognizance of when considering the introduction or expansion of computer technology in her service.

Nurses need to be wary of systems in which the nurse has to enter data that do not benefit the nurse or the patient but which are only useful to other health-care members — eg physiotherapists or dietitians.

When the nurse has decided that the data which must be entered are of benefit to the patient she should analyse and negotiate whether a nurse is the appropriate person to enter the data. Nurses spend 40–60% of their time on non-nursing activities and data entry would add to this. Nurses therefore need to evaluate carefully whether the time spent in entering the data could be accounted for in relation to the appropriate contribution it would make to the nursing care of the patient (Woolery 1990: 50).

The nursing profession should become actively involved in determining criteria for the design of the computer system and in laying down professional standards for the creation of nursing information systems. If nurses simply sit back, non-professional people will develop nursing information systems for nurses. Such systems need to be validated by knowledgeable nurses.

Nurses must also learn to ask questions from computer-generated reports. There is a real risk of nurses making decisions on data and reports generated by computers where the data actually fit the principle of 'GIGO' — 'garbage in, garbage out'. Nurses should thus learn to scrutinize, criticize, interpret, and evaluate the output from computers carefully in order to get meaningful information which can reduce the time they spend on non-nursing activities and which can increase the quality of patient care (Woolery 1990: 52–3).

The patient's right to privacy, and the security of his records, can easily be violated when a mainframe computer system is in place with terminals in each unit or section. The use of identification numbers by the hospital's personnel members in order to access the system safeguards the data on the computerized patient records. These numbers indicate a person's status in the organization and determine the information which that person may retrieve. For example, clerical staff might be able to have access to data concerning the patient's identification — eg age, address, next of kin, etc. — but not to the nurse's or doctor's progress notes (Tappen 1989: 259).

IMPACT ON THE SOCIAL AND POLITICAL STRUCTURE OF THE ORGANIZATION

Computer information systems may change the patterns of social interaction within an organization. The computer provides a medium for rich interpersonal collaboration across departmental boundaries because the network supplies access to new, timely, relevant information for each section, department, or unit. People can utilize this computer network to communicate with each other without having to get together in a meeting. This type of communication encourages participation on a more equal basis by removing personality factors such as a very timid nurse or an overpowering nurse manager. These networks thus promote more input from reticent nurses who would not dare to oppose a proposition made by a dynamic nurse manager in a meeting. More ideas are thus exchanged regarding an issue, and openness is promoted in the organization, thereby facilitating a greater exchange of ideas and collaboration across vertical and horizontal boundaries (Sinclair 1990: 67).

Timely, relevant information helps the nurse manager to identify and address problems relating to nursing care and management on time. Effective planning and control is made easier. It thus prevents unpleasant surprises and decreases the nurse manager's need for crisis management or crisis-driven behaviour (Sinclair 1990: 68).

Another effect of computer information systems is the diffusion of knowledge throughout the organization. Knowledge is power because the more knowledge a person possesses the more powerful he feels. When the organization's staff members are all informed, top management will not be able to lead or to manage by simply decreeing a policy. The managers will be forced to consult ever more widely with their informed subordinates before organizational goals are formulated, and they will have to use persuasion to get their subordinates to follow the set path. When information is made widely available, the competent decision-maker, wherever he/she may be found in the organizational structure, will become known and respected. This reappraisal of worth based on decision-making ability may disrupt a hierarchical system of authority. For example, the competent sister in ward A may become just as powerful as, or more powerful than, the nurse manager of section B because of her decision-making abilities (Sinclair 1990: 70).

The computer, in assuming repetitive, routine functions, frees the nurse to attend more to direct patient care or nursing management tasks. The individual has more control over her job performance when the computer is used extensively to take over non-nursing and routine tasks. This should lead to an increased sense of accomplishment and job satisfaction (Sinclair 1990: 72).

CONCLUSION

The computer has become a valuable tool for management in general, as well as for the efficient nursing service manager. Utilization of the computer and the appropriate software programmes to their fullest extent should enable her to present correctly-calculated submissions to higher authorities, and these submissions would carry the necessary weight to ensure that the nursing department gets its rightful proportion of budgeted funds. It should also enable the nurse manager to have more time available to do first-hand observational data-collecting concerning the organizational climate in her service by walking around more often on rounds.

She will need to understand the effects a computer information system will have on the organizational culture in general, and will need to be aware of ethical and other issues which must be addressed when instituting such a system.

References

Coetzee, M. (1984). Rekenaars as 'n hulpmiddel in verpleegkundige administrasie. *Curationis,* volume 7, number 4, pp. 38–40.

Coetzee, M. (1985). 'n Rekenaargesteunde wissellys. *Curationis,* volume 8, number 2, pp. 50–6.

Coetzee, M. (1985). Gehaltesorg en koste-effektiewe dienslewering deur middel van 'n geoutomatiseerde pasiëntklassifikasiestelsel. *Curationis,* volume 8, number 1, pp. 44–8.

Cox, H. C., Harsanyi, B., and Dean. L. C. (1987). *Computers and Nursing.* USA: Appleton and Lange: Norwalk, Connecticut/Los Altos, California.

Culpepper, R. C. (1984). Computers for quality care — what can they do? *Computers in Nursing,* volume 2, number 3, pp. 85–7.

Finkler, S. A. (1985). Microcomputers in nursing administration: a software overview. *JONA,* volume 15, number 4, pp. 18–22.

Fitzpatrick, T., Farrel, R. Y. and Richter-Zeunik, M. (1987). An automated staff scheduling system that minimizes payroll costs and maximises nurse satisfaction. *JONA,* volume 5, number 1, pp. 10–13.

Hanson, R. L. (1982). Applying management information systems to staffing. *JONA,* volume 12, number 10, pp. 5–9.

Lombard, S. (1989). The need for information systems in the private sector. *Nursing RSA,* volume 4, number 9, pp. 14–17.

McNairn, J. A. 1986). The choice is yours. *Nursing RSA,* volume 1, number 8, pp. 43–7.

Scholes, M., Bryant, Y., and Barber, B. (eds.) (1983). *The Impact of Computers on Nursing.* Elsevier Science Publishers: Amsterdam.

Shipham, S. O., Hay, J. T. and Fallick, P. M. (1989). Role of strategic management in the design of a hospital information system. *Nursing RSA,* volume 4, number 5, pp. 12–19.

Sinclair, V. G. (1990). The impact of computer support on social and political dynamics in health care organizations. *Nursing Administration Quarterly,* volume 14, number 3, pp. 66–73.

Tappen, R. M. (1989). *Nursing Leadership and Management: Concepts and Practice.* Davis: Philadelphia.

Werley, H. H. and Lang, N. M. (editors) (1988). *Identification of the Nursing Minimum Data Set.* Springer Publishing Co: New York.

Woolery, L. K. (1990). Professional standards and ethical dilemmas in nursing information systems. *JONA,* volume 20, number 10, pp. 50–3.

CHAPTER 29

INDUSTRIAL RELATIONS AND QUALITY OF WORK LIFE

M. Bezuidenhout

CONTENTS

INTRODUCTION

Industrial relations has become an issue of immense importance in South Africa during the last decade. Complex industrial relations and the involvement of trade unions are a fact of life today, and their importance will become even greater because of the social, economic, and political problems facing the country.

Control, in a management setting, involves the ability of management to direct and influence the actions taking place in an organization. Management determines an organization's input, processing, and output, and directs employees at each stage.

Industrial relations is concerned with the association of employers and employees — the joining of the two groups for one purpose. In health care that purpose is to provide patients with care, and clients with service. Industrial relations involves a people-oriented process which includes regulations, contractual agreements, negotiations, organizational policies and procedures, and the personal interests and whims of all the people concerned in the enterprise. It is important to recognize that, today more than ever before, the nurse manager needs an understanding of the relevant legislation, the basic principles of disciplinary action, the solving of grievances, collective bargaining, arbitration, and the settlement of disputes.

Inevitable confrontations must be managed in a way that permits nurses and nurse managers to deal with issues and the impact of those issues without destroying goals shared by the profession and the organization (Marriner 1982: 260). The importance of non-formal interpersonal relations and knowledgeable management conduct cannot be overemphasized.

DEFINING INDUSTRIAL RELATIONS

According to the Department of Manpower, the term *industrial relations* refers to all aspects and matters connected with the relationship between employer and employee. The term encompasses matters relating to negotiations in respect of remuneration and other conditions of employment, the prevention and settlement of disputes, the application, interpretation, and effect of laws administered by the department, and the management of the affairs of trade unions, employer's organizations, federations, and industrial councils (Manpower Training Act No. 56 of 1981, Section 1, xxi).

Industrial relations is especially concerned with the relationships established between employers, employees, and the state, while engaged in economic activity in an industrial setting. According to Bendix (1992: 4) the sphere of industrial relations encompasses the following: relationships, the work situation and the working man, the problems and issues of modern industrialized society and of certain processes, structures, institutions, and regulations, all of which occur within a specific social, political, economic, and historical context, and none of which can or should be studied in isolation. The primary objective of industrial relations is to achieve peace in the workplace by developing and maintaining an acceptable system of interaction between the employer and the employee.

Non-formal industrial relations

The non-formal relationship is usually an interpersonal relationship that exists at the micro-level on the work floor. It develops between the manager or supervisor and the subordinate because they are in constant interaction with one another due to the functions and common objectives of the work environment. This relationship includes actions such as the giving of instructions, receiving feedback, the pursuance of service objectives, planning, and control (De Beer 1987: 3). Close co-operation between the supervisor and subordinates is important if goals are to be achieved.

It is important to distinguish between *informal* and *non-formal* relations. Informal relations accentuate social interaction while non-formal relations indicate the work relationships that need to be maintained to a certain extent in order to create a healthy work environment within which organizational goals may be achieved (De Beer 1987: 3). The manner in which the supervisor gives instructions, and the way in which her subordinates experience those orders, the attitude displayed by the supervisor towards taking disciplinary action and the experience of the subordinate in these matters, are important examples of the non-formal relationship while they have nothing to do with informal relations.

The way that the power and influence inherent in management positions are used is of great concern to employees. According to Brannigan (1989: 4) one of the main sources of conflict in the employer–employee relationship currently stems from the process of management. Wade (1985: 7), and Muller and Coetzee (1990: 27) are of the opinion that nursing management is generally inclined to be autocratic. Managers are so accustomed to speaking to people as subordinates, making snap decisions, issuing instructions, and maintaining absolute control, that subordinates lose interest and initiative and stop thinking for themselves because there is no need for independent thought (DiVincenti 1977: 58).

Autocratic leaders frequently exercise power with coercion. Sullivan and Decker (1988: 214–5) describe their personalities as firm, insistent, self-assured, often dominating, and they like to constantly be the centre of attention. Such leaders are assumed to be self-centered, indifferent to the needs of the organization, resistant to change, and lacking in creative potential. The formal authority that they possess gives them the right to give commands to subordinates, and they depend upon this authority and use it to get the performance that they require.

DiVincenti (1977: 58) postulates that because an employee finds it necessary to adopt an attitude of obedience to her autocratic leader as a constant reminder of management's power to hire and discharge, the employee assumes a dependent attitude.

On the other hand, if managers and the organization as a whole, are responsive to employees' concerns and needs and accept the right of every individual to have the opportunity to participate in creating the system under which she works, employees may view the working relationship as co-operative. The achievement of organizational goals will then meet the personal goals of both management and staff because the efforts and benefits are shared.

Characteristics of a good non-formal relationship are loyalty, a positive, supporting attitude, and affection for one another. These aspects of a working relationship cannot be enforced by regulations. According to de Beer (1987: 4) the psychological contract that exists between the manager and the employee is the cardinal means of regulating the non-formal relationship. During the continuous interaction between these two parties the contract is either confirmed and strengthened or dismantled and weakened. The attitude of subordinates towards management is usually a good indicator of the existing quality of non-formal relations within an enterprise.

Poor non-formal relationships will give rise to work dissatisfaction because many lower level employees experience satisfaction on the interpersonal level. Dissatisfaction usually leads to the need to organize and act collectively. Marriner (1982: 259) supports this view by stating that, in the absence of shared efforts, benefits, and respect, employees seek ways in which they can exercise control over the direction of the organization, often through the process of collective bargaining.

The employee's perceived need for collective bargaining stems from industrial relations practices by management that have not met employees' expectations. Labour unrest usually starts from poor non-formal relationships on the floor. It is generally accepted that when critical levels of suspicion, distrust, and disloyalty are reached in the non-formal relationship, this is the first phase of the conflict cycle (De Beer 1987: 7). Conversely, if the non-formal relationship between management and the subordinates is healthy, it can contribute greatly to the quality of service and the prevention of employee dissatisfaction, even though environmental conditions may be poor.

UNIONS AND EMPLOYER REPRESENTATION

Analysis of the labour relationship reveals that the power of an employer is best matched by a combination of workers who, by collective action, obtain concessions which would not otherwise have been granted and, in doing so, attempt to improve their position both at the workplace and in society as a whole. It is this collective organization which forms the basis of trade unionism (Bendix 1989: 41). Just as workers can belong to trade unions, so employers can join employers' associations.

Trade unions

It is accepted that it is legitimate for employees to join formal organizations in order to express their interests and seek to influence management decisions in order to achieve their goals (Salamon 1989: 30). The legal definition of a trade union is 'any number of employees in any particular undertaking, industry, trade or occupation, associated together for the purpose, whether by itself or with other purposes, of regulating relations in that undertaking, industry, trade or occupation between themselves, or some of them, and their employers or some of them' (Labour Relations Act no 28 of 1956).

While the objective of trade unions is to protect and promote the particular goals of individual workers or groups of workers, the employers' interests, on the other hand, are to maximize their return on investment for shareholders, which means making the maximum profit which seems fair and reasonable to all parties concerned, including the employees.

A union representative, or shop steward, is selected by a majority of the employees in a particular unit (Marriner 1982: 268). Provision should be made for the accommodation of shop stewards and their role should be clearly spelt out. It is the shop steward who represents workers when grievances are lodged or when disciplinary action is taken. He acts as a link between the employees, the employer, and the trade union itself. The role that the shop steward plays in the enterprise is of cardinal importance in the promotion of harmony between the enterprise and the trade union. As Nel and Van Rooyen (1991: 150) point out:

> ... the primary role of the shop steward is to ensure and maintain the equilibrium in relations between management and labour within the framework of existing rules, regulations and customs.

The main objective of a union is to protect and promote the interests of members with regard to the employer–employee relationship, so unions should not be seen as synonymous with strikes. Although the ultimate weapon of the union is to withhold labour, the idea is that workers should become organized to negotiate for a better deal. According to Brannigan (1988: 2) the three main areas of trade union involvement in nursing centre around unresolved grievances involving wages, unfair dismissals, or discipline.

Potgieter (1992: 87) gives examples of unfair disciplinary action. The services of a professional nurse in a management position at a private hospital were terminated after eleven months in this position. She received a letter informing her that she was unable to cope with management tasks, that her dismissal would take immediate effect, and that she would receive the additional payment of one month's salary. According to Potgieter the nurse did not receive any prior warning, reprimand, or remedial disciplinary action in order to improve her management skills. She was thus unaware of her so-called unsatisfactory behaviour until she received the letter of dismissal. In another example, Potgieter (1992: 103) states that a professional nurse in a top management position at a newly established private hospital was informed, even before there were any patients admitted to the hospital, that she would probably not be able to keep up with the pace of work. The nurse felt that she had the right to complete her trial period before being judged, and informed management to this effect, after which she was informed that her position had already been promised to another and that she could only stay on in a subordinate position.

Such action from management leads to much hardship and damage to an individual's self-image and confidence and causes discontent amongst the other employees because they share the feeling of insecurity when disciplinary matters are not handled fairly. In an attempt to receive fair and just treatment, employees seek assistance from a third party which, in the case of nurses, may be either the South African Nursing Association (SANA) or a trade union of their choice.

No person in South Africa may be prevented from belonging to a union which he or she chooses to belong to. However, public servants and those employed in essential services may not use the industrial conciliation machinery in the Labour Relations Act in the event of a dispute. They have to resort to arbitration. According to Brannigan (1988: 3) this means, in essence, that nurses employed in the public sector may not strike in terms of the Labour Relations Act.

Both the South African Nursing Council (SANC) and SANA emphasize that nurses will always have an ethical responsibility towards their patients, regardless of what legislation allows or does not allow. SANA states very clearly that a patient should never be used as a bargaining tool to improve the socio-economic status of nurses (*Nursing News,* volume 15, number 11, 1991: 1). According to a policy statement regarding strike action by nurses, SANA:

- is of the opinion that a strike by a nurse is a violation of the patient's right to safe and continuous nursing care;

- believes that a nurse should never be placed in a situation where she feels there is no option open to her other than to resort to strike action.

SANA believes that the nurse therefore has a right to:

- fair and equitable employment practices;

- reasonable conditions of employment;

- a fair dispute resolution procedure which must be negotiated by, and agreed between, the employer and the representative organization for nurses, and which should exclude strike action but include compulsory arbitration;

- SANA believes that nursing services should be declared an essential service in terms of the Labour Relations Act, thus entrenching the right to arbitration;

- it will not condone, nor utilize, strike action as a means of dispute resolution between employers and employees;

- it believes that strike action by nurses, where the patient's rights to safe and continuous nursing care are endangered, constitutes unprofessional conduct (*Nursing News,* volume 15, number 9, 1991: 4).

The nurse's behaviour should at all times be a credit to the profession. Neglect in maintaining the health of a patient under her care may be considered as negligence and may lead to disciplinary action by the SANC. Despite the nurse's acceptance of the professional and ethical code, entailing that she should place the interest of her patient before self-interest, she still has rights as a human being and as a citizen. Sound industrial relations practices therefore need to be developed — especially compulsory arbitration — so as to prevent nurses having to go to the extreme measure of striking in order for grievances to get the necessary attention.

Employers' associations

Individual enterprises may consider whether or not to join an employers' organization. Employers' associations can consist of any number of employers in a particular undertaking, industry, trade, or occupation, who associate for the purpose of regulating relations between themselves and their employees in that industry.

According to Gerber et al. (1992: 391), participation in employers' associations and finally in the industrial council system means that collective bargaining can take place on behalf of the institution by means of employers' representatives, and that specialists in negotiation and collective bargaining can perform this task on behalf of the institution.

COLLECTIVE BARGAINING

The principle of freedom of association, the process of collective bargaining, and some measure of joint decision-making, is considered by Bendix (1989: 15) as an accepted means by which to achieve a balance of power between the various participants in the industrial situation.

A collective action may be as simple as two people going together to management to discuss their wishes, or it can be as complex as a union-negotiated agreement (Marriner 1982: 260). Increasingly, employees are trying to join together in a single organizing unit to gain greater influence from larger group numbers. Collective bargaining is the negotiating of terms and conditions of employment, or other issues of mutual aid or protection. It need not necessarily be carried out in the context of a union.

Both management and labour are bound to conform to the legal requirements for the collective bargaining process. The law requires that those engaged in collective bargaining must meet at reasonable times, confer in good faith, and put their agreements in writing if either of the parties request it. Brannigan (1988b: 1) gives the prerequisites for effective handling of the process of collective bargaining:

1. Parties should have enough power to persuade each other, but not enough to force total surrender. It must be kept in mind that the survival of the employer is essential for the employee to receive an income.

2. Both parties must be willing to move from their original positions, indicating their willingness to make a compromise.

3. Both parties must have a mandate enabling them to know how far they can negotiate or compromise. They must have clear guidelines giving them leeway to move within the predetermined limits set by their respective parties on the particular matter.

4. Equality, mutual respect, and good faith between the negotiating parties are essential prerequisites for effective agreements that satisfy both parties.

The purpose of collective bargaining is to apply pressure on the employer to redress perceived inadequacies in the conditions of employment and to regulate conflict arising out of management demands.

Decisions on health care have traditionally been made largely by management, so power has rested with management. Employees and trade unions frequently wish to bargain about patient care issues, and management has been hesitant to discuss this area to any great extent since it, rather than the union, traditionally has held the responsibility for the health care outcomes of the institution (Marriner 1982: 267). Unions have become more and more involved in the health industry, causing great concern due to the effect this has on nursing practice. Some examples of such instances given by Brannigan (1987: 4) are:

- A registered nurse working in industry chastised her nursing auxilliary for suturing a three-day-old human bite. Before she knew what was happening, she had been called before a union 'kangaroo court' and had been disciplined by the union for what is considered by nursing and medical staff as fair action, but what the union decided was unfair practice.

- A matron in an old age home was chastised by the union for allowing her nursing assistants and even registered nurses to do certain cleaning duties such as cleaning urine and blood off of the floor. As far as the union was concerned, that is the specific duty of the cleaners and may not be done by anybody else.

Brannigan (1988: 4) reiterates that nurses must do what needs to be done — nurses must decide on practical, educational, and service issues, and on the future of nursing. She further states that nurse managers have an obligation to ensure that the quality of patient care and the decisions about nursing in South Africa remain in the hands of nurses, rather than allowing non-nursing trade union leaders to make the decisions and determine the future of patient care.

Collective bargaining is an internationally accepted modus operandi for handling conflict in the workplace, so nurses and nurse managers must examine their attitudes toward nursing and the impact of the chosen bargaining structure on nursing and the work setting. The process of collective bargaining should be seriously considered by the nurse manager who is earnest about maintaining good industrial relations within her service.

FORMULATION OF CLEAR POLICIES AND PROCEDURES

According to Brannigan (1989: 4), primary triggers for union intervention in health services are unsatisfactory salaries, unresolved grievances, and unfair discipline. The last two aspects, in particular, are areas for great concern. Grievance procedures are lengthy, involved, and sometimes difficult to implement. Brannigan indicates that in many instances the communication channels are blocked and individuals are severely victimized for raising genuine grievances. This view is supported by Potgieter (1992: 132) who states that often grievances are brought to the attention of management, but management ignores them. According to Critical Health (1988: 60), during 1987, 400 nurses at a training hospital in the Transvaal participated in strike action as their complaints about the quality of food, discrimination, intimidation by hospital security personnel, and racist behaviour by management were ignored. Grievances that were brought to the attention of Cape Provincial Authorities in 1990 included poor wages not keeping up with inflation, and the lack of job security as 'some categories of workers are barred from becoming members of the permanent staff, even after three or four decades of service, and they still do not qualify for pensions' (Potgieter 1992: 38).

This leads to dissatisfaction and gives rise to industrial action by nursing personnel. Potgieter (1992: 42) concludes that nurse managers appear to be unskilled in the handling of grievances as the same mistakes in this regard are made repeatedly at the same hospitals. This approach is unacceptable, and is not conducive to creating or maintaining good non-formal relationships. Appropriate planning and preparation by nursing management will have to be carried out in order to handle the labour situation effectively whilst retaining control of services. Cunningham (1990: 37) is of the opinion that the basic principles of democracy and fairness will have to be maintained within nursing management, as is expected in general industry. He confirms this view by stating:

> ... if industry sets a precedent of what is to follow in the health service, all those involved in health care will have to realise that certain principles they may hold, which are incongruent with the ideology of freedom and democracy, will have to be compromised if work relations are to be constructive.

Disciplinary procedures

Any enterprise, irrespective of its nature, structure, or objectives, needs to have a set of rules and a code of conduct. These rules determine permissible and acceptable behaviour for all the employees in the enterprise. A disciplinary procedure outlines the formal process adopted whenever an employee breaks the rules of the undertaking or commits any other act which might be in breach of her contract of employment.

Salamon (1987: 503) defines formal discipline as 'action taken by management against an individual or group who have failed to conform to the rules established by management within the organization.' Such action often proves to be an emotive and contentious issue, particularly when it results in the ultimate sanction of the dismissal of an employee. It not only involves subjective concepts such as 'fair' and 'reasonable', and 'right' and 'wrong', but it also concerns the power, authority, and status of management.

Contrary to the opinion of many employees, a disciplinary procedure is not intended merely to ensure that they are properly disciplined. It is introduced to prevent the irrational disciplining of employees. In her study involving nurse managers in private and public hospitals, Potgieter (1992: 133) found that disciplinary action was not always applied in a fair and just manner. Potgieter (1992: 109) states the case of a professional nurse in the public sector whose annual salary increase was denied due to disciplinary action. The matter was not re-evaluated again for the following four years, until the nurse sought help from SANA in 1988. Several written inquiries directed at her employer, over a two year period, received no reply. Eventually the matter received attention at the end of 1990; management conceded to reinstate her annual increase as from 1989, and stated that they would allow her to continue her career with a clean record providing she kept to the rules! The result of this specific disciplinary situation was not only the employee's financial hardship, and the continual threat of her 'past behaviour' being mentioned, but it clearly indicated management's failure to implement a fair and progressive disciplinary procedure, taking into account its responsibility to take remedial action where employees need help to adjust their unacceptable behaviour.

Bendix (1989: 258) motivates the need for proper procedures by noting that the use of disciplinary procedures ensures that all employees are treated in the same manner, that an employee is not disciplined or dismissed at the whim of a manager or supervisor, that the employee is afforded the opportunity of a fair hearing before dismissal occurs, that a transgression of the same kind is treated in the same manner by all managers, that employees have a degree of certainty regarding the type of treatment they will receive, and that managerial representatives also obtain certainty about their actions and decisions.

In order to ensure consistent and fair discipline in the institution, and to promote disciplined behaviour among all employees, it should be the institution's policy to vest disciplinary action and accountability in line management (Gerber et al. 1992: 399). The objective should be to ensure that disciplinary action is taken immediately in response to a transgression, that it is progressive in nature, that it settles the disciplinary matter at the lowest possible level, and that it is consistently applied.

In the hospital situation the ward sister is considered to be 'first line' management; she would consult and refer aspects regarding disciplinary matters to middle management (usually the zone matron). If the matter can not be resolved at this level it should be referred to the nursing service manager as soon as possible to comply with the prerequisites for effective disciplinary action.

Inadequate and inconsistent handling of disciplinary matters, and the resulting grievances, have a negative effect on employees, causing anger, disappointment, and distrust. In addition, employees' self-image, confidence, and professional image are adversely affected in the process (Potgieter 1992: 134). It must be noted that disciplinary action also aims at helping the employee to improve or correct her unacceptable behaviour, so follow-up action and guidance by management are essential.

Ground rules for disciplinary action

In order for disciplinary action to be fair and just, certain ground rules need to be established and thoroughly implemented in the institution, setting the goal posts for both management and subordinates.

According to Bendix (1989: 259) the principles and requirements in formulating disciplinary codes, procedures, and actions are:

1. A disciplinary code should be comprehensive and complete. It should list all types of offences which may occur, and should specify the disciplinary measures to be applied in each case.

2. The disciplinary procedure must be clear and accessible to employees. Explanations ought to be worded in simple language which all employees can understand, and the procedure must be known to employees.

3. The procedure should conform to the principles of natural justice. This means that the incident should be investigated, the punishment should match the offence, an employee must be fully informed of the reason for the disciplinary action against her, she must be provided with an opportunity to present her case, she should be allowed a representative, the circumstances should be taken into account, there should be consistency in disciplinary measures, and there should be a right of appeal or review.

4. Discipline should be progressive in nature. Generally, no disciplinary action is taken before an informal warning has been given. If such a warning has no effect, a written warning is handed to the person concerned, who is requested to sign this document for the following reasons given by Gerber et al. (1992: 400): to ensure that the employee understands the validity of what has been written, so that it can be used as evidence at a later stage if necessary, to notify the employee that the disciplinary procedure has been set in motion, and to bring to the employee's attention the fact that the document will be included in his personal file.

5. There should be a clearly-stated policy as to the duration of retention of recorded warnings on personal files of an employee after he has rectified his behaviour. SANA issues the following guidelines on the retention of warnings on an employee's file:
   - a recorded verbal warning will be removed from an employee's file and destroyed after six months;
   - a written warning after 12 months;
   - a final warning after two years (*Nursing News,* volume 15, number 11, 1991: 12).

It should also be noted that progressive disciplinary action should be for a specific offence and that disciplinary action cannot be taken on a cumulative basis involving different indiscretions.

Disciplinary and grievance procedures are aimed primarily at interaction between the supervisor and employee on the shop floor (see table 29.1). It is at this level that the foundations are laid for good interpersonal relations. These structures aim to minimize conflict between the employees and management by setting clear expectations, procedures, and actions, which apply to both management and the employee.

THE GRIEVANCE PROCEDURE

Employee grievances are wide-ranging and vary from general dissatisfaction about wages and working conditions, dissatisfaction regarding promotion and training, complaints about a lack of facilities or inadequate equipment, to unhappiness on the part of an employee regarding unfair treatment, unreasonable orders, unrealistic expectations, and blatant discrimination. Bendix (1929: 283) defines a formal grievance as:

> ... a complaint, other than demands formulated by a collective body, which is related to the employee's treatment or position within his daily working routine and which, because it may result in a dispute, warrants the formal attention of management.

According to the Hospital and Nursing Year Book of Southern Africa (1991: 228) the purpose of the grievance procedure is to lay down policy for dealing with grievances lodged by employees, in order to achieve the following:

- consistency and fairness for all employees;
- to resolve the grievance at the lowest possible level, but creating a structure for access to the highest authority if necessary;
- to resolve the grievance as expeditiously as possible;
- to entrench the right to be represented/assisted by a fellow colleague/representative.

There is no doubt that the grievance procedure can be well applied to deal with conflict in the workplace. Written grievance procedures obviate the need for management to become involved in arguments with labour, as mutually accepted procedures are set and applied. A grievance procedure fulfills the following functions (Bendix 1992: 283):

- it creates the opportunity for upward communication from employees;
- it ensures that complaints are dealt with effectively by management;
- it creates awareness of employee problems or of problem areas which could be subjected to further investigation;
- it prevents disputes from arising;
- it renders the disciplinary procedure more acceptable, since employees can object to management performance;
- it emphasizes management's concern for the well-being of employees.

These objectives will only be achieved if the grievance procedure functions effectively and is properly utilized by both employees and management (refer to table 29.1).

Managers need to realize that the key to a successful grievance procedure is *prompt action*. A delayed or neglected grievance is often the origin of a new grievance. If specific time limits are laid down in the procedure, employees are usually prepared to allow the process to take place, and will also be satisfied to wait longer if facts are difficult to establish. This means, however, that they need to be kept informed. Gerber et al. (1992: 398) state that an effective grievance procedure is an integral part of the enterprise's total communication system, and it keeps both workers and managers aware of each other's needs, desires, attitudes, opinions, values, and perceptions.

Table 29.1: Grievance, disciplinary, and retrenchment procedures

GRIEVANCE PROCEDURE

1. Definition
1.1 A grievance is defined as any feeling of injustice or dissatisfaction which arises out of the employer/employee relationship and which requires the attention of management.
1.2 Management should not attempt to prescribe or restrict the nature of grievances. However, the following do **not** fall under this procedure:
  1.2.1 appeals against disciplinary action, as there is provision for this in the disciplinary procedure;
  1.2.2 any issues which do not relate directly to the working environment or the employer/ employee relationship, e.g. personal, social or family problems.

2. **Purpose**
The purpose of this procedure is to lay down policy for dealing with grievances lodged by employees, to achieve the following:
2.1 consistency and fairness to all employees;
2.2 to resolve the grievance at the lowest possible level, but creating a structure for access to the highest authority if necessary;
2.3 to resolve the grievance as expeditiously as possible;
2.4 to entrench the right to be represented/assisted by a fellow colleague/representative.

3. The grievance procedure
STEP ONE
1. An employee should bring the grievance to the attention of her immediate supervisor by filling in the GRIEVANCE REPORT FORM.
2. When presenting the grievance, the employee may be accompanied by her representative.

3. The supervisor shall attempt to resolve the grievance **within 2 working days** (or longer if agreed to by the employee) and shall record such attempt on the grievance report form.
4. If the grievance is resolved, this is recorded on the form and the form is then filed.

STEP TWO
1. If the grievance is not resolved at stage one, or the employee is unhappy with the outcome, the form is then handed to the next level of authority.
2. This process shall continue up the line of command until the form is handed to the highest official in the organisation.
3. The maximum time for processing the grievance at each stage shall be **2 working days** unless agreed to otherwise by both parties. All attempts at resolution shall be recorded on the form.
4. If the grievance is resolved, this is recorded on the form and the form is then filed.

STEP 3
1. If the grievance is not resolved at stage two, the highest official, on receipt of the grievance report form, shall attend to the grievance within **5 working days.**
2. If the grievance is resolved, this is recorded on the form and the form is then filed.

STEP 4
1. If the grievance is not satisfactorily resolved, the matter shall be raised at the next meeting of the management.
2. If the grievance is resolved, this is recorded on the form and the form is then filed.

STEP 5
1. In the event of all grievances, the decision of the highest official will be final. The management may at its

discretion, however, delegate authority for a final decision for an individual grievance to the highest official.

2. If the grievance is not satisfactorily resolved after the above procedure has been fully exhausted, the grievance will become a matter of dispute and be dealt with in terms of the provisions of the Labour Relations Act, Act 28 of 1956.

DISCIPLINARY PROCEDURE AND CODE

1. Definition

1.1 Disciplinary action can be seen as any action initiated by management to maintain discipline and to act when breaches of discipline occur.

1.2 It is the sole responsibility and authority of management to maintain discipline and to act when breaches of discipline occur.

2. Aim

2.1 The action is initially aimed at correcting or changing the employee's conduct or working performance, rather than being punitive.

2.1 This procedure and code aims at standardising and formalising disciplinary practice so that:

— it is applied consistently and fairly;

— it is applied promptly at the lowest possible level;

— the employee may be represented by a colleague/ representative of his choice;

— the employee is put on notice that his behaviour or performance is unacceptable;

— the action taken matches the severity of the offence;

— there is support for the decision

to terminate his services if necessary.

3. The Disciplinary Procedure

When a complaint has been received or there is an apparent offence requiring disciplinary action:

3.1 The employee shall be advised by her immediate supervisor that disciplinary action may be warranted.

3.2 The nature of the offence and the relevant proof should be presented to the employee.

3.3. Section A of the **Disciplinary Report Form** shall be completed in all instances, even if the appropriate discipline is a verbal warning as this must be recorded in the employee's file.

3.4 Timeous arrangements shall be made for disciplinary hearing for all disciplinary cases, except where verbal warnings are given. Adequate notice of such hearing shall be given to the employee concerned. The employee should also be advised of her right to be assisted in representing her case.

3.5 The hearing will be conducted by those authorised to discipline and the employee, with her representative if she so chooses, shall be provided an opportunity of defending herself at such hearing. Witnesses, as required, may be called by either party.

3.6 Once all the relevant facts have been heard and investigated, disciplinary action shall be decided upon by the individual conducting the hearing. The following factors should be taken into account:

— the severity of the offence;

— mitigating circumstances;

— previous record (reference should be made to previous records only when the guilt of the person has been proven);

— length of service.

The person presiding at the hearing shall

be guided by the Disciplinary Code. If the level of discipline required is beyond her authority, the relevant authority shall be consulted.

RETRENCHMENT PROCEDURES

1. Definitions

1.1 'Retrenchment' means the termination of the employment contract because of financial difficulties of the employer, recession, etc.

1.2 'Redundancy' means the termination of the employment contract due to technological changes, automation, etc. where the specific post held by the employee becomes superfluous.

For the purpose of this document, the word 'retrenchment' will be used to cover termination of employment, regardless of whether it is for reasons of retrenchment or redundancy.

2. Purpose

2.1 The purpose of this procedure is to lay down mutually acceptable policy which will determine principles/ criteria to be considered in finally deciding which employees will be retrenched.

2.2 The decision to retrench employees is that of the employer, but the employer recognises the right of the employee and her representative Association to be informed about such retrenchment, and to make representations in this regard.

3. Principles for retrenchment

3.1 An initial attempt should be made to **avoid** retrenchment. The following aspects should thus be considered in consultation with the representative Association before retrenchment:

3.1.1 Natural attrition trends, i.e. posts that become vacant should not be filled.

3.1.2 Overtime should be stopped.

3.1.3 Short-time where feasible, so that no-one loses his or her job.

3.1.4 Transfer to other departments, even if this entails retraining or changing jobs.

3.1.5 A reduction in casual or temporary employees first.

3.1.6 Early retirement for those nearing retirement age.

3.1.7 Voluntary agreement to retire or leave.

3.2 Once the above aspects have been considered, certain principles for selection of those who must be retrenched should be considered:

3.2.1 Where objective criteria exist for assessment of performance and productivity, such factors shall be taken into account.

3.2.2 Protection of certain groups, e.g. breadwinners, should be considered.

3.2.3 After all the above have been considered, the principle of last in, first out will be applied.

(From *Hospital and Nursing Year Book of Southern Africa 1991*, published by H. Engelhardt and Co. Reprinted with the kind permission of the publishers.)

Being sensitive to potential causes of dissatisfaction and eliminating them, will prevent the need to apply the grievance procedure. The prevention of grievances is more important than handling them, so poor managerial practices have to be eliminated and managerial behaviour must be adjusted to improve worker morale.

The grievance procedure in practice

Bendix (1992: 283–5) is of the opinion that there are no steps which have to be adhered to at all costs in the establishment of a grievance procedure, but the following general rules apply:

1. The employee should be granted the opportunity to bring her grievance to the attention of top management.

2. She should be permitted representation, if so desired.

3. Management at the various levels should give careful consideration to the grievance and should make genuine attempts to resolve it.

4. Time limits should be established for each stage of the procedure.

5. The grievance will not be seen as resolved until the employee declares herself satisfied.

6. The employee has the right, if the grievance remains unresolved, to declare a dispute.

7. Grievances should, whenever possible, be handled by line management, but staff management, in the form of the personnel department, may act in an advisory capacity.

Grievance procedures can be structured in various ways and stages which will depend on the size and complexity of the enterprise, but their operation should be fair and just, from the point of the employee's interaction with his immediate supervisor up to the point where the grievance is lodged with the nursing service manager. It is also essential that all steps and actions taken must be carefully documented for record and reference purposes.

The following are the recommended steps to be followed when handling a grievance in the health services (*Nursing News*, volume 15, number 10, 1991: 14; Hospital and Nursing Year Book of Southern Africa 1991: 228):

Step 1

1. An employee should bring the grievance to the attention of her immediate supervisor by filling in the grievance report form.

2. When presenting the grievance, the employee may be accompanied by her representative.

3. The supervisor should attempt to resolve the grievance within two working days (or longer, if agreed by the employee) and should record this attempt on the grievance report form.

4. If the grievance is resolved, this is recorded on the form and the form is then filed.

Step 2

1. If the grievance is not resolved at stage one, or the employee is unhappy with the outcome, the form is then handed to the next level of authority.

2. This process should continue up the line of command until the form is handed to the highest official in the institution.

3. The maximum time for processing the grievance at each stage should be two working days, unless otherwise agreed by both parties. All attempts at resolution should be recorded on the form.

4. If the grievance is resolved, this is recorded on the form and the form is then filed.

Step 3

1. If the grievance is not resolved at stage two, the highest official (the nursing service manager), on receipt of the grievance form, should attend to the grievance within five working days.

2. If the grievance is resolved, this should be recorded on the form and the form is then filed.

Step 4

1. If the grievance is not satisfactorily resolved, the matter should be raised at the next management meeting.

2. If the grievance is resolved, this is recorded on the form and the form is then filed.

Step 5

1. The management may at its discretion, however, delegate authority for a final decision to the highest official (head office in the public service, or the managing director in a private institution). The decision of the highest official will be final.

2. If the grievance is not satisfactorily resolved after the above procedure has been fully exhausted, the grievance will become a matter of dispute. The nurse may then declare a dispute by means

of her SANA representative or shop steward, in the case of trade union membership, and the matter will be dealt with in terms of the provisions of the Labour Relations Act, Act 28, of 1956.

Disputes

If a grievance procedure runs its course without any agreement being reached between the employees and management, and the employees will still not accept the decision of management, a dispute situation arises (Gerber et al. 1992: 392).

A dispute procedure prescribes the action to be taken by both parties during the interval between the establishment of a dispute situation and a possible work stoppage or, even worse, a strike. Gerber et al. (1992: 392) indicates that the different procedures/ negotiating platforms — eg SANA's trade union leg, industrial council and conciliation boards — function under the Labour Relations Act.

Negotiating platforms

SANA has different platforms for negotiation for its various groups of members, ie the Public Service Joint Forum for members employed in government services, and recognition agreements in the private sector. There are some platforms, however, where SANA has had no access because it has not been registered as a trade union — eg the industrial councils for local authorities (where over 11% of SANA's members are employed) and conciliation boards (*Nursing News,* volume 16, number 8 1992: 10). It is for this reason that the members of the nursing profession voted for the registration of a trade union leg of SANA during 1992.

SANA trade union leg

The registration of this leg enables SANA to gain access to negotiating platforms in order to adequately represent its members. Just as SANA had to gain recognition as a staff association with the Commission for Administration to represent its members in the public service, so a part of the association had to register as a trade union with the Department of Manpower to represent other members (*Nursing News,* volume 16, number 8, 1992: 10) where their negotiating platform is an industrial council or conciliation board.

Industrial council

An industrial council consists of trade unions that have been registered with the Department of Manpower and employers' associations in a specific trade or occupation, where collective bargaining takes place and agreements are reached, which are gazetted and legally enforceable in places of employment falling within the ambit of the industrial council (*Nursing News,* volume 15, number 9, 1991: 8).

The duty of an industrial council is to maintain industrial peace between all employers and employees over whom it exercises jurisdiction. It also endeavours to prevent disputes and settle those that have arisen. Where no industrial council has jurisdiction, the Director-General of the Department of Manpower can establish a conciliation board to settle a particular dispute (Gerber et al. 1992: 392–3).

Conciliation boards

Where a dispute arises between an employer and employees, or their representative organization, and these parties are not members of an industrial council, the dispute can be referred to a conciliation board. This is a temporary body established in terms of the Labour Relations Act. Once the dispute is resolved, the conciliation board is disbanded. Conciliation boards can, in certain instances, also be used for negotiation purposes (*Nursing News,* volume 15, number 9, 1991: 8).

Although provisions are laid down by law for the settlement of disputes by either industrial council or conciliation boards, unionized and non-union employers sometimes bypass the legal procedures established by law. In these cases the only other way is for management to take the initiative and establish a recognition agreement in co-operation with the employees and a representative body for the employers.

Recognition agreements

A recognition agreement is a document signed by an employer and an organization representing employees, where the employer acknowledges that the organization (SANA or a trade union) has the right to represent the employees concerned and to bargain on their behalf. It usually also contains agreed procedures — eg grievance and disciplinary procedures — which assist in the conduct of this relationship (*Nursing News,* volume 15, number 9, 1991: 8).

SANA deals with private sector employers, either formally (by way of recognition agreements), or more informally on an ad hoc basis. At this point in time approximately 30 recognition agreements have been entered into between SANA and private employers to look after the interests of members employed by these private enterprises. The recognition agreement gives formal recognition to SANA as the representative body for nurses, and allows for SANA representatives to be trained and for SANA to negotiate salaries and conditions of services. One of the main provisions of most of the recognition agreements is compulsory arbitration in the event of a dispute (*Nursing News,* volume 16, number 8, 1992: 10). This means that an independent arbitrator is called in who listens to both the employer's and SANA's side of the problem and then makes a decision which is binding on both parties. The person who may act as an arbitrator may be decided upon during the drawing-up of the recognition agreement or may be decided upon later and will vary depending on the specific kind of dispute involved.

Dialogue between management, employees, and sometimes a third party needs to be maintained in order to prevent a work stoppage. Procedures aimed at resolving the conflict situation may vary from mediation to voluntary arbitration or compulsory arbitration.

Mediation

In terms of the Labour Relations Act, an industrial council or conciliation board may, if they are of the opinion that mediation will promote settlement of a dispute, apply to the Minister for the appointment of a mediator who is acceptable to both parties. The mediator will confer with both parties, investigate the subject matter of the dispute, and attempt to bring about a settlement (Bendix 1992: 524). However, Gerber et al. (1992: 393) state that there is no obligation on the part of either party to accept the mediator's proposals. It is therefore in the interests of both the employer and the employees to appoint a mediator who will be acceptable to both parties and who will maintain his role as a neutral and objective person, so that both parties will want to accept his proposals.

The process of mediation has not often been used in the nursing profession as the mediator's proposals are not binding on the parties and may thus be rejected by either or both of them.

Arbitration

Arbitration is a procedure in terms of which an independent and impartial third party hears both the employer's and the employee's side of a matter or dispute and gives a binding decision. Where arbitration is undertaken in terms of the Labour Relations Act, it can be voluntary or compulsory. In the event of disputes in essential services, arbitration is compulsory.

Voluntary arbitration

Voluntary arbitration can be set in motion by an industrial council or conciliation board. If a council or a board has a dispute, it may be referred for arbitration, and it may further decide whether the arbitration is to be conducted by a single arbitrator, by an even number of arbitrators and an umpire, or by the industrial court. The industrial council or conciliation board can also decide who the arbitrator, arbitrators, and the umpire should be (Gerber et al. 1992: 429).

Compulsory arbitration

Compulsory arbitration takes place in respect of disputes occurring in essential services. The procedures followed in compulsory arbitration are the same as those followed in voluntary arbitration. However, the decision made by the arbitrator will be enforced and all parties are bound by it (Gerber et al. 1992: 429).

Essential services, as defined in Section 46 of the Labour Relations Act, are those services where employers and employees are not entitled to enter into industrial action (eg strikes and lockouts) and they have to resort to compulsory arbitration for unresolved disputes. Local authorities, light, power, water, sanitation, passenger-transportation, and fire-extinguishing services are classified as essential services (*Nursing News,* volume 15, number 9, 1991: 8). Health services are currently not included in this definition. In this regard, SANA has already made a submission to the Department of Manpower for nursing services to be declared an essential service (*Nursing News,* volume 15, number 11, 1991: 1). SANA's argument has always been that nurses should not need to strike; the creation of a mechanism of compulsory arbitration in all nursing services will ensure a means of resolving deadlocks in the negotiating process or in the case of disputes (*Nursing News,* volume 16, number 8, 1992: 10). Compulsory arbitration has been utilized by SANA in cases of unfair disciplinary action and unfair dismissals.

Strike action

During the conduct of industrial relations, sanctions may be imposed by either of the parties. The purpose is to express disagreement with the goals, intentions, or actions of the other side, or persuade the other side to relinquish its position in negotiations and to move closer to one's own position.

Sanctions may be of an individual or collective nature. Individual sanctions by an employer may include the disciplining or dismissal of an employee, while collective sanctions involve unilateral rules or conditions relating to employees. Employees, in turn, may impose individual sanctions by repeated absenteeism, resigning from their positions, or by industrial sabotage. Collective sanctions by employees may take the form of strike action, a go-slow, a work-to-rule, and community and/or international pressure.

Since the benefit that an employee may derive from individual action is less than that of the employer, employees and unions engage in the imposition of collective action. Strike action is often viewed as the main collective sanction (Bendix 1992: 240). During the process of negotiating, the threat of strike action is used to pressurize the other party into making concessions in order to enhance the position of the employees.

SANA defines a strike as a concerted cessation, retardation, or obstruction of work by employees, usually to compel their employer to settle their grievances, to agree to their demands concerning conditions of employment, or to employ, suspend, or dismiss a person (*Nursing News,* volume 15, number 9, 1991: 8). Bendix (1989: 213) sees strike action as

> ... a temporary, collective withholding of labour, its objective being to stop production and thereby to oblige the employer to take cognizance of the demands of the employees.

When considering the rights of workers, Gerber et al. (1992: 380) stipulate that employees have the right to strike as this right is protected by the Labour Relations Act. A strike is usually effective only if undertaken collectively, regardless of whether or not workers are unionized. Practice has shown, though, that unionized workers usually stage the most effective strikes.

The state has imposed certain limitations on strike action, and a differentiation exists between legal and illegal strikes. Legal strikes are those which are instituted within the parameters set by government legislation, whereas employees engaged in illegal strike action do not follow or adhere to the legislated procedures or regulations.

Section 65 of the Labour Relations Act sets out a number of circumstances under which a strike is prohibited and prescribes a specific procedure to be followed if a strike is to be legal. Gerber et al. (1992: 432) explain the matter as follows: workers may not strike during the time in which any award, agreement, or determination is binding on them, or if the workers are involved in essential services, or if there is an industrial council with jurisdiction, unless the matter has been considered by the industrial council and the industrial council has not arrived at a solution within a fixed period of time, or, where there is no industrial council, where a conciliation board cannot arrive at a solution within a fixed period of time. Finally, workers may not strike if an industrial council or conciliation board has referred the matter for arbitration. If all these conditions have been met, the strike is legal.

However, employees sometimes take the right to strike upon themselves, without the approval of government or union officials.

Bendix (1992: 241) states that, ultimately, no legislation and no criminal sanctions can entirely preclude a large group of employees from jointly withholding their labour. Employees who engage in strike action in contravention of the law, however, may have little chance of legal recourse should the employer initiate counter-action against them, but this does not negate their ability, or even their right, to engage in strike action.

The NEHAWU strike of 1992, involving employees from the public sector, was considered to be an illegal strike action as the Public Service Act prohibited its employees from participating in strike action. This resulted in the dismissal of many employees in the public sector, causing great dissatisfaction and hardship amongst the employees belonging to the union.

Possible causes of strike action among nursing personnel

As previously stated, the most common causes of strike action by nursing personnel are grievances that have not been satisfactorily resolved. These grievances basically centre around mistakes made with salaries, overtime payment, and problems related to the taking of leave and performance appraisal. It can therefore be said that conditions of service are an important predisposing cause of strike action by nurses (Muller 1991: 38).

Grievances resulting in student strike action at the Baragwanath Hospital in 1985 were:

- aspects related to the nursing residence — eg gates that were closed too early, the quality of the food, and security personnel who allegedly molested nurses;

- student requests for transport for specific occasions, such as outings;

- students wanted a democratically-elected student body;

- complaints of victimization and discrimination in disciplinary matters and during selection for post-basic courses;

- discontent about salaries;

- failure to acknowledge trade unions and the lack of facilities for trade union meetings (Brannigan 1988: 24).

Muller (1991: 38) states that sympathy strike action involving nurses occurred during 1990, and it appears that nurses experienced victimization in this regard.

Handling strikes

When it is apparent that a group of employees intends to withhold its labour or to refuse to continue working, management should react in the manner which is most likely to resolve the issues as speedily as possible, focusing on the origin of the problem and taking all reasonable precautions to prevent injuries to personnel and damage to property.

In order to achieve these objectives, a contingency plan must be drawn up in advance. This will only be possible through proactive planning, organizing, and decision-making in order to ensure appropriate and uniform behaviour on the part of management. According to the IPM Fact Sheet No. 106, managers could adopt the following procedures in the event of a strike:

- Maintain a chronological diary of events.

- Responsibility for the overall situation should be allocated to one person, usually the superintendent or most senior nursing service manager.

- There should be no police involvement if possible as it often inflames the situation. However management should liaise with the police and reach agreement on their respective roles and responsibilities in case of violence.

- A reliable two-way channel of communication should be opened with the striking workers. Negotiation at mass meetings should be avoided, and an attempt should be made to identify representatives with whom management can communicate.

- Report-back facilities and time schedules should be agreed upon. Management must carefully listen to, and take note of, any grievances or demands.

- The Department of Manpower should be informed. Their role is to provide advice and information on legal procedures and not to intervene.

- A single spokesman should be appointed to liaise with the press. The media should be kept informed, and distortion of facts should be avoided.

- Normal facilities such as food, accommodation, and transport should be provided where possible. Any form of potential confrontation should be avoided.

A strike or stoppage develops a personality of its own and management should acknowledge such a personality and should not immediately attempt to suppress the strike. A statement from management that the striking workers should cease their striking before negotiating is a contradiction as it implies that the workers must forfeit their bargaining power in order to bargain. Such a request is not likely to be successful (Gerber et al. 1992: 395–6).

Once the strike has ended and the workers return to work, management has a responsibility to follow- up the matter. This responsibility includes the following (Gerber et al. 1992: 396):

- Promises made should be carried out.

- Managers and supervisors must be briefed and requested to be tactful and firm without relinquishing essential controls over issues such as promptness and maintaining standards.

- All non-strikers should be informed of what happened and should be commended for their responsible decision not to strike.

Speedy consideration should be given to the following issues:

- The time and cause of the strike.

- The role communication played in causing and/or quelling the strike.

- Current procedures for handling discipline and grievances.

- The mistakes that were made and the lessons learned.

- Adjustment to plans in order to handle strikes better in future.

- The labour relations policy may have to be reviewed.

It is a well-known fact that strikes in the health services have a disruptive and negative effect on patient care. However it is a legitimate collective action within the ambit of industrial relations, and managers have to prepare themselves in order to handle strikes as effectively as possible and be prepared for much work in rebuilding relationships and eliminating the issues that caused the strike.

UNFAIR LABOUR PRACTICES

Legislation with regard to unfair labour practices has been amended since 1979 and is currently regulated by the Labour Relations Amendment Act, No 9, of 1991. The definition of unfair labour practices, according to this amendment, is as follows (Bendix 1992: 537–8):

> Unfair labour practice means...
> (a) any act or omission, other than a strike or lockout, which has the effect that:
> (i) any employee or class of employee is or may be unfairly affected or that his or their employment opportunities, work security or physical, economic, moral or social welfare is or may be prejudiced or jeopardized thereby;
> (ii) the business of any employer or class of employers is or may be unfairly affected or disrupted thereby;

(iii) labour unrest is or may be created or promoted thereby;

(iv) the labour relationship between employer and employee is or may be detrimentally affected thereby; or

(b) any other labour practice or any other change in any labour practice which has or may have an effect which is similar or related to any effect mentioned in paragraph (a).

The above definition is open to wide-ranging interpretation. It can incorporate almost everything regarding labour situations which has affected the welfare of employees, the business of an employer, and industrial relationships in a negative way. SANA has handled cases involving unfair disciplinary action, unfair handling of grievances — especially involving humiliating and degrading behaviour towards subordinates and unfair dismissals. The majority of cases brought before the industrial court have centred on dismissals or retrenchments. Bendix (1992: 538) list the following causes that may give rise to unfair labour practices:

- victimization;

- failure to bargain with a representative union;

- dismissals for strike action;

- dismissal for disciplinary reasons without furnishing a valid reason;

- unfair discrimination on the basis of race, creed, or sex;

- the use of insulting and disparaging terms;

- unilateral implementation of new terms and conditions of employment;

- unilateral change in the bargaining forum;

- unfair unilateral suspension of employees;

- differential and discriminatory terms and conditions of employment;

- body searches;

- refusal to work overtime;

- disruptive action by union organizers;

- refusal to grant access to trade union officials;

- any act of intimidation of an employer or employee;

- failure to abide by the terms of an agreement.

As the definition is wide and non-specific it was left to the industrial court to establish guidelines as to the nature of unfair labour practices. The court relies upon cases brought before it, so, general guidelines may be established but no binding precedents have yet been set.

As far as the handling procedure is concerned, an alleged unfair labour practice is first brought before the industrial council or conciliation board, and the council or board has to resolve the unfair labour practice. If a decision cannot be reached, the matter is referred to the industrial court.

QUALITY OF WORK LIFE

The quality of work life indicates the degree to which employees are able to satisfy their important personal needs by working in an institution. This depends on certain factors within the institution. Quality of work life means different things to different people. Dessler (1984: 429) indicates that it may mean a fair day's pay, safe working conditions, being treated with dignity, opportunities for advancement, creative tasks, or a successful career, depending on the personal needs and development level of the employee.

Work serves many purposes. Its economic function, for producing goods or services, is its most obvious value. The employee is paid for her services, enabling her to purchase food, clothing, shelter, and other necessities as well as luxuries. Some social needs are also met in the workplace. One's job connotes a certain social status both for the employee and her family, it contributes to an employee's self-esteem by reflecting a contribution to the work group, department, or company (Beach 1985: 320). It is also not uncommon for an individual's occupation to shape her sense of identity.

Enhancing the quality of work life

In order to enhance the quality of work life for each employee, an institution has to take into account each employee's needs and values, the extent to which these needs are being satisfied, and the extent to which the values are being conformed to. Gerber et al. (1992: 350) indicates that the institution will have to become involved in activities aimed at satisfying needs that are regarded by the employees as being important.

Walton, the most widely quoted author on the quality of work life, explains the requirements that constitute a good or desirable quality of working life in terms of eight broad conditions of employment (Beach 1985: 325–6; Gerber et al. 1992: 352):

- *adequate and fair compensation:* this includes adequate payment and fringe benefits so as to enable the employee to maintain an acceptable standard of living while working within the institution;

- *safe and healthy working conditions:* these apply to both the physical and psychological environment within which the employee functions;

- *opportunity to utilize and develop human capacities.* This means that the employee is granted as much autonomy in her work as possible. It also means that the work should be made stimulating and interesting by involving the employee in the planning phases of projects, by delegating tasks in their entirety and not just in parts, by delegating tasks that require a number of skills, and by supplying the employee with the necessary information and management perspectives in order for her to recognize the value and place of her work in the organization;

- *future opportunity for continued growth and security:* this involves expanding one's capabilities, the opportunity to use new knowledge and skills, promotion opportunities, as well as job and financial security;

- *social integration in the work organization:* opportunities should be created for social interaction with other employees;

- *the right to privacy and freedom of speech within the enterprise —* employees are to enjoy dignity and respect, and are to be treated like adults in the work environment;

- *work and total life space* is a balanced relationship between an employee's working time and her time away from work to spend on her family life;

- *social relevance of the work* refers to the principle that the employee's job must be to the benefit of all in the institution and for the community in which the employee operates.

Dessler (1984: 430) adds the following to Walton's list:

- fair, equitable, and supportive treatment of employees;

- open, trusting communications between all employees;

- an opportunity for all employees to take an active role in making important decisions that involve their jobs.

It is clear that the quality of work life involves all facets of the employee's functioning in an institution. Optimal utilization of an employee, and her satisfaction in her work environment, are essential to the achievement of a high quality of work life in an enterprise. Because of individual differences among people, and because of differences in the opportunities for satisfying needs in different departments, considerable variation in the satisfaction experienced by employees can be expected within the same institution.

Strategies to improve the quality of work life

Chris Argyris, a behavioural scientist, made an in-depth study of the emotional health of workers. Basically he argued that, as people mature into adults, they develop needs for independence, broader interests, and the power to control their own destinies. An institution that is characterized by autocratic leadership, absence of teamwork, lack of trust, lack of commitment, victimization, discrimination, and discourteous behaviour would obviously not enhance the quality of work life for employees. Good communication, team efforts, challenging work, and equal and fair treatment, on the other hand, would enhance the quality of work life.

Various methods can be used to improve the quality of work life. These include aspects such as management and supervisory style, opportunities for decision-making, job satisfaction, a safe physical environment, satisfactory working hours, and meaningful tasks. The following methods may be used to improve the quality of work life:

1. Participative management. This is a system of management in which employees participate in the making of management decisions that affect them and their jobs. Typically it involves a departmental supervisor conducting meetings with her immediate subordinates to make plans and decisions regarding such matters as the staffing of units, the distribution of tasks, the handling of problems, and working conditions. This process increases employee motivation, generates ideas, and reduces resistance to new methods and processes. It helps meet the human needs for autonomy, achievement, and self-expression (Beach 1985: 326).

2. Management by objectives (MBO). MBO involves three psychological foundations, namely goal-setting, feedback, and participation. It is known that employees who have clear goals usually perform better than those who do not. Clear, attainable goals help channel energies in specific directions and let subordinates know the basis on which they will be appraised and rewarded. Employees who receive frequent feedback concerning their performance are usually more highly motivated than those who do not. Feedback that is specific, relevant, and timely, helps satisfy the need most people have for knowing where they stand and exactly what is expected of them. Allowing subordinates to genuinely participate in setting their own goals can increase their commitment to those goals and improve their performance. It also makes them feel more involved, and this appeals to their higher-level needs, resulting in a feeling of self-worth and positive contribution.

3. Effective leadership and supervisory behaviour. Administrative justice ensures that disciplinary and grievance-handling

proceedings are carried out according to recognized principles (Beach 1986: 330). Employees like to work for supervisors who show consideration for them, who are supportive, and who are fair and just in their treatment of others. The supervisor should create an atmosphere of approval in interpersonal relationships with their subordinates, as their perception of the quality of their working life is heavily affected by the treatment they receive from their supervisors. The supervisor must be able to organize and direct people in order to enable them to reach the organizational goal of quality patient care, and she should possess the technical knowledge and other skills needed in order to diagnose difficulties or problems within the service units. She should set challenging but attainable performance standards, she should be available when she is needed, but she should leave enough room for independent thought and the use of initiative when subordinates have the potential to be creative and independent. According to Beach (1985: 328), another important dimension of effective leadership and supervision is the development of teamwork among employees. The supervisor should generate an appropriate degree of participation in day-to-day decisions, so that employees care about their work because they are highly involved.

4. Quality circles. In recent years the emphasis has shifted from controlling quality of health care to assuring high-quality health care. As part of that shift of emphasis, health agencies have used quality circles to motivate employees to improve the quality of nursing care that is delivered to patients (Gillies 1989: 529).

5. Job enrichment programmes. Job enrichment can be defined as the purposeful restructuring of a job to make it more challenging, meaningful, and interesting for an employee. This process assumes that the employee is able to do a job at a higher level, carry more responsibility, and that she will react positively for being given the opportunity to function at a higher level. Gerber et al. (1992: 355) argue that the following conditions must be met for an employee to react favourably to job enrichment:

   • the job must offer variety, indicating that a number of different skills will be used;

   • the employee must understand the job in its entirety;

   • the job must be meaningful so that the employee will feel that she is performing an important task;

   • the employee must have independence and freedom so that she can make her own decisions regarding her job;

   • there must be sufficient feedback on the job she is doing.

Job enrichment may be achieved in various ways. First, work groups may be formed where each employee is allocated a specific section/responsibility of the total number of tasks that need to be done. As a task becomes her own responsibility, she is allowed to plan and make decisions with respect to that task, resulting in a sense of achievement and authority. She can then identify with that section of work. Secondly, tasks may be combined so that one employee will be responsible for different aspects of a process. Thirdly, vertical loading may be instituted. This means an employee will plan and control her own work. Fourthly, channels need to be introduced so that faster and better work methods can be communicated to the employee without delay (Gerber et al. 1992: 355).

6. Career development. To fully utilize people's potential, to help employees realize their career ambitions, and to enhance their feelings of achievement and recognition, management needs to implement a systematic career planning and development programme aimed at guiding and developing subordinates. The principle components of a comprehensive career programme within an institution are (Beach 1985: 328):

   - human resource planning;

   - communication of job opportunities and career path information to employees;

   - career counselling, both by the supervisor as part of performance appraisal and by the personnel department;

   - provision for the education and training of employees both within and outside the organization; and

   - special broadening and stimulating job assignments and job rotation.

   Some institutions also have formal assessment centres to analyse and evaluate the capabilities and potential of the personnel.

7. Alternative work schedules. Employers are continually trying to introduce more flexible work arrangements which will give employees more freedom of choice in their working hours. Such schedules presently appear in three different forms namely flexitime, part-time employment/job sharing, and shorter work weeks.

   - Flexitime is a system in which the workday is divided into *core time* and *choice time*. The worker is able, within certain predetermined limits, to begin and end her workday as it suits her. Core time is defined as the predetermined number of hours during which all staff assigned to a shift must be on duty.

- Part-time employment is especially attractive to working mothers and pensioners who have other commitments and do not wish to work a full eight-hour day every day of the week. The concept of job sharing means that two people share a full-time job. This may be especially useful in times of economic recession where it can prevent people from losing their jobs (Gerber et al. 1992: 358).

- Shorter working weeks involve accomplishing a full week's work in less than five days. In nursing practice 12 hour shifts have become popular, resulting in a four day work week with a longer time off duty.

CONCLUSION

Industrial relations have become a prime concern for nursing managers in the rapidly changing socio-economic and political situation in South Africa. Management is always concerned about the extent to which a union may attempt to control and influence their institution. This is a valid concern, but management can influence the work setting by creating an atmosphere in which employees are treated fairly and by establishing reasonable working conditions and an atmosphere of shared benefits as a positive means of preventing collective action.

In order for management to be effective in their handling of industrial relations they need to acquire skills and knowledge relating to certain procedures and principles such as disciplinary action, the handling of grievances and disputes, collective bargaining, and strike action. They must also be aware of the factors that may lead to unfair labour practices.

Institutions have to take care of their employees by offering a good quality of work life. Management can purposefully plan and implement certain strategies enabling employees to experience a higher quality of work life, depending on their specific personal needs. Most of the programmes discussed constitute attempts to increase employee satisfaction and performance through intrinsic motivation. Programmes such as participative management, management by objectives, and quality circles seek to involve employees more thoroughly in decision-making and activities related to their jobs, resulting in a feeling of participation, commitment, satisfaction, self-actualization, security, and high self-esteem.

References

Beach, D. S. (1985). *Personnel: the Management of People at Work*. Fifth edition. Macmillan: New York.

Bendix, S. (1989). *Industrial Relations in South Africa*. Juta: Cape Town.

Bendix, S. (1992). *Industrial Relations in South Africa*. Juta: Cape Town.

Brannigan, E. (1987). *Trade Unions and the Nursing Profession*. Unpublished paper presented at the National Symposium of the Department Health and Welfare, House of Assembly: 'Verpleegadministrasie en die hedendaagse Gesondheidsdienste'.

Brannigan, E. (1988[a]). *Trade Unions and the Nursing Profession*. Unpublished talk presented at Kimberley.

Brannigan, E. (1988[b]). *Collective Bargaining as a Conflict Resolution Strategy*. Unpublished paper presented at the University of the North.

Brannigan, E. (1989). *Labour Relations in the Nursing Services*. Unpublished paper presented at the symposium 'Labour relations in the Health Services — Key to Peace'.

Critical Health. (1988). No. 24. Doornfontein: Editorial Collective.

Cunningham, P. (1990). Labour pains. *Nursing RSA,* volume 5, Number 9, pp. 35–8.

De Beer, J. J. (1987). *Nie-Formele Arbeidsverhoudinge*. Departement Personeelbestuur, Universiteit van Pretoria. Ongepubliseerde referaat.

Dessler, G. (1984). *Personnel Management*. Third edition. Reston: Virginia.

Die ABC van arbeidsverhoudinge. *Nursing News,* 1991, volume 15, number 10: p. 14.

Disciplinary procedures. *Nursing News,* 1991, volume 15, number 11: p. 12.

DiVincenti, M. (1977). *Administering Nursing Service*. Second edition. Little Brown: Boston.

Engelhardt, H. (ed.) (1991). *1991 Hospital and Nursing Year Book of Southern Africa*. Engelhardt: Cape Town.

Gerber, P. D., Nel, P. S. and Van Dyk, P. S. (1992). *Human Resources Management*. Second edition. Southern: Johannesburg.

Institute of Personnel management. (Undated) IPM Journal. Fact Sheets Supplements, numbers 103–7.

Lockhart, C, and Werther, W. B. (1980). *Labor Relations in Nursing*. Nursing Resources: Wakefield.

Lombard, B. U. and Swart, S. M. (1979). Arbeidsbetrekkinge. Unisa: Pretoria.

Marriner, A. (1982). *Contemporary Nursing Management*. Mosby: St Louis.

Muller, M. (1991). Stakings deur verpleegpersoneel. *Nursing RSA,* volume 6, number 10, pp. 37–41.

Muller, M. E. and Coetzee, L. (1990). *Verslag oor die Ondersoek na die Verpleegberoep.* Saamgestel en uitgegee deur die SAVV.

Nel, P. S. and Van Rooyen, P. H. (1991). *South African Industrial Relations: Theory and Practice*. Second edition. Academica: Pretoria.

Nursing News (1991). A patient should, and could, never be used as a bargaining tool. *Nursing News,* volume 15, number 11, p. 1.

Nursing News (1991). The ABC of industrial relations. *Nursing News,* volume 15, number 9, p. 8.

Nursing News (1992). The trade union leg of SANA and other negotiating platforms. *Nursing News,* volume 16, number 8, p. 10.

Potgieter, S. (1992). *Griewe Hantering deur Verpleegdiensbestuurders in Hospitale.* Verhandeling voorgelê ter vervulling van die vereistes vir die M.Cur Graad aan die Randse Afrikaanse Universiteit.

Republic of South Africa. Labour Relations Act No. 28 of 1956. Cape Town.

Salamon, M. (1987). *Industrial Relations Theory and Practice*. Prentice Hall: New York.

Slabbert, J. A. (1987). *Vakbondwese en Arbeidsverhoudinge*. Digma-Publikasies: Roodepoort.

Sullivan, E. J. and Decker, P. J. (1988). *Effective Management in Nursing*. Second edition. Addison-Wesley: New York.

Verpleegsters mag nie staak nie. *Nursing News,* 1991, volume 15, number 9, p. 4.

Wade, V. (1985). *The Position of the Nursing Administrator with Regard to Labour Organizations*. Unpublished paper.

APPENDICES

APPENDIX 1: NOTE ON FINANCE

Whatever system is used for planning, the availability of finance will be the limiting factor.

The private sector

In the private sector:

- the profit motive applies;
- shareholders' money is involved;
- business principles apply to finance;
- working with business units cost or pool budget.

The state system

The state system is non profit-making, but:

- public money is involved;
- public administration principles apply to finance;
- there is a centralized financial management system.

Basic procedure for allocation of finance

1. The amount of finance available for the branch is finalized in May/June (note: 'branch' refers to the branch hospital and health services of a provincial administration.).

2. Physical planners provide lists of three needs:

    - facilities;
    - equipment;
    - personnel.

Figures are then put into the lists.

3. This submission is re-prioritized and incorporated in the request for a guideline allocation of finance.

4. The request is submitted in June for the financial year fifteen months later.

5. In June of the same year, a provisional guideline allocation is provided for the financial year nine months later.

6. The organization is requested to draw up a budget outlining the required capital expenditure on a new project, as well as the finance for existing services.

7. The maintenance of existing health services will be the branch's priority. If there is adequate finance available, plans and request for a new facility will be considered.

8. The budget is drawn up and submitted through the branch to the Provisional Executive Committee, then to Treasury, and to National Health.

9. If it is approved by these three organizations, a final guideline amount is determined.

10. A budget is drawn up in December for the financial year three months away.

11. The planners provide the following for the Department of National Health: schedules of facilities, with planned equipment schedules, and the planned establishment of posts. Financial estimates are attached.

12. If finance is available, the project may go through in the next financial year.

13. The human resource plan is submitted to the Branch Hospital and Health Services of the particular provincial administration.

14. Once approved, the project moves into stage 2 of human resource planning; development of the human resource plan (see figure 1.1). This will commence as soon as the commissioning team has been established.

APPENDIX 2: IMPORTANT HEALTH LEGISLATION

- Health Act No. 63 of 1977
- National Policy for Health Act No. 116 of 1990
- Defence Act No. 44 of 1057
- Acts relating to the professions, eg Nursing Act No. 50 of 1978; Medical, Dental and Supplementary Health Service Professions Act 56 of 1974; Pharmacy Act No. 53 of 1974.

Important laws concerning industrial relations

- Labour Relations Act No. 28 of 1956
- Manpower Training Act No. 56 of 1981
- Wage Act No. 5 of 1957
- Machinery and Occupational Safety Act No. 6 of 1983 and/or Mines and Works Act No. 27 of 1956 and amendments
- Basic Conditions of Employment Act (Act No. 3 of 1983 as amended by Act No. 27 of 1984)
- Guidance and Placement Act (Act No. 62 of 1981)
- Workmen's Compensation Act No. 30 of 1941
- Unemployment Insurance Act No. 30 of 1966
- Disability Grants Act No. 27 of 1968
- Fund Raising Act No. 107 of 1978 amended
- Act No. 41 of 1980 amended; Act No. 19 of 1981 amended; Act No. 57 of 1988.

APPENDIX 3: GUIDELINES FOR WARD AND ICU DESIGN

Ward design guidelines

Abbott, G. R. (1983). *Briefing and Design Guide: General Ward. Pretoria: CSIR.*

Cowan, D. and Abbott, G. R. (1984). An economical approach to the provision of hospital beds and the design of wards. *World Hospitals,* volume 20, number 1.

Curry, I. (1980). Towards a better ward design. *Nursing Times,* 3 January, pp. 38–9.

Scher, P. (1989). Nucleus appraised — the pros and cons. *Hospital Development,* January 1989, pp. 33–7.

Tatton-Brown, W. (1978). Owed to the nightingale – 2: ward evaluation. *Nursing Times,* 3 August, pp. 1279–84.

Tatton-Brown, W. (1978). Owed to the nightingale. *Nursing Times,* 3 August, pp. 1273–8.

Williamson, N. (1983). A ward with a view. *Nursing Mirror,* 27 April, pp. 24–7.

ICU design guidelines

South African Society of Anesthetists (1990). *Guidelines for Practice.* Crest Health Care Technology (Pty) Ltd: Maraisburg.

Task force on guidelines (1988). Recommendations for critical care unit design. *Society of Critical Care Medicine. Critical Care Medicine,* volume 16, pp. 746–806.

APPENDIX 4: ROOM DESCRIPTION

Department: surgical ward

Room: procedure room

Function	*Facilities and equipment*
1. Assist ambulent/wheelchair patient onto couch.	Couch with lockable wheels Bedsteps Cubicle curtains around couch Door width 200 mm Space for ±2 assistants around couch
2. Sterile procedures that may be performed include: wound dressing/irrigation, urinary catheterization, lumbar punctures, fluid aspirations, sigmoidoscopy.	Space for 1 to 2 surgical trolleys around couch with sterile sets of equipment. Procedures are usually performed from the patient's right side. Bar stool. Examination lamp, mobile, electricity supply. Two socket outlet at bedhead.
3, Support patient on continuous oxygen and suction when needed.	Oxygen and vacuum outlet at bedhead.
4. X-ray viewing prior to or during a procedure.	Two-plate X-ray viewer, placed opposite the operator.
5. Handwashing.	Basin with elbow operated taps. Soap and towel dispenser. Pedal action bin.

Note: the design team will extract the items provided in the contract. The equipment must be ordered by the institution/DHS.

APPENDIX 5: ACTIVITY DATA SHEET

ACTIVITY DATA SHEET

DEPARTMENT

ROOM

REFERENCE

ROOM NO.

AREA AVE. MAX.

OCCUPANTS

DAYTIME DAY/EVENING 24 HR.

RELATIONSHIPS

COMPILED

REVISED DATE

CONFIRMED USER

PCU

FUNCTIONS
SPECIFIC, CLERICAL, STORAGE, ETC

FINISHES

WALL — STANDARD / SPECIAL

FLOOR — STANDARD / NON-SLIP / SPECIAL

DOOR — SINGLE / DOUBLE / ONE & HALF / SPECIAL

WINDOW — ESSENTIAL / DESIRABLE / OPTIONAL / UNACCEPTABLE / BLACKOUT / OBSCURE GLASS

FITTINGS

PINBOARD

WRITING BOARD

WORKTOP — STANDING 600 DEEP / SITTING 750 DEEP / FORMICA

SPECIAL

STORAGE

CUPBOARDS LOW / CUPBOARDS FULL HT / CUPBOARDS WALL

SPECIAL

SHELVING — DEPTH 200 / 400 / 600

STANDARD

SLATTED

STAINLESS

SPECIAL

SERVICES

POWER — 15 AMP / 3 PHASE / SPECIAL / SPECIFY NO. / EMERGENCY

COMMUN. — INTERNAL / EXTERNAL / PUBLIC / NURSE CALL / SPECIAL

ALARMS

COMPUTER

RADIO

TELEVISION — CCTV / DOUBLE

X-RAY VIEW — SINGLE

PIPED SERVICES SPECIFY NO. WALL / PEND. / BENCH / FUME CAB.

O₂

N₂O

VAC

AIR (LP)

AIR (HP)

CO₂

LPG

SPECIAL

SPECIAL

ENVIRONMENTAL STANDARDS

AIR-COND — RETURN AIR / EMERGENCY POWER / 100% FRESH / SPECIAL

VENTILATION

TEMP — COMFORT / SPECIAL

LIGHTING — STANDARD / EMERGENCY POWER / DIMMABLE / NIGHT / EXAM-WALL / EXAM CEILING / SPECIAL

SOUND — NORMAL / SPECIAL

SANWARE
QTY WATER / ASST. HOT / COLD / STD. / ELB / LAB / TAPS

SURGEON BASIN

STANDARD BASIN

SS SINK SINGLE

SS SINK DOUBLE

SS SINK DEEP

SS SINK BELFAST

BEDPAN WASH

WC

BIDET

SHOWER

BATH

URINAL

SLOPHOPPER

SPECIAL

FIXTURES

SOAP DISP STD — SOAP DISP CLIN

SOAP DISH — CLOTHES HOOKS

TOWEL RAIL — TOWEL RING

TOWEL DISP — TOILET ROLL HLD.

MIRROR STD — MIRROR LONG

GRAB HANDLE — GRAB RAIL

EQUIP RAIL — DRIP RAIL

CUBICLE TRACK — SHOWER TRACK

OTHER

FRANKLIN GARLAND GIBSON AND PARTNERS   TEL 3096784
PRINCIPAL AGENT   FAX 3454427

NDAH

Index

Alphabetical arrangement is word-by-word. Page references in italic indicate illustrative material. The term *passim* denotes that the references are scattered throughout the pages indicated.